The Optometric Profession

PRINCIPLES OF⟨◎⟩PTOMETRY SERIES

VOLUME ONE

The Authors

MONROE J. HIRSCH, O.D., Ph.D.

Lecturer, School of Optometry, University of California; President, American Academy of Optometry; Editor, *American Journal of Optometry and Archives of American Academy of Optometry;* Author: *Refractive State of the Eye* (Editor). Recipient, The Silver Medal of the Distinguished Service Foundation of Optometry; F.A.A.O.; F.A.A.A.S.

RALPH E. WICK, O.D., D.O.S.

Lecturer, School of Optometry, University of California; Past President, American Academy of Optometry; Advisory Research Council, American Optometric Foundation; Alumnus Member, Armed Forces National Research Council, Committee on Vision, National Academy of Science; Recipient, The Silver Medal of the Distinguished Service Foundation of Optometry; F.A.A.O.; F.A.A.A.S.

The authors have co-edited *Vision of the Aging Patient* (1960) and *Vision of Children* (1963), both published by the Chilton Book Company.

THE
OPTOMETRIC
PROFESSION

MONROE J. HIRSCH, O.D., Ph.D

&

RALPH E. WICK, O.D., D.O.S.

School of Optometry, University of California
Berkeley, California

CHILTON BOOK COMPANY

PHILADELPHIA   NEW YORK   LONDON

To emphasize the future—
this book about yesterday, today,
and tomorrow is dedicated
to our sons

GEOFFREY A. HIRSCH
and
BRUCE C. *and* BARRY G. WICK

PREFACE

This book, in part at least, is an anatomy of the profession of optometry. An analysis is made of the structure of optometry in the United States. Comparative studies are made with other professions and with the optometric service in other countries. But the analysis goes beyond mere structure. To understand the profession, one must study its development. For this reason the history of optometry is presented.

As a craft, optometry is as old as spectacles. Soon after spectacles were invented, men began to manufacture spectacles, to supply them to the public, and to help people obtain the proper spectacles. This was a form of optometry, and to this extent, optometry is over 700 years old. But as a legalized profession, optometry is only as old as the present century—that is, about 65 years old.

At the time optometry was recognized by the first state of the United States in 1901, it was possible to learn to practice optometry in a two-week course. During the phenomenal growth and development of the optometric profession, the course of study increased to six months, one year, two years, three years, four years, five years, and now six years. There are men alive today who studied optometry for each of these lengths of time. As a general rule, it may be noted that a year has been added to the optometric curriculum about every decade.

Educational increases went hand in hand with an expansion of the scope of optometry. The present-day optometrist practices in a manner and with knowledge much more sophisticated than the optometrist at the turn of the century. The development of optometric *science* was a worldwide occurrence, and the development of the optometric *craft* was primarily a European phenomenon; the development of the optometric *profession,* however, is mainly an American contribution. The development of the profession and the delineation of its boundaries were affected markedly by the social structure of the United States. Optometry developed to fill a need among people. Increased education and scope came in response to the needs of the populace.

vii

As this book was being written, an important milestone had been reached in the development of optometry. The various universities at which optometry was taught had just increased the course to six years and had begun to grant the doctorate degree. In fact, this book was written as a text for such curricula. In all optometry schools, the student begins professional courses after at least two years of pre-optometric basic science courses. He remains in the optometry school for four years. During the first year, along with basic sciences, he receives a course of optometric orientation. This course is the first exposure to optometry for many students. This book was written to meet the needs of the student in such a course.

We do not feel, however, that the usefulness of the book is limited to beginning students. Because optometry is a profession that is growing rapidly, the practicing optometrist who has been away from school a few years will benefit from this consideration of the present scope and traditional background of his profession. Perhaps seeing optometry in its true perspective and in relation to current social trends may give the practicing optometrist a renewed faith in his mission and in the service he is offering.

In speaking to the neophyte optometrist directly, but aiming also at the practicing optometrist, we are using a technique as old as Shakespeare. In *Hamlet,* Polonius offers advice to his nephew in a famous recital. But through this, Shakespeare has spoken to all men for over 300 years. When Polonius tells his nephew: "This above all, to thine own self be true," Shakespeare is offering the same advice to all who listen. In describing optometry as we see it, we direct our comments to beginning students, who we hope will be helped; but we are also looking beyond the students to practicing optometrists.

Optometry is a unique profession. Although it has obvious similarities with other health professions, it is nonetheless *itself* more than it is anything else. There are those who feel they must describe optometry as applied physiological optics or applied psychophysics. To be sure, optometry is sometimes one of these, sometimes the other; but for the most part, "Optometry is optometry, is optometry, is optometry" (Morgan, 1954).

Just what is this elusive uniqueness? The emergence of optometry as a profession has been so rapid that its scope or sphere is still changing. Several things optometry is not. It is not, as has been sometimes claimed, a limited form of medical practice. Although some of the tests optometrists perform are also performed by physicians, optometry is not a part of medical practice. It is also not merely the fitting and selling of eyeglasses, although a few regressive members of the present optometric group still offer their clients little more than this. Because so much of a child's education is received through his visual sense, the optometrist has some knowledge in the field of learning; but optometry is not a part of education, nor even psychology.

Optometry is a separate and independent health profession. It has traditions and codes of ethics and conduct similar to those of other health professions. But there are enough differences so that optometry is not a *part* of any of the other health professions.

The need for delineation and description of the scope of optometry has been felt by many. The visual psychologist who has played a part in the education of optometrists, S. Howard Bartley, has recognized the need for a literature that describes what optometry is. He, more than any other person, has encouraged the authors to undertake this volume. He argued that, because optometry is so new a profession, and because it means so many things to so many people (including the currently practicing optometrists), the need is all the more pressing. Although we cannot say in a word what optometry is, to this question this volume is addressed. It is our hope that the reader, when he has completed it, will have some notion of what the optometric profession is in 1968 and how it got to be what it is.

Bartley's recognition of the need for a book of this sort suggests another area of usefulness. In addition to new and older optometrists, the members of other health professions and those interested in health planning need a description of this newest health profession. Because health care in the future must be a team effort, the members of the team (and its directors) must know the characteristics of each of the team members. We have tried to keep the material free from the technical aspects of optometry so that this book might help any interested person who might wish an answer to the question "What is optometry?"

The authors have tried to describe the various parts of optometry as impartially as possible. However, mere description is not enough. Attempts are made at an interpretive view of optometric history. We realize our interpretation will not meet with the approval of all optometrists, nor would we want it to do so. A book of this kind must challenge, as well as instruct; must interpret, as well as state facts; and must, above all, develop a sense of pride in the accomplishments of the profession.

Sociologists who have studied the social structure of professions in the United States and throughout the world have agreed that all professions go through certain basic steps in arriving at full maturity as a profession. Optometry is traced through this process in this book.

The present text has been written at a period in history during which the American people are becoming greatly interested in a re-evaluation of their social structure and of their place in the world. Increased interest by government in health and medical care is part of this period. The authors could not help but be influenced by this environment. They could not help but ask where optometry fits into the picture of health professions, not only in the United States of today, but also in the world of tomorrow. Thus, within the framework of today's social structure, the role of optometry, its makeup, its raison d'être, its history and traditions, and its hopes and aspirations all are the subject of this text.

As the authors studied and wrote, two facets of the subject were constantly and forcibly brought to their attention. First, one cannot study the optometric profession without being amazed at its phenomenal growth. Within 65 years, optometry in the United States has come from meager beginnings to the status of an independent profession recognized by all states, and, of equal importance, recognized as a doctorate program at major universities. During this period, other health professions have emerged—physical therapy, for example. But there is a major difference. Optometry is the only *independent* health profession to emerge during the present century and to gain academic acceptance. Physical therapists do not practice independently. Pharmacy has attained the university doctorate level relatively recently, but it had its beginnings far earlier than optometry. Thus the phenomenal development of optometry within so short a time has been a constant source of amazement. The authors sought more deeply for the reasons why optometry has grown so rapidly and so well. Has it been the dedication of individuals? Has it been the happy circumstance of history—that is, has it happened at the right time? Has it been something inherent in the nature of optometry? Or has it been a combination of these factors? The observation of rapid growth and the questions it has suggested continued with us through the writing.

The second thread that ran through our period of study of the optometric profession was the realization of the tremendous job still to be done. For despite this amazing development, optometric service is still denied or unavailable to most of the people of the world. The challenge of the optometric profession is one faced by any service to humanity the technology of which has reached a high level of competence—how to bring this service to bear on the problems of people. And being clinicians who daily see the effect of optometric service on people, the authors could not help being impressed by this phase of the problem.

It is customary in a preface to give thanks to those who have helped in the preparation of the manuscript and to disclaim for them any responsibility for errors. Both of these things we do willingly—for we have received a great deal of help, and we recognize fully that the nature of the subject demands judgments the burden of which the authors alone must bear. We are grateful to the American Optometric Foundation and its board of trustees for a grant to cover manuscript preparation expenses. Help in this regard was also received from the School of Optometry at the University of California, where all our requests for office help and supplies were willingly met.

Several typists helped in preparing the manuscript, offering editorial help, as well as simple typing. We are indebted to Maggie Mahan, Wini Hirsch, Cara Woodford, Margaret Lorensen, and Karen Walker, each of whom was responsible for several chapters. We are grateful for the encouragement and intellectual stimulation offered by the staff at the School of Optometry, University of California, and particularly Dean Meredith W. Morgan, who did everything possible to aid us in our work. Our colleagues, Dean Morgan and Professors Merton C. Flom and Henry B. Peters, have read sections and offered valuable comments; they are responsible for many improvements in the text but not for any errors of style, content, or judgment that must inevitably be present in a book such as this one. We owe our publishers, The Chilton Book Company, a great deal. Their cooperation has been inspiring—their patience boundless. Although Chilton gave help in many forms, the most important was the making available to us of the services of Mrs. Grace Weiner, librarian at the Los Angeles College of Optometry. Throughout the writing, Grace has been the "silent" third author. In addition to amassing the bibliography, checking each reference, and obtaining permissions for quotations, she has read the manuscript, offered editorial suggestions, and drawn on her tremendous knowledge of optometric literature to improve the manuscript. We are indeed grateful to Mrs. Weiner for her assistance as editorial bibliographer, her official designation, but much more for the help she was not required to give but did. Truly, in this effort, she played the key role. To each of these people and organizations we offer thanks for the aid we have received, and to ourselves alone we attribute the shortcomings of this biography of a profession.

The present text is intended to be one volume in the series *The Principles of Optometry*. Perhaps the fact that a series of many volumes to be written by many authorities is even contemplated is more striking evidence than anything we have written of the present status of optometry. Clearly, this youngest of the health professions has come a long way in 65 years.

MONROE J. HIRSCH
Ojai, California
and
RALPH E. WICK
Rapid City, South Dakota

May 1967

CONTENTS

The Optometric Profession

CHAPTER 1

INTRODUCTION

Optometry is the art and science of vision care. This customary definition recognizes the two facets of any health profession—skill and learning. It tells us what is encompassed by the optometric service—namely, vision care. Such a definition, however, lacks a description of the optometric group of practitioners. Such a definition describes the optometric field of study and proficiency but not the sociology of optometrists as a group, collectively referred to as the optometric profession.

Optometry is an independent, legalized health care profession offering a unique and unified service for the maintenance and enhancement of good vision and the amelioration of vision defects. Such a definition has many elements in it that describe the optometric group. It is an independent group; as a group it has achieved legal recognition; the service has unity.

A textbook describing the specific knowledge and skills of the optometrist would be based on the first definition. A book such as the present one, which is a view of the history, sociology, and philosophy of the optometric profession, depends on a definition such as the second one. The topics discussed in later chapters are based on the elements of this second definition.

Specifically, we shall consider (1) how the profession developed into its present form, (2) the precise nature of this unique optometric service, (3) why modern society requires the service and how it fits into the overall scheme of health care, and (4) what the future may be expected to hold for this form of service. Each of these points is introduced briefly in this chapter and discussed in depth in later chapters.

HISTORY—*An Overview*

Just as our definition of optometry contained several elements, so there are several aspects to the history of optometry. First, there is the history of the service itself. Although the term *optometry* to describe a health care profession is less than 100 years old, the service itself, in

1

one form or another, has been rendered for a much longer period.

The history of the legalization of optometry in the United States is a second aspect; this occurred during the short period of a quarter of a century. The earliest law governing optometric practice was passed in 1901 in Minnesota; the last of the existing states adopted optometric regulating legislation within a quarter of a century after Minnesota passed hers.

Optometry as a profession is a third aspect. This history began at the turn of the present century and is still being written, for optometry as a profession has not yet reached its ultimate state of development. The simplest definition of "profession" is any vocation that is not purely commercial or mechanical. By such a criterion, the earliest suppliers of the optometric service were not professional people. In recent years, the purely commercial act of selling spectacles has been replaced by a service and skill offered on a professional basis: a body of knowledge about eye defects and their correction has developed, and a learned profession has evolved.

In the evolution of optometry, there were three chronological periods, which may be characterized briefly as follows:

1. Pre-optometry (before 1300 A.D.). Before spectacles were invented and put into use, man tolerated his vision defects. Some eye diseases were recognized and treated by the physicians of the time, but vision defects were neither understood nor ameliorated. The historical event that ended the first period and began the second was the invention of spectacles, the major device for correcting vision defects.

2. Early "Optometry" (about 1300 to 1900). During these 600 years, the principles of optics and spectacle lenses were enunciated. The contributors to this science were not optometrists as we know them today but were astronomers, physicists, mathematicians, and other scientists. Just as modern medicine owes its scientific basis to anatomists, physiologists, chemists, biochemists, and bacteriologists, so optometry is indebted to the early physical scientists.

Along with scientific advancement, the craft of spectacle making developed. Each year an increased number of spectacles were produced. These were sold by the lens makers, by street peddlers, and by shopkeepers such as haberdashers. These people were the first to supply an optometric service.

Spectacles were available for almost 600 years, during which time the concept of testing a patient for proper lenses evolved very slowly. During this time, although spectacles were available and although eye defects existed, spectacles were supplied by commercial means and not as part of a health service. Physicians were the only health practitioners of the time, and few of them became interested in the problem of correcting defects of the eye.

3. Modern Optometry (about 1890 to the present). It is a well known principle in the history of science that the time between succeeding significant contributions decreases geometrically. This principle is well illustrated in optometry. The pre-optometric period encompasses tens of thousands of years; the early "optometric" period, 600 years; the modern period, a mere 75 years. Although this phenomenon characterizes all history, it is nonetheless impressive. There is a much greater similarity between the optometrists of 1700 and 1900 than between the optometrists of 1900 and 1950. Change occurs with increasing rapidity as years pass.

The period of modern optometry began with the legalization of the profession in the United States during the first quarter of the twentieth century. But professionalization has been a much more subtle and gradual process.

Increasingly during the last 75 years, optometrists have placed more emphasis on the service aspect of optometric care than on the device supplied for correction. The customer for spectacles has become a patient seeking advice and care. The optometrist of the earlier period supplied spectacles and helped his customers to select them; emphasis was on the spectacles. The modern optometrist also supplies spectacles and also assesses visual capacity, but he stresses vision testing, and advisory and service aspects rather than the spectacles themselves.

As one reads history, he sometimes gains the erroneous notion that there has been an orderly progression, each event leading to improvement and each idea receiving universal acceptance. But this is not the case, either in the history of any science or idea or in the history of optometry in particular. Moreover, ideas have achieved different degrees of acceptance in various parts of the world at different times. Optometry at present has reached a different level in the United States from that in other countries.

Optometry as a professon has reached its highest development in the United States. It has reached almost as high a state of development in several other English-speaking countries, particularly Great Britain, Australia, Canada, and New Zealand. In some European countries, such as Germany, Switzerland, and Denmark, it is only beginning to emerge as a profession. In other European countries, such as France, Holland, and Belgium, the optometric services are offered by a group of men, but the practice is a trade and cannot be called professional. In more than half the world, optometry is unknown.

In some areas, optometry is unknown because all health services are at a very low level. In other areas, Russia for example, there is no optometric profession, but optometric service is available on a limited basis to people through other professions. As a general rule, the more highly industrialized a nation and the more complex the civilization, the more highly developed is its optometric service.

No field of thought develops in a vacuum, and here again optometry is no exception. Optometry is described as an independent profession, which denotes that it is *not* a specialty of general medicine. In this regard, it is very similar to dentistry, which in the United States is also an independent health profession. The comparison of optometry to dentistry is interesting because dentistry has also reached much higher development and refinement in the United States than in any other country. Although optometry is independent, it has developed and exists as a health profession among other health professions. In studying the place of optometry in the complex social structure of the health professions, it is therefore sometimes necessary to describe optometry relative to other professions.

Optometry, in summary, has been practiced differently during different periods of history and also at any moment of time in different countries. Furthermore, optometry is only the sum total of the day-to-day practices of a group of men—the practicing optometrists.* Optometrists as a group are no more homogeneous than any other group of men practicing the same art and vocation. Thus, even in the United States at this moment, optometrists practice differently. Some recognize the full scope of their profession, while others practice within a very limited sphere. The majority recognize the professional characteristics of optometry, but a few still relate to their "customers" much as did the "optometrists" of 600 years ago.

In the light of these differences in time, in place, and in individuals, how may we describe optometry, for that is the task of this text? The optometry we describe here is that of the majority—the mainstream of optometry in the United States. Fortunately, the practice that is best for the patient is in this mainstream. But no interpretation can be made that this mode of practice will be best in the future. Change is inevitable; throughout this book, we discuss the directions in which change may be expected and the direction that will, in the authors' opinion, be most desirable.

VISION DEFECTS

Part of the definition of optometry offered at the beginning of this chapter referred to the amelioration of vision defects. Although a complete description of such defects, their life cycle, cause, physical

---

* This same concept was used in 1967 by the SCOPE committee of the California Optometric Association. The scope of optometry was described as being delineated by "what optometrists do in their daily practices."

characteristics, symptomatology, and correction, is an essential part of the curriculum in optometry and beyond the scope of this book, a very brief synopsis may prove helpful.

Vision is a highly complex process. Light, reflected or originating at the object being perceived, enters the eye and forms an image (is focused) on a layer containing chemical pigments that react to luminous energy. As chemical reactions occur, luminous energy is converted to nerve impulses, which are transmitted to the brain, where perception occurs. Despite the exquisite complexity of this system, the sharpness of vision depends to a great extent on the clarity of the image. Almost no eyes form a theoretically perfect image; almost all are subject to defects in focusing light to form an image. Whether an individual is affected by the blurred image or not depends greatly on the degree of imperfection.

If the condition of being out of focus is marked, one of three reactions will occur: (1) The individual may see distant objects as blurred and lacking in fine detail. This occurs in myopia and sometimes in astigmatism. (2) The eye, through its own mechanism of focus, may clear the blurred image, but the individual will suffer discomfort from overuse of the focusing mechanism. This occurs in hypermetropia. (3) The eye may attempt to focus the image and fail to do so, leading to both blurredness and discomfort. This occurs in astigmatism.

Overcoming the effects of such defects of focus common to almost all eyes is a major function of optometry. A second type of defect occurs in the focusing mechanism. Within limits the eye can change focus, thereby enabling a normal eye to see objects clearly at both near and far distances. However, this ability may be developed poorly in an individual or may deteriorate. It may be either insufficient or inefficient. The result is either blurred vision or discomfort when viewing objects at certain, but not all, distances.

Because the ability to change focus declines with age, most persons over forty encounter difficulty; by age fifty, few can focus both near and far objects clearly. At one or the other distance, most usually at close range, blurred vision is encountered. Hence, few persons past middle age can read small type unaided. This defect of the eyes is called presbyopia.

Man has two eyes, and it is necessary that the activities of the two be coordinated. A third type of defect is that in which the two eyes do not act in harmonious relationship with each other. The two eyes may not point directly at the object being regarded, or they may do so only with the exertion of undue effort on the part of the individual neurovisual system.

Of great importance is the fact that the focusing mechanism of the eyes and the mechanism subserving coordination are related to each other. Hence, a spectacle lens that corrects a defect of focus may have a desirable or an undesirable effect on coordination. Human visual systems may have defects of focus, defects of coordination, or defects of the relationship between these two.

Defects like those just described are *not* diseases of the eye. For their alleviation, they require neither surgery nor medication. They can be recognized, diagnosed, and remedied by nonmedical procedures. Two major procedures for alleviating these disorders are lenses or spectacles, and vision training or exercises. The recognition, diagnosis, and remediation of defects of this type comprise the major optometric service.

Eyes are not only subject to defects such as those just described. They may also have diseases. The microorganisms that attack other parts of the body sometimes attack the eyes. The eye is also subject to degenerations or abnormalities that require surgical correction. Cataract, for example—a state in which the lens within the eye becomes opaque—can be remedied by the removal of the now useless occluding lens from the eye. The eye is also subject to disturbances of the normal physiological relationships; the pressure of the eye, for example, may become elevated. This abnormal situation is one of the clues to the diagnosis of glaucoma, a disease that requires treatment by medication or surgery to prevent blindness.

Such abnormalities, requiring for their alleviation either medicine or surgery, traditionally and properly have been a part of the practice of medicine. The treatment of these diseases of the eye, like the treatment of disease in general, is part of the practice of medicine and is not within the scope of optometric service.

Just as diseases of the eye were historically treated within the province of medicine, so defects of focus and coordination were for the most part historically ignored and neglected by medical practitioners. As late as the middle of the nineteenth century, physicians who dealt with eye diseases did not test for defects of focus or coordination; they even advised against the use of spectacles for alleviation of such defects. From this unfulfilled need, modern optometry began.

We have differentiated here between eye diseases that require surgery or drugs, both medical procedures, and defects of focus or coordination that, for their alleviation, require spectacles, eye training, or other forms of nonmedical therapy. The reader should not get the impression that the incidence of one type of defect is as great as that of the other. There is anything but an equality of incidence. Defects of focus or coordination are quite common among human visual systems; diseases are relatively rare. Furthermore, during the past thousand years, several factors have contributed to the further disparity in incidence.

Diseases of the eye are becoming increasingly rare. With increased preventive hygienic measures and the success of public health measures, many diseases of the eye are gradually disappearing. Ophthalmia neonatorum, a major cause of blindness in the past, has all but disappeared from modern civilizations. This disease, caused by an organism transmitted to the newborn by the mother at birth, may be avoided by the instillation of a drug in the eye of all newborn infants, a procedure widely practiced where public health is understood and practiced. Trachoma, another major cause of blindness among the ancients and societies with poor hygiene, is now extremely rare in countries such as the United States.

On the other hand, while defects of focusing or coordination are probably not increasing, our intolerance to such defects is. Increased longevity, universal literacy, and the visual demands of a more complex society have increased the need for optimal vision and visual coordination. The inability to watch television without getting a headache or to drive an automobile safely are problems that were unknown fifty years ago. With our entry into the space age, more and more demands for maximal vision, efficiency, and visual comfort are being placed on us. Thus, the need for correcting vision defects has increased throughout history and is continuing to increase. This increasing need for correction of moderate vision defects is a very important concept in understanding the role of optometry in modern society.

WHY MODERN MAN REQUIRES OPTOMETRIC CARE

The preceding discussion of vision defects suggests why modern man requires optometric care. He requires such services for the amelioration of the results of these defects, and modern man requires such care far more than did his forebears. There are four major reasons why people today find it more necessary than ever before to seek optometric care and to wear spectacles or receive vision training exercises:

1. The most common reason for wearing spectacles today is to enable persons past the age of forty or so to read and to do fine, close work. As we have already noted, the ability to change focus decreases with increased age; by middle age, most people require spectacles to see close objects clearly. This need was not as important to man a thousand years ago for several reasons.

Little reading has been done by man until very recently. While literacy has reached a high level in the United States today, there are countries in the world where less than ten percent of the population is literate. Clearly, the need for reading spectacles does not exist except in a literate society. It was not just coincidence that the invention of movable type in printing and of methods for making paper inexpensively occurred about the same time as the introduction of spectacles. The need for spectacles and the mass production of reading materials occurred at about the same period in history.

Increased literacy and mass-produced reading materials are the major reasons for the great need for spectacles today. They are not, however, the only reasons. Early man lived a much shorter life than modern man; relatively few of the ancients lived long enough to experience the decline in focusing ability that occurs with increased age. One characteristic of modern society is the increasing proportion of older people in it.

In earlier times, age carried with it respect by the young and a degree of prestige. The close or fine work required of an older person was often delegated to a younger relative. Many of the tasks for which older persons wear spectacles today were in former times performed for them by relatives and friends. The productive or working period of life, particularly in pursuits that require reading and close work, is longer today than formerly.*

Finally, in presbyopia, vision is poorer at lower levels of illumination. If one among our ancestors did live to an old age and did need to do close work, he did so in daylight. Bright light causes the pupil to contract; a small pupil offsets some of the effect of an out-of-focus eye. Modern man, however, does a great deal of his close work under artificial illumination. Indoor illumination rarely attains the high levels of intensity that outdoor daylight does, and as a result, modern man, working under artificial illumination, notices the effects of presbyopia at an earlier age than did his forebears.

The need for spectacles for close work, the major cause for wearing spectacles, has been increased by each of the factors just discussed—namely, mass production of printed materials, increased literacy, the need to work under artificial illumination, increased longevity, and the lengthened productive life of older people.

* Morgan (1967) offers an interesting observation in this regard. He noted, while traveling in Spain, that the workers (artisans) making Toledo jewelry were mainly children. The work was held so close to the eye that only a person under the age of thirty or so could maintain his eyes in focus comfortably at such a task. The use of child labor in former years, Morgan has suggested, may not have been solely an economic and social need of society, but may have been brought about partly by physiological causes; without spectacles, only the young were capable of performing fine work.

2. Another reason people require an optometrist's service is to enable them to see clearly at a distance. Older people with marked farsightedness cannot see distant objects clearly, persons of any age who have marked astigmatism also do not see clearly, and defects of coordination of the two eyes can sometimes cause distant objects to be blurred or indistinct. The major cause of distant objects being seen as if in a fog or a haze, however, is myopia (nearsightedness).

There are all degrees of myopia, and persons afflicted with only slight degrees can see distant objects *almost* as clearly as those with perfect vision. They can recognize a human form at a great distance, even though they may not distinguish all the facial features quite as readily as an unafflicted individual can.

Therefore, a defect such as myopia to a farmer or stonemason was no great handicap in the past; it is a serious handicap to a modern man who drives an automobile at sixty miles an hour and who must perceive details of the roadway as clearly and rapidly as possible. Nearsightedness was not a handicap to the child in the past who helped work the family farm and tend the animals or who helped the women weaving; it is a serious handicap to the present-day child who must read small symbols on a chalkboard in an artificially-illuminated room or who must watch educational films in a dimly-lighted classroom.

Myopia, like presbyopia, is worse in dim illumination. Modern optometrists all know of patients who have only slight degrees of myopia and who use their spectacles only for such activities as night driving or viewing motion pictures or television. Thus, myopia of moderate degree was not the same handicap to ancient man, who was less likely to require sharp vision after sundown, as it is to modern man, who at day's end, views a television screen at some distance or bowling pins at a greater distance. A moderate degree of blurriness or fogginess was probably taken in stride by our ancestors; they simply lived with it.

Myopia of marked degree causing greatly diminished vision is another story: all too often early man died because of it. In 1632, King Gustavus Adolphus of Sweden, at the Battle of Lützen during the Thirty Years' War, became lost, was separated from his guards, and was slain. Some historians attribute the catastrophe to the king's nearsightedness. It occurred on a foggy morning, which undoubtedly further reduced his vision. Whether this story is apocryphal or not, surely many an ancient man lost his life to wild animals or human enemies because he could not see clearly. Many more died of starvation because they lacked the vision to obtain food for themselves in a hunting society.

3. Man today seeks the optometrist's skills to enable him to use

his eyes without discomfort. Errors of focus or of coordination can cause headache or pain in the eyes. An individual may have noted that use of his eyes for certain tasks causes discomfort, and he thus may knowingly or subconsciously avoid these tasks. The difficulty, however, is the same; the eyes do not function comfortably.

Ancient man with difficulties of this sort either avoided tasks requiring critical seeing (just as modern man sometimes does), or he learned to live with the discomfort. However, the tasks he was called on to perform were very different from those performed by modern man. The same eye defect that causes a present-day accountant in the period before income tax filing time to seek visual correction lest his "eyes fall out of his head" had little effect on the farmer of long ago.

Even though the critical seeing that causes errors of focus or coordination to bring pain to modern man was rarely required of early man, there are records going back several thousand years to show that man did suffer visual discomfort. For most men of those times, such discomfort was probably taken as part of man's lot. One characteristic of those times is the number of lesser aches and pains that ancient man had either to learn to avoid or to bear.

Defects in vision such as those discussed may also cause eyes to be red, to burn, and to water; or they might cause the individual to rub his eyes or to squint. As a result of poor hygiene and rubbing the eyes, sties can be caused. In the past, these discomforts were not understood to be associated with defective vision and were either accepted stoically by ancient man or were treated as primary afflictions by the methods of the day. Today, spectacles or orthoptic exercises usually prevent these symptoms.

4. Finally, modern man seeks optometric care because he has a lack of coordination between the two eyes great enough to cause the eyes to appear abnormal, that is, cross-eyed or wall-eyed. Operationally, this is not as great a handicap as one might believe. Man can function very well in most situations with the vision of only one eye. If the other eye turns away from the object being seen or if it loses vision, the individual is not greatly handicapped. The cosmetic effect is another matter, and ancient man was not one to allow deviations from the average to go unnoticed or unpersecuted.

The individual who had crossed eyes was often considered to be bewitched. Interestingly, this same attitude is still held among many people throughout the world. A cross-eyed person is feared in such widely separated areas as Assam in northeast India and the countryside of rural England. Oddly enough, the same abnormality was considered to be attractive by the Mayan Indians. Koch (1949) notes that between 800 and 1400 A.D. Mayan mothers in Guatemala, Honduras, and Yucatán attached small balls of red wax and feathers between the eyebrows of newborn babies to cause the eyes to cross.

The individual of the past who had eyes that did not appear to be aligned normally did not suffer greatly from the visual aspects of his anomaly, but in most cultures, he may have suffered socially from the problem. We might note here for the first time a theme we shall reiterate throughout this book. The modern optometrist offers more than just spectacles or orthoptic exercises. One of the most important contributions he makes is toward enlightenment. Some disorders must be tolerated, even in the present state of our knowledge. An understanding of vision and the engendering of an enlightened outlook are major contributions made by the optometrist.

THE FUTURE

The defects of the human eye just described will remain with man in the foreseeable future. Although efforts to arrest the development of certain of these defects are being made, current research has yielded no greatly encouraging results. Some defects, to be sure, can be prevented. For the most part, however, the major defects of astigmatism, presbyopia, myopia, hypermetropia, and muscle imbalance are not readily preventable. Research will continue, but it is reasonable to conclude that man will be subject to these defects for many more years.

New techniques for neutralizing these defects may develop, and have been developing at a rapid rate. Contact lenses are now used routinely in place of conventional spectacles by millions of people in the United States. Improved methods for administering vision training exercises are constantly being researched and incorporated into the optometrist's armamentarium. The defects themselves, however, will probably continue to be present for quite some time, despite efforts at prevention.

Man's need for sharp vision and his unwillingness to settle for less than an almost perfectly functioning visual system will not diminish in the future. If the visual demands of our times are greater than those of man a thousand years ago, the demands of the space age on vision will be even more so. In the space age, devices to increase the power of the visual system beyond its normal capacity may be required. Comparing contemporary man to his ancestors, we note that he requires perfect vision in order to drive an automobile, something his horse-and-buggy-driving forebear did not require. Space man, however, may well require better than normal vision. Devices for increasing ability may become as commonplace as the devices now used to bring vision up to maximal normal efficiency.

The optometrist will be needed increasingly by the society of tomorrow; the optometric service will be needed by an increasing number of people. The definition of optometry today contains the phrase "maintenance and enhancement of good vision and the amelioration of vision defects." The word "enhancement" suggests that optometry of tomorrow may increase vision beyond its present scope when this is required for exceptional environmental situations.

The pressing problem today is and will be for some time the making of optometric service available to all who need it. The traditional system for obtaining health care in the United States has been one in which the patient is solely responsible for obtaining care for himself. This situation is rapidly changing. Now government, insurance companies, employers, trade unions, and others are helping the patient to obtain care. These trends will have a marked influence on all health services. Optometry is no exception. We shall, therefore, in subsequent chapters discuss at some length means for making optometric service available in changing times.

This introduction began with a definition; it ends with a challenge. The problem of maintaining a high level of health service while making the service available to all people is the challenge faced by all health professions. This challenge is being faced by optometry today and is the responsibility of every optometrist.

CHAPTER 2

THE OPTOMETRIC SERVICE

Independent optometric service in the United States is rendered to millions of patients by approximately 17,000 optometrists. The most satisfactory method of describing the total service is to describe its parts in much the temporal sequence that the patient, the recipient of the services, encounters them. This chapter is a discussion of the procedures and elements of the optometric service; it describes the daily workings of the optometrist with a patient.

THE CASE HISTORY

An outstanding characteristic of the optometric service is that it is communicative. The patient communicates with the optometrist by stating what it is that bothers him, that is, the symptoms that led him to consult the optometrist. The optometrist communicates in several ways. He may request further information from the patient. Ultimately, the optometrist will wish to explain the nature of the visual problem to the patient and the means that will be used to correct the defect. But there is communication even beyond this. Many of the testing methods themselves are communicative. The optometrist states what perceptual judgments he wishes the patient to make; the patient responds with a description of how he sees the various items in the testing situation. Thus, communication begins the moment the patient and optometrist meet, and it does not end until the total service has been completed.

The discussion between the patient and the optometrist, which is the first step in the optometric service, is called the case history. There are several reasons for this preliminary discussion. The optometrist by direct questioning attempts to identify the patient's problem. Although he may not ask his questions in these words, the optometrist seeks an answer to the question, "Why are you consulting me *now?*" He wishes to know what visual symptoms the patient is manifesting. He also wishes to know what made the patient choose this moment to seek optometric care—in other words, is the patient describing a recent or long-standing disturbance?

One characteristic of health services and health care, particularly in the United States, is that the patient usually makes a tentative diagnosis before he seeks care. In medical practice, for example, the patient with a pain who consults a physician has already made a partial diagnosis; he has decided that the pain is not a minor occurrence of no significance. Most people have minor aches and pains from overexercising or from some other physiological cause. When the patient consults a physician about a pain, it is because it is more severe or more persistent than the common aches. He has thus decided that this particular pain is different from others, and in doing this, he has made a preliminary and partial self-diagnosis.

This same phenomenon occurs among patients who seek optometric care. If the patient consults the optometrist because he has headaches, he has already made a tentative diagnosis. He has decided that his headaches *may* be due to impaired vision. He is not sure; often patients wish to consult the optometrist to determine if a headache could be due to the eyes or other causes. In such a case, the patient has decided that he may have to see more than one health practitioner, but will consult the optometrist first because he thinks his vision is the most likely source of the headaches. If a patient does not see clearly, he also may seek optometric service. He assumes the most likely cause of poor vision is the refractive state of his eyes.

Patients do a rather good job of self-diagnosis. People in the United States seem to be more health conscious than those in many other countries, and certainly they are among the most enlightened people in the understanding of modern health procedures. This has resulted in the maxim that the best way to determine what is wrong with a patient is to ask him—and to listen when he speaks.

The first aspect of the case history, then, is asking the patient what problems, pains, or symptoms he is encountering that have led him to seek optometric consultation. Part of the technique consists of allowing the patient to speak in his own words and manner, part in asking further direct questions. If the patient notes that his vision is blurred, the optometrist may ask him at what tasks it is blurred, at what distances, and under what illumination. If the patient reports a headache, the optometrist will want to determine if it is associated with use of the eyes, what part of the head hurts, how long the pain lasts, the length of time the patient has been having the headache, what measures usually relieve the headache, and what course it usually follows. Some clinicians adopt a method of personal shorthand that enables them to differentiate between information the patient has volunteered and that elicited by direct questioning.

The first aspect of the case history is the identification of the patient's concept of his visual problem. The patient is encouraged to state why he seeks optometric care. This is another way of asking the patient what he expects to receive as a result of coming to the optometrist. When the optometrist asks "Why are you consulting me now?" he is mentally noting what he will need to do at the end of the service in order for it to have been a satisfying encounter for the patient. It is important to determine with some accuracy what is really bothering the patient. Frequently, the patient will say one thing and mean something very different.

An elderly patient, for example, often will state that he is consulting the optometrist because he can no longer read. This patient may have no desire to read but is using this frame of reference to express his fear that he is going blind. He says, "I can no longer read," but he means, "Is the fact that I am losing the ability to read an indication that I shall soon be in complete darkness?" The optometrist's role in taking a case history is not only to listen to the patient's recital and to ask appropriate questions, but also to interpret what the patient is saying. This is truly a communicative skill that must be developed through experience with people.

A second aspect of the case history is that discussion with the patient enables the optometrist to get to know him as an individual. This is the time when the optometrist begins to determine how this patient will accept various forms of therapy. The optometrist wants to know what mental outlook this patient has. What are the patient's hobbies, vocation, likes and dislikes? What are his habits, and how readily does he accept change? Here again the optometrist should lead the conversation into channels and then listen. Sometimes he will ask direct questions; sometimes, rely on the patient to introduce information. The net result will be a judgment formed by the optometrist as to the sort of person with whom he is working.

In addition to listening, the optometrist learns to observe the patient while he is taking the case history. Is the patient nervous? Does he sit at ease or on the edge of his chair? Does he tilt his head? How do his eyes appear on casual inspection? Does he smile and laugh a great deal, or is he very serious?

The case history can also be used as a diagnostic tool by a skillful optometrist. Certain anomalies are best diagnosed by the patient's symptoms. An example of this is migraine headaches, which are diagnosed solely by the patient's report. Thus, if a young patient reports that he "gets headaches" and "sees bright lights," the optometrist will ask several direct questions. If the headaches are unilateral, are preceded by such visual sensations as streaks of lightning, colored balls, wavy lines, or blind areas in the field of vision, and if they appear periodically, or are followed by nausea, the patient has classic migraine. The diagnosis is completed from the patient's recital of the course of events in his periods of headache.

If a patient reports that he sees double, such factors as how long he has noted the double vision, the conditions under which it appears, and the degree of separation of the two images are useful in differentiating the cause of the phenomenon. Thus, a third aspect of the case history is its diagnostic utility. Some anomalies can be identified solely on the patient's report. Other types of anomalies can be differentiated on the basis of the patient's experience.

While the case history is being recorded, the optometrist should be able to answer for himself the questions: Why did this patient consult me? What does this patient expect me to do for him? What sort of a person is this patient? What anomalies might he have?

During this time, the patient has not been a passive information-yielding machine. He too has been receiving information, and this is a fourth aspect of the case history. The patient has had an opportunity to learn that the optometrist is interested in his problem and will attempt to solve it. He is placed as much at ease as possible so that in the ensuing tests, which also are communicative, he will be able to do the best possible job. From the patient's point of view, the case history enables him to decide what sort of an individual the optometrist is. The degree and quality of rapport that is established during the taking of the case history determines how good this optometrist-patient relationship will be.

Several times in the preceding discussion, optometry has been described as communicative or markedly influenced by the field of communication. This is true; however, the communication does not end the moment the optometrist and patient leave the consultation room to enter the examining room. Rather, the communication is continued and improved throughout the total experience. Any test the optometrist subsequently performs might suggest further questions to ask the patient.

The observation of an anomaly in the patient's eye, which could either be recent or of long standing, might lead the optometrist to ask if any former examiner had noted its existence. The finding of reduced vision might lead the optometrist to ask the patient if he drives an automobile and when his license was obtained or last renewed. The finding of a deviation of an eye from perfect alignment might lead to the question of whether the patient has not observed double vision in the past. Thus, the case history is never completed. As the optometrist's relationship with the patient continues, new data may at any time be added to those already obtained.

The first step in the optometric service—communication with the patient—is a continuing process. True, the taking of the initial formal case history is usually concluded in a few minutes, but the process continues. Optometrists differ in the completeness of the case histories taken by them. The best clinicians are usually those who spend considerable time in this preliminary discussion with the patient. But just as optometrists differ, so do patients. In some instances, the end of the fruitful period of the case history has been reached after a minute or two; in others, the patient is best served by a preliminary discussion lasting as long as fifteen minutes. The determination of how much good may be derived from continuing the discussion is a decision each optometrist must make for each patient.

RULING OUT PATHOLOGICAL CONDITIONS

Most patients who consult an optometrist believe that they require optometric care. They are usually correct in their assumption, for patients usually do a good job of tentative diagnosis. However, the optometrist has the responsibility to confirm the patient's tentative diagnosis in this regard. He must determine that optometric therapy will in fact benefit the patient *and* that no other service is required. In short, the optometrist must determine whether the patient has an anomaly of vision, a disease of the eye, a general disease with symptoms similar to those of visual defects, or some combination of these.

Many patients are also aware that the differentiating of disease from defects of vision is part of the optometric service, and they consult the optometrist for this reason. The detection of eye disease is performed by the optometrist not only to determine which patients he may proceed with along optometric lines, but also because it is actually a part of the optometric service. This acceptance of the responsibility for recognizing disease has not always been a part of optometry, nor is it as integral a part of optometry in other parts of the world as it is in the United States and other English-speaking countries. In some European countries, the optometrist is specifically forbidden to examine the eye to determine whether it is healthy.

Optometric relationship to disease is sometimes not easy to understand. The optometrist does not treat diseases of the eye and does not attempt to make difficult, definitive, differential diagnoses between two diseases. The question might then arise as to why the optometrist attempts to discover disease, since he does not treat disease. The answer is to be found in the sociological aspects of health care in the United States.

Every patient with any symptom that he believes requires professional care must make a decision as to which professional man to consult. If he has a toothache, he consults a dentist. In the earlier part of the twentieth century, most physicians practiced general medicine. Individuals had a family doctor who usually had brought them into the world and who was consultant to the entire family for a multitude of ills. If the family doctor recognized that a problem was beyond his capacity to solve, he referred the patient to a specialist. Medical specialties, in general, were based on physiological systems—for example, genitourinary, cardiovascular, and respiratory. Some specialization was based on the procedure that would be used—such as surgery and radiology.

Under such a system, the patient who had any symptom of illness usually consulted his family doctor first, but the trend is away from this system. Today, there are far more medical specialists than there are general practitioners, and the gap continues to widen. More and more the patient himself is making tentative diagnoses and selecting specialists who he thinks will be appropriate.

Thus, the optometrist is often the first member of the health professions to see the patient. As this happens more and more, the optometrist has increasingly accepted the responsibility that goes with this confidence on the part of the patient. The optometrist has evolved as the general practitioner in the eye field, not as a specialist. A major characteristic of the general practitioner was that he saw all patients first, cared for those whose ailments fell within his realm, and referred to specialists patients whose ailments were more complex. A major characteristic of the specialist was that he received patients who had previously been screened and had been found to require special services. The optometrist, seeing patients first, is then truly a general practitioner for patients who have symptoms associated, or believed to be associated with, vision. He too cares for patients whose ailments fall within his realm, and he accepts the responsibility for referring those whose ailments are more complex or outside his realm.

Although optometry developed within the social structure that made it a general practice profession, this need not have been the case. If the sociology of health care had been such that all patients first saw a trained screener, whose sole responsibility was to make the tentative diagnosis that the patient now makes and to refer the patient to various specialists, optometry might have developed as a specialty. But this did not happen, and recognition of disease, of necessity, became a part of optometry and a very important part. Today's optometrist spends much time in his training learning to differentiate between healthy and diseased visual systems so that he may fulfill his obligation as a general practitioner to his patient. He also learns to recognize visual symptoms of general disease so that he may also fulfill his obligation as the first member of the health professions who sees a patient.

Optometrists are very fortunate that they are able to retain the role of general practitioner in the eye field. At one time, more physicians were general practitioners. Many physicians regard the trend from general practitioner to specialist with regret. Although medical advances caused the trend, these doctors believe that something is lost with the disappearance of the general medical practitioner. The image of the friendly family medical advisor is being replaced by that of an impersonal specialist. Optometry, on the other hand, because its scope is circumscribed, can retain for its members the role of general practitioner. As practiced in the United States, optometry is a profession whose members are advisors on all visual problems. Perhaps no aspect of optometry's development is as satisfying to its members as its ability to retain the role of general practitioner.

Because the optometrist is the general practitioner in the field of vision, and because the optometrist is usually the first health professional to see the patient who has a visual complaint or symptom, he must do an adequate job of ruling out the existence of disease. More and more, optometrists have added tests and procedures to their armamentarium to enable them to meet their responsibility. Thus, one major part of the optometric testing procedure is designed to ascertain whether the patient has a healthy visual system and whether any general disease may be manifesting itself in visual symptoms.

The specific tests the optometrist employs are many. Their administration and interpretation take up a good part of the optometric training program in schools of optometry. Several of the procedures that optometrists perform on most patients are described in the following paragraphs.

EXTERNAL EXAMINATION

Patients who have visible anomalies of the lids and outer coat of the eyeball often associate them with optometric care. Furthermore, some visual defects can cause or aggravate changes of the lids and eye. Thus, the optometrist inspects these external tissues under magnification and good illumination.

FUNDUS EXAMINATION

The ophthalmoscope illuminates the inside of the eye for inspection. The situation is much like looking through the keyhole of a door into a dark room beyond. If the observer places his eye to the keyhole, he sees only darkness. If he places an ordinary flashlight to the keyhole, he has no place for his own eye. The ophthalmoscope introduces illumination as though it came from the same point as the observer's eye. The optometrist can thus study the inside, or fundus, of the patient's eye.

From this examination the optometrist can learn many things. Primarily, he is interested in determining if the eye is free of disease that might require special attention. In most patients, the eye is healthy. It may have minor physiological variations correlated with advancing age or improper development. The optometrist notes these variations and calls them to his patient's attention. When manifestations of eye disease or general disease are noted, the optometrist obtains special attention for his patient.

Some of the general diseases the presence of which may be suggested by changes in the fundus of the eye are diabetes, kidney disorders, hypertension, arteriosclerosis, brain tumors, and some of the diseases caused by microorganisms, such as tuberculosis and syphilis. Optometrists study enough about these and other diseases to recognize their eye manifestations. They do not attempt to complete a definitive diagnosis, recognizing that this is a part of the practice of medicine.

The difference between optometric and medical responsibility to the patient may be clarified by an example. If an optometrist observes a hemorrhage in the fundus, he recognizes that it may be due to any of the diseases already enumerated. It also may have resulted from a vascular accident or from undue capillary fragility. The important consideration for the optometrist, however, is that he see and identify the hemorrhage. It is his responsibility to refer the patient to the appropriate medical practitioner for diagnosis and treatment of the disorder. The optometrist's understanding about disease is sufficient to recognize the various diseases that can cause hemorrhage. He does not attempt to differentiate between them. Medical technology has advanced so greatly in the past few decades that there are now many laboratory tests the physician can use in making the correct diagnosis. Disease is diagnosed by many procedures. The appearance of the eyeground is only one of them.

SLIT-LAMP BIOMICROSCOPY

The slit-lamp biomicroscope is used to examine several of the transparent layers of the anterior segment of the eye. The instrument consists of a bright source of illumination and a microscope. Many abnormalities of the anterior eye not visible without magnification can be discerned with this procedure.

VISION FIELDS

When a person with normal vision looks at an object, he sees it clearly. He also sees objects around the fixated point, but he sees these less clearly. Even objects some distance from the center of fixation are seen. The total picture seen by an eye is called its visual field. The various peripheral areas are served by separate nerve fibers. If some of these fibers have been damaged, the subject will see the object being viewed clearly, but part of the peripheral field might be without vision. Such defects frequently are not brought to the patient's attention in his everyday life, especially if they are small. As long as he sees clearly that which he is looking at, he may be oblivious to the disappearance of parts of the peripheral field.

An investigation of the patient's total field of vision is of value in detecting any disease that may have affected some of the nerve fibers. Because a fairly large area of the brain is involved in visual perception, a hemorrhage, tumor, or disease in the brain that affects just a few fibers may be detected through determination of the visual fields. In such testing, the patient fixates an object in the center of the field, while another object of appropriate size and color is moved about in his field of indirect vision. The disappearance of this test object from the field of indirect vision indicates nonfunctional nerve fiber units. The examiner then attempts to delineate the area of visual loss. Certain eye diseases also show up in their early stages through characteristic loss of vision in the periphery.

If only the middle 30 or so degrees of the visual field are investigated, a tangent screen is used. This instrument—a black square suitable for recording changes—has a central fixation target.

If the total field is investigated, a semicircular arc called a perimeter is used. Several instruments for measuring the field of indirect vision other than perimeter or tangent screen are used, but they are all modifications of the two basic types. In the function of ruling out pathological conditions, the optometric service includes an investigation of the field of indirect (peripheral) vision as well as measurement of central vision.

TONOMETRY

The human eye is a sphere containing fluids and gels the pressure of which is maintained within certain limits. Fluid is constantly formed and at a given pressure leaves the eye. If the pressure rises above a safe level, the eye may lose vision. One test of visual function therefore is some assessment of the pressure of the eye. If the pressure is found to be outside the normal limits, the patient may require medical procedures to prevent loss of vision. Such an assessment of pressure—called tonometry—is part of the optometric service.

In recent years, great advances in tonometry have been made by optometrists. An electronic instrument that is rapid, safe, and accurate was developed at the School of Optometry of the University of California as part of that institution's optometric research program.

Techniques for using standard tonometers for assessment of the intraocular pressure have also been perfected by optometrists.

The inclusion of tonometry in optometric service is relatively recent and has been adopted primarily in the United States. It resulted from the optometrist's understanding of his responsibility for the detection of pathological conditions among his patients. In the brief period of about ten years, tonometry has become a part of the optometric service.

Five of the procedures the optometrist uses for the detection of pathological conditions have been enumerated. The optometric student spends a good deal of time learning to perform such techniques and to interpret and understand them. In his student training and later in his practice, however, the optometrist limits himself to identifying the patient who requires medical attention. As the general practitioner in the eye field, the optometrist recognizes that the medication required for treatment of disease and the use of surgery are medical specialties. He also recognizes the responsibility of a general practitioner to refer patients whose conditions require specialized attention.

OPTOMETRIC CLINICAL PROCEDURES FOR REFRACTION

The determination of the vision that the patient has in each eye and what lenses or training procedures might improve the vision in each eye is only one part of total optometric service. It is, however, the oldest part of optometry and remains the core of optometric service. Even today, in places where optometry is practiced in its most limited form, this aspect is common to all optometrists. In some European countries where optometrists do not attempt to rule out disease, measuring refraction and supplying spectacles are the totality of optometry. Even when optometry is practiced to its fullest extent, however, refraction remains the optometrist's heritage and his forte.

In refraction, the optometrist determines how well each eye sees and which errors of focus may be present—that is, myopia, hypermetropia, or astigmatism. In refraction, the optometrist also determines the precise optical lens that, when placed before the eye, will neutralize the error and give the patient optimal vision.

One characteristic of the tests the optometrist performs is that each is related to one or more other tests. Thus, the datum sought in the administration of the test is only part of the information the optometrist receives. In the present discussion, we shall not be able to discuss all the interrelationships that exist—that essentially is the study of clinical optometry. However, we may use visual acuity, a basic measure in optometry, to illustrate this phenomenon.

VISUAL ACUITY

Visual acuity is a measure of how well the individual sees. The customary letter chart is one with which most Americans are familiar. They have been asked to read the smallest letter they could in school vision tests conducted by nurses, have been tested for automobile driving licenses, have received physical examinations from a physician or for military service, and probably have seen the chart many other times. The basic datum is the size of the smallest letter that can be read on the chart. But the test tells the optometrist many other things.

If vision with lenses was formerly normal but no longer is, one of several diseases is suspected. Thus, even such a basic vision test as acuity can sometimes become a test for the presence of disease. As another example of extra information obtained from a simple acuity test, a patient looking at a line of letters may report that he is unable to read them, but when single letters of the same size are presented to him, he can read them, and he can also read single letters several sizes smaller. This finding, especially if present in one eye only, suggests a form of functional vision loss—amblyopia—that may be amenable to vision training for its improvement. Or, as a third example, a patient might report that, when he looks at a line of letters with both eyes, the acuity is poorer than with either eye alone. This would suggest that some aspect of coordinating the vision of the two eyes is abnormal.

This same phenomenon is true of most of the tests that the optometrist performs. The interrelationship of tests is critical. Individual optometric tests have their major value when interpreted along with other optometric tests. Taking tests and recording the numerical values to describe the results are only a small part of optometry. When we consider what parts of the testing procedure may be delegated to technicians, we must keep this fact in mind. The significance of this concept may be illustrated by considering several medical laboratory tests and comparing them to optometric tests. A medical technician may draw a sample of blood and perform such procedures as determining the sedimentation rate, the red blood cell count, and the white blood cell count. These data are given to the general physician or internist, and he is aided in his diagnosis by them. The value of the numerical data is the same whether the physician does the tests or whether his technician does the tests.

In optometric tests, however, because they are subjective and because the subject's responses have qualitative as well as quantitative aspects, information may be lost if the diagnostician (optometrist) does not conduct the test himself. Optometric tests give information *other than* the recorded numerical result. Acuity tests can tell not only *what* the patient sees but also *how* he sees. This factor is characteristic of most optometric testing. These tests often are not simple physical measurements, but are arrived at through communication between tester and patient. This communication is capable of yielding information beyond the simple numerical result being sought.

Thus, each simple optometric test could be delegated to a technician for its administration. Data could be accumulated and turned over to a diagnostician for analysis. However, if this procedure were followed, much information would be lost—information not available from the simple numerical findings. Optometrists are aware of this fact and often state that a satisfactory diagnosis of a patient's vision problem cannot be achieved through analysis of "cold" data. This concept in optometry is important to understand when we consider the analysis of optometric data. Systems of analysis of data that depend on the numerical relationship of the findings to each other have been devised. However, these are recognized as only first approximations. No system is a satisfactory substitute for the integrated communicative experience of examiner and patient.

In testing refraction and acuity—that is, how well the patient sees and what lens helps—several tests may be used. Some, such as the acuity test, are subjective and depend on communication. Others are simple physical, objective tests. Even in the physical tests in which objective data are sought, however, the optometrist is trained to note the patient's reactions to the tests themselves. The fact that a patient positions himself at the instrument with a head tilt may be significant. Also significant would be the observation that the patient winces when a bright light is used. These and other observations may give clues to the total vision problem.

KERATOMETRY

A great deal of the eye's total power depends on the curvature of the front and most readily accessible surface—the cornea. This curvature may be assessed accurately by studying a magnified image of the reflection of test patterns from this surface. The instrument that presents a test pattern and a telescope for observing the magnified image of this pattern is called an ophthalmometer, or keratometer. Most astigmatism is due to the curvature of the cornea; this instrument enables the optometrist to measure astigmatism due to the cornea. It serves, therefore, as a starting point for subsequent measurements.

Even this simple measurement, however, has significance beyond its obvious interpretation. For most patients, the corneal astigmatism determined by this instrument will be similar in degree to the total astigmatism of the eye. However, this sometimes is *not* the case, and this fact in itself has great significance. If there is marked disagreement between corneal astigmatism and the total astigmatism of the eye, then some other factor must be causing astigmatism. For example, the lens of the eye may be tilted—a diagnosis made indirectly through the disparity of findings.

Information obtained from the keratometer has another use. In addition to measuring astigmatism, it also measures the contribution of the cornea to the total refraction of the eye. Lenses that correct refractive errors are made up of two refracting surfaces—front and rear—the algebraic sum of which is the power of the lens. Thus, a lens of power +1.00 may be made with a +6.00 front and a −5.00 rear. The same power can also be produced by a +3.00 on one surface and a −2.00 on the other. Both lenses have the same power: +1.00. Which combination of lens surfaces should be used to obtain a power sometimes assumes importance. Decision of which combination to use depends on many factors, one of which is the keratometer readings.

Here, then, is a situation in which data (keratometer readings) are accumulated and used later in a totally different context. Even though we have not detailed the optics of this example, it serves to demonstrate the unity of the service mentioned earlier. The individual who has the clinical data should be the same individual who designs the form of the lens to be used. If the total optometric service is fragmented, as sometimes happens, the design of the corrective device may not be optimal.

Because contact lenses fit on the cornea or front surface of the eye, an exact measurement of this surface is important in fitting. Keratometry has value beyond that for the original fitting. It may be used subsequently to diagnose the effect that the contact lens is having on the cornea. Irregularities in the central cornea, which may be the result of contact lens wearing, can be observed and their importance assessed. Keratometry before and during the fitting of contact lenses is an essential part of the overall fitting procedure.

RETINOSCOPY *

This procedure is the most frequently used objective clinical method for determining refractive state. During the test, accommodation is relaxed by having the subject direct and maintain fixation on a distant object. Through the aperture of the retinoscope—a hand instrument that shines a beam of light through the pupil of the sub-

---

* This section on retinoscopy and the following one on subjective testing are cited almost verbatim from Hirsch and Morgan (1965).

ject's eye—the examiner observes the illuminated retina. As the retinoscope is rotated, the beam of light traverses the fundus and a shadow is observed to move. The direction in which this shadow moves tells the examiner whether myopia or hypermetropia exists. Its speed indicates the degree—the faster the motion, the less the refractive error.*

Noting the speed and direction of the shadow as he rotates the instrument, the examiner introduces appropriate lenses of known power before the eye. Lenses are added until a neutral (infinitely fast) motion is produced. As appropriate lenses are added, light coming from the fundus as a secondary source is brought to a focus closer to the aperture in the retinoscope. The closer the focus comes to the aperture, the more rapid the motion of the reflex. When neutrality is reached, the motion is infinitely fast, and the examiner recognizes this infinitely fast motion as the moment when the lens before the subject's eye is equal to the refractive state plus the "working lens." A correction is made for the distance between the subject's eye and the examiner's eye by subtracting the "working lens."

During the test, lenses may be introduced before the eye by means of a lens bar, by individual trial lenses, or by a device with disks containing many lenses (phoropter).

It has taken about a minute to read the description of this test; it takes a clinician about as long to perform the test on one subject. It takes many years of practice, however, before the clinician can develop sufficient mastery of the technique to depend on these results.

SUBJECTIVE TESTING

This is the other major method of determining the refractive state of the eye clinically. The same procedure of introducing various lenses of known power in front of the eye is used. In this method, instead of the examiner noting the appearance of the eye as he brings the eye closer to best focus for a distant object, the subject is asked to report the appearance of test letters placed twenty feet from him. Systems of test charts and such psychophysical methods as bracketing are used to lead the examiner ultimately to the single lens that brings the eye into best focus.

The number of subjective techniques is legion. Each clinician learns to depend on a battery of perhaps half a dozen techniques that he uses routinely. He knows a hundred more if these fail to elicit a response he deems valid.

The art of subjective refraction is applied communication. The examiner tells the subject which form of discriminative judgment he

* This statement is true if, as is customary, a "working lens" placing the examiner at optical infinity is introduced before the patient's eyes.

wishes the subject to make and aids the subject in communicating his conclusions. During the entire procedure, conditions are altered slightly, and the subject's responses are elicited. Each response suggests another comparison for the examiner to present.

Retinoscopy is a testing skill that is acquired slowly by clinicians. The performance of a subjective test is a skill that requires an even longer time to master. Only after much practice does the clinician become competent in this combination of applied psychophysics and communication. At one time or another, the examiner resorts to just about every one of the psychophysical methods.

In the case history, communication was established between the optometrist and the patient. Subjective testing is also a communicative experience, and to some extent, it is an extension of the total communicative process. The two separate phases—case history and subjective testing—may even be brought further together by the optometrist. For example, if in the case history the patient noted that he had seen a blur or fog in the distance, and the examiner finds during the subjective examination that a lens is indicated, the examiner may show the patient the chart with and without the lens, asking: "Is this the blur you were telling me about?" "Is your vision with this lens free of the blur you have been experiencing?" Or the examiner may bring the two bits of information together and begin to think in terms of correction by asking: "Is the blur you see without the lens eliminated by the lens? Is it enough blur, and does it bother you enough, to warrant wearing a lens like this to get rid of the blur?"

Again we stress the interrelationship of the various aspects of the total optometric service and the inseparability of the parts. Although optometric tests may be described and discussed separately, they are really part of a total service designed to determine, correct, and explain the patient's problem. The procedure is not one of taking tests and analyzing them at a later time, but rather a continuous communication between patient and examiner to reach a satisfactory solution to the patient's problem.

ACCOMMODATION

Were the eye a single focus instrument not capable of changing to bring objects at different distances from it into focus, no tests of refraction other than acuity, retinoscopy, and subjective responses would be needed. But the eye is not a static organ; vision is dynamic. The human eye is capable of changing focus for objects at different distances—a process known as accommodation. Therefore, this function of vision must be tested and measured.

The function of accommodation declines with age almost throughout the life of the individual. During the first 40 years of life or so, this slow decline in accommodation is not of great significance for most people because they have more than enough power of accommodation to see objects clearly at their customary near position, as for example in reading. However, about the age of 40 and thereafter, the decline in accommodation is sufficient either to make it impossible for the individual to see close objects clearly or to require such undue effort of the accommodative mechanism as to cause discomfort, such as headaches or pain in and around the eyes.

Accommodation is tested for most patients. In the young, it is tested to determine whether some abnormality in accommodation exists that may interfere with normal functioning of the eyes in seeing close objects. In the patient over 40, the accommodation is tested to determine whether the normal aging process has advanced sufficiently to interfere with near vision.

Perhaps the simplest test of accommodation is one in which the acuity is again measured at distances close to the individual. Another test is to determine how close an object may be brought toward an individual before he notes a blur. There are perhaps half a dozen other tests, all of which assess the amount of ability the individual's visual system possesses for changing focus. Optometrists use one or more of these tests for each patient.

The speed and facility with which a patient may accommodate for a close object is also of importance, because speed and facility of accommodation are characteristics of the *quality* of accommodation, contrasted to the *quantity,* which is measured by amplitude tests. Sometimes the patient's report is sufficient to establish a diagnosis of poor quality of accommodation, again illustrating the interrelationship between case history and testing procedures. Thus, a patient may report that after reading he notes that distant objects blur for several seconds before they clear up. Or he may mention the reverse—that when he first looks at a printed page, it blurs but clears ultimately. Such a patient may have sufficient ability to change focus, but he does so slowly and with great effort.

Because patients past the age of 40 begin to have difficulty with the amount of accommodation they possess, they require lenses for reading different from those they use to see distant objects. The two different lens formulas may be combined into a single lens with two different foci—thus the name bifocal. With increased longevity, there are more and more people who wish to see objects clearly at several different distances. These patients and this aspect of vision have come to demand an increasingly large amount of the optometrist's time.

In this section, we have discussed the measurement of visual acuity, of refractive errors, and of the ability to accommodate. This phase of the total scope of optometry represents the narrowest practice of optometry. Optometry began with the measurement of vision and the designing of spectacles to correct its errors; even today in some countries and among some optometrists in the United States, this is the totality of optometry. To most modern optometrists, however, this heritage and birthright is the cornerstone of their practice, but it is not total optometry.

TESTS FOR BINOCULAR VISION

If man had one eye only, or if the movements of the two eyes were always perfectly coordinated, then the previously described monocular tests might be the total optometric procedure. But man has two eyes. Sometimes these are perfectly coordinated, but often they are not. Some eye movements are so poorly coordinated that only one eye sees at a time, the other eye pointing either in, out, up or down, but *not at* the object being viewed by its fellow eye.

Such disorders are not simple mechanical failures of the musculature. Rather, the visual system has developed in an anomalous fashion. Normal reflexes are absent or faulty. Anomalous patterns have developed in place of normal responses.

For every patient whose eyes actually deviate, there are several whose eyes, although straight, *tend* to turn from perfect alignment. Such patients function binocularly but with great effort. The strain of maintaining single vision and straight eyes produces symptoms of discomfort or causes the individual to avoid certain tasks. Occasionally, the patient has double vision. Because such anomalies exist, the optometric examination must include tests for binocular function.

Because of the complexity of the subject, listing the dozens of individual tests of binocular function is beyond the scope of this book. A large part of the optometric curriculum deals with the anatomy and physiology of both the visual and nervous systems. The geometric aspects of binocular vision and the psychology of perception are equally important. Several optometry courses deal solely with the theoretical and practical aspects of binocular vision, its basis, its anomalies, and the tests and treatment for them.

Even though dozens of tests for binocular vision exist, all of them are not performed for any one patient. Rather, the optometrist follows the same procedure described in subjective testing for refractive error. He performs enough tests either to satisfy himself that binocularity does not present a problem for the individual being examined *or* to delineate the binocular anomaly. For some patients, only two or three tests establish that normally functioning binocularity exists, and no further testing in this regard is necessary. As always, the information gleaned from the earlier communicative experiences with the patient tends to dictate the procedures. The patient who has no apparent signs or symptoms of binocular vision anomalies will receive fewer tests than the patient whose symptoms indicate binocular problems. The patient for whom binocular remediation in the form of orthoptic exercises or special lens correction is anticipated will receive more and different tests than the patient who is presumed to have only a simple refractive error.

The extreme case, the child with crossed eyes, will receive an entire battery of tests—a *squint work-up,* which may require one or more hours to complete. The symptom-free patient with apparently normally functioning eyes may require only two or three minutes of actual testing to confirm his expected normality.

Optometric testing does not employ the same sequence of individual tests for every patient. Rather, testing is continued as long as meaningful information is lacking. Some tests may suggest the need for other tests. To practice optometry with a predetermined routine to which every patient is subjected is to misunderstand the very nature of optometry.

Binocular vision has another important aspect. The reflexes that mediate the turning of the eyes and direction of gaze of both eyes at the same object are associated with the reflexes that mediate the changing of focus. This relationship between convergence and accommodation is important in the practice of optometry. From a practical point of view, it indicates that the lenses that correct a refractive error may induce or alleviate a binocular problem. Thus, not only must the optometrist ascertain that a binocular problem does not exist initially, but he must also understand what effects his correction of vision may have on binocular vision.

As in refraction tests, those for binocular vision may be either subjective or objective. In subjective tests, several devices are used to test binocular function. In the simplest type of test, the patient views an object with each eye. He reports the distance that separates the two images, and prismatic lenses are introduced until he reports superposition of the images seen by the two eyes. In objective tests, the movements of the eyes are observed as various procedures are followed.

Each single test is in itself simple. Each yields an important datum. The optometrist does not have to memorize a vast series of tests, however. Once he understands binocular vision and its theoretical basis, he understands the data he may wish to obtain. The testing procedures themselves then become understandable. Here, as in other phases of optometry, the importance of theory to practical application becomes clear. It is a myth that the *practical* thing to do is to learn a series of tests and their interpretation. Rather, when one understands the theory of binocular vision thoroughly, he understands the tests used for it and is ready to apply them intelligently. Moreover, the optometrist may improvise new tests. As long as he understands the physiology of binocular vision, he can improvise questions and situations to present to the patient that will produce meaningful needed information.

THE DECISION

In describing the optometric service, we have discussed the case history that imparts the patient's problem to the optometrist, the ruling out of disease, and monocular and binocular clinical testing. Having completed these four phases of the procedure, which may require as few as a half dozen, or as many as 50, individual test items, the optometrist must decide what to do. He does not arrive at this point without constant reappraisal. Throughout the procedure, the optometrist has been adjusting his testing as the end point has become more narrowly defined. He has performed the tests that he thought appropriate for the individual patient. He arrives at the time of decision with some idea of what will be needed. If there is still doubt, the testing continues. The decision to terminate testing is an indication that the optometrist knows the solution to the patient's difficulty.

When optometry is practiced as the true art that it is, the optometrist analyzes data and approaches a decision as he administers tests. This method was not always practiced by optometrists. Nor can a student learn to practice in this manner until he masters the necessary fundamentals. Interestingly, the student in optometry first learns much as optometrists of an earlier day practiced. He keeps in mind, however, that the necessities involved in the teaching situation result in artificial conditions. He learns in this way until he has mastered the fundamental concepts. As the entire picture fits together, he learns to practice expertly. In a sense, students in the learning process recapitulate the evolutionary phases of the profession. This being so, it is fitting to review the various methods of analyzing optometric data in chronological sequence.

When optometry was very young in the United States, examination of the eyes for refractive errors was almost the total scope of the optometric service. The lens that appeared to give the patient the best vision in each eye was sought. When this was determined, the service was ended. Then, owing to advances in learning, the physiological aspects of binocular vision became understood, and their clinical applications were worked out. It became necessary to teach these new concepts to an entire group of men already in practice. It was neither practical nor feasible to take these practicing optometrists back through courses in theoretical physiological optics in order to bring them up to date. Simplified systems of practical application had to take the place of basic knowledge. Optometry went through a phase of "analysis of data," the assumption being that data accumulated in a vacuum could later be analyzed for meaningful applications.

One early system of data analysis very widely used was that of the Optometric Extension Program.* The optometrist was taught to perform each of a specified battery of tests. The specific number of tests, first 18 and later 21, was to be performed on every patient. The program supplied optometrists with a list of normal, or expected, values for each of the tests. These norms were the average values obtained for each of the tests on a group of symptom-free patients. Thus, data for the individual patients could be compared to the normals or averages. For each test, an individual would have a score higher or lower than the average.

The optometrist was supplied with a series of formulas in which he substituted the values obtained for the individual patient. If a certain pattern was observed, this indicated a certain type of anomaly. The process of substituting individual findings in the formulas was called "chaining and typing." A specific kind of therapy was indicated for each of the types.

For the optometrist who, before the appearance of this program, had been doing no binocular testing, this was a marked advance. The system was simple to learn, was completely mechanical, and offered cook-book procedures that produced answers not formerly obtained. In the absence of an understanding of physiological optics, this was the best that could be hoped for. It was a marked advance because the optometrist now considered the effects of binocularity, in addition to determining refractive error. However, it had the same limitations that all formula learning has in any endeavor, as opposed to conceptual learning in the same endeavor.

Although optometry has progressed far beyond this system, elements of formula learning are useful in teaching. Students may be taught to perform at least a minimum number of tests by mere de-

* The Optometric Extension Program system for optometric data analysis was described in the monthly papers distributed to members during the 1930's. It was described by Skeffington (1931) in a book copyrighted by the author. Morgan (1944d) wrote: "The most lucid and readily available account of this particular system of 'analytical refraction' is to be found in Dvorine's book . . ." (1939). The system has also been described by Lesser (1933) and most recently by Manas (1965).

scription of the tests. They also learn the general function that the test purports to measure and the average value of the test. Thus, while few optometrists today take seriously the older formulas and chaining and typing, students still begin their optometric experience by learning tests and the average expected values.

The fallacy of comparing individual findings to averages—in fact, the fallacy of dealing with averages at all—soon became apparent to many optometric scientists. More sophisticated systems were introduced to optometrists, at first in the schools and later to the men in practice. Not only were the systems more sophisticated, but so were the optometrists who were learning them. Knowledge of physiological optics was becoming a part of optometric training.

Morgan (1944a, b, c, d), for example, elaborated the concept that any average value was derived from a frequency distribution that had variability. He determined the standard deviation for several of the binocular clinical tests and suggested that a value of two standard deviations from the mean might be abnormal. He offered no system of applying the data to formulas, assuming that the optometrist understood the basic nature of the test, and that if he found abnormality, he could arrive at conclusions without a cook-book system. The student today also learns the distribution of data for the various visual functions along with the averages.

Another way of analyzing optometric data is that of graphic analysis. In this method, the data of several functional tests are plotted on a graph. If the data hold certain relationships to each other, the patient is presumed not to have a binocular vision problem. Clearly, this system, like Morgan's, gets away from average values. The data for the individual are compared to other data for the same individual rather than to norms.

The graphic system is based on material first presented by Donders (1864). Percival (1892) gave the clinical applications of the graphic analysis system and in fact offered several graphs of patients' visual functions.* To Maddox (1893) is attributed the first rational

---

* Percival's early descriptions were quite clear, but there was a time lag of 30 years before other visual scientists recognized the usefulness of his method. Twenty additional years would elapse before the method was widely used by optometrists— a lag of fifty years between the first description and appreciable application to patients. Percival (1928) wrote: "My definition of the area of comfort was published in the *Ophthalmic Review* in 1891 [actually published in 1892] and since that time I have seen nothing to alter in my original communication. Some of my original diagrams are given below." The diagrams he presents are not greatly different from those used in modern graphic analysis.

Weymouth, Brust, and Gobar (1925) seem to have recognized the importance of Percival's work, and wrote: "Percival's (1892) conception of an 'area of comfort' occupying the middle third of the zone of relative accommodation and convergence is, we consider, a very valuable one, and our figures are in accord with the main features of his."

theory of accommodation, convergence and its components, and the relationship between accommodation and convergence (Morgan 1944d). In the 1920's, the system of graphic analysis of optometric data was studied by Weymouth, Brust, and Gobar (1925) and Sheard.* The system was modified and brought to optometrists' attention through the work of Fry (1937, 1939, 1943) and Hofstetter (1945).

The systems of the Optometric Extension Program, of Morgan, and of graphic analysis are still used as teaching aids. As a student today learns how to perform each of the tests for binocular function, he learns first what its basis is and what the physiological aspects of the test are. Then he learns the average value for this test (OEP); he learns the standard deviation for this test among the population (Morgan); and he learns where this finding would be plotted on a graph of binocular function, thus enabling him to visualize its relationship to other data.

The student of optometry today learns through these methods, each of which in the past had many optometric adherents. The tests give him familiarity with the data with which he will be working. The student develops a "feel" for optometric testing. As he works with patients during his years in the college clinic, he discovers the relationships between tests. He learns that certain tests for certain patients offer no meaningful new information. The student begins to anticipate how certain tests will result. As testing becomes almost automatic, he can direct his attention to aspects other than the mechanical administration of the test. He begins to think in terms of the end result *while* he is testing. He no longer tests and then analyzes, but analyzes while he is testing. As he develops this skill, he gains a great deal of diagnostic capacity, for experienced clinicians insist that tests analyzed *in vacuo* or from "cold data" lack information.

Thus the optometrist of today knows not merely tests but the physiology of the function being tested, the psychophysics of testing, the interrelationship of functions and tests to each other, and the implications of the test. Most important, he does not even perform a test unless it will yield him a bit of information he requires to arrive at a solution of the patient's problem. Early optometrists first performed a routine or specified battery of tests and then analyzed the results. Students today learn by this method until they have the necessary skill and maturity to analyze as they examine.

---

* Sheard presented this paper at the seventh annual meeting of the American Academy of Optometry in 1928. It was printed as an original paper twice—once in the *Transactions of the American Academy of Optometry* (1929) and once in the *American Journal of Optometry* (1930).

OPTOMETRIC THERAPY

The communicative experience that began with the patient's recital of his symptoms during the case history and that continued through the testing procedures administered to gain information about the patient's visual problem also continues into the therapeutic phase. The optometrist may have decided that lenses and orthoptic training will solve the patient's problem. He will then explain to the patient the procedures that should be used. If the optometrist has decided that the patient requires the services of a member of another health profession, he will explain this fact to the patient. If he has decided that the patient's visual environment requires modification through better illumination or shorter periods of sustained use of the eyes, he will discuss and describe this modification to the patient.

Resolution of the patient's initial problem and subsequent explanation of what should be done are important parts of optometric service. If optometric procedures will help, they are explained to the patient and instituted. If optometric therapy is not the solution for the patient's symptoms, then some other decision in solving the problem is required.

The optometrist is the general practitioner in the field of vision. In discussing optometric therapy, it is useful to compare it to that used by the general practitioner in medicine.*

When a patient consults a physician for some symptom of illness, the physician will perform tests to determine the exact nature of the ailment. Like the optometrist, he knows hundreds of tests but performs only those likely to identify the cause of the patient's complaint. The physician most frequently can and does alleviate the patient's symptoms by drugs or medication. The optometric analogue of a drug is a lens. Thus, the optometrist will most frequently prescribe a lens. Nor does the analogy cease there. Just as there are thousands of drugs, so there are countless lens combinations. Just as certain drugs are used more frequently than others, so certain lens combinations are used more frequently than others. Just as drugs are sometimes used to aid diagnosis—that is, experimentally to determine if the symptoms respond to them—so lenses are used for diagnostic purposes. Just as some drugs alleviate while others cure, so

---

* Because optometry is not a branch or part of medical practice, the reader may wonder why the analogy with the medical general practitioner is used here. The authors feel that this will be a useful teaching aid, since most readers will have a fair idea of the generalist concept in medical practice.

some lenses neutralize an error and thereby alleviate symptoms, while other lenses have a desirable effect on a visual function and its future use. Lenses are to the practice of optometry what drugs are to the practice of medicine.

A second form of medical procedure is described by the broad term physical therapy. In order to rest a sprained part, the physician might recommend and fit a patient with a sling; optometrists in similar situations use an eye patch to force a fellow eye to work. The physician might have the patient come to his office to lie under a heat lamp or diathermy equipment; the optometrist gives vision training or orthoptics on much the same basis. On the other hand, the physician may prefer to have the patient obtain a heat lamp and treat himself at home, just as the optometrist may recommend that the patient obtain a simple apparatus for giving himself orthoptic exercises at home.

Again, the analogy is closer than one might believe at first glance. Physicians in general practice find that patients assigned to do certain tasks at home rarely follow advice, just as optometrists find that in-office orthoptic training yields better results than that administered by the patient to himself at home. Or, the physician may find that rather than relief of a symptom through exercise and similar physical means a patient may prefer a pain-killing drug; optometrists find that many patients prefer to wear lenses to alleviate their symptoms rather than to spend time and effort with eye exercises to alleviate the symptoms. Because the results depend on patient cooperation, many physicians limit their therapy to drugs, offering physiotherapy to occasional patients only; optometrists often regard the lens or orthoptics alternative in a similar manner.

A third course of action the general physician might follow is to advise the patient how he may help alleviate his symptom and how he may prevent its recurrence. He might suggest improvements in diet, more exercise, more sleep, or similar general hygienic measures. The optometrist as a general practitioner also offers advice about illumination, rest periods, length of time to use the eyes, distance to hold objects from the eyes, or similar measures designed to enable the patient to use his eyes with minimal discomfort.

A fourth function of a general practitioner is the recognition of problems that demand the attention of a specialist. The optometrist recognizes problems that require the skills and training of surgeons or other specialized people. When the general practitioner of medicine refers a patient to a surgeon, he still retains an interest in that patient's well-being. It is not uncommon for the general practitioner to visit the postsurgical patient in the hospital and attend to needs of the patient that are not related to the surgery. Similarly, the optometrist, having referred a patient for surgery, retains an interest in the patient's well-being and cooperates in the postsurgical care of the patient. Just as the general practicing physician is often trusted by the patient to recommend the surgeon, so the optometrist as a general practitioner in the eye-care field is often requested by the patient to choose the surgeon. This activity is part of the responsibility of the general practitioner.

Another function of the general practitioner is to recognize those anomalies best left untreated. This is an important part of the professional judgment that the patient expects his generalist to exercise. The optometrist may decide that a child with ocular deviation of small angle whose anomaly is not amenable to surgery, exercise, or any other therapy is best served if the parents are advised not to institute therapy. The optometrist will then explain carefully why he believes that refraining from therapy is the best solution for this patient, and he will explain that the anomaly is not too great a handicap. The optometrist may discover a very early cataract in a very elderly patient. He may believe that the patient's age makes it almost certain that the cataract will not develop within the patient's lifetime. The optometrist may obtain a concurring opinion from an ophthalmologist. The important point to recognize here is that often the procedure that will serve the patient best is to do nothing. Refraining from treatment must be regarded as an important form of treatment.

Finally, the general practitioner is a family counselor. The optometrist frequently is consulted on genetic and other problems. Optometrists are expected to understand hereditary and genetically determined conditions associated with the eyes. The attitude of the general practitioner is one of acceptance of the responsibility for his patient's well-being. The readily available counselor is a necessary part of any good health program.

Counseling by both the optometrist and the general medical practitioner is one of the most important functions either one performs. Many patients who consult the general medical or general eye practitioner have minor symptoms or physiological variations that require no treatment other than the understanding of their nature. The word *doctor* stems from the Latin word for teacher. The general practitioner often must teach his patient how to live with minor symptoms. The optometric patient who notes floating spots when he looks at the sky requires only a description of the nonpathological nature of this phenomenon to set his fears at rest. The patient whose headache is caused by tension requires a description of the phenomenon and an understanding of his reactions to tension. Optometrists see many patients who are worried by normal, nonpathological phenomena, and as general practitioners, they teach such patients how to live with these phenomena.

Even when therapy is instituted, it is accompanied by advice and teaching. The general medical practitioner who has a patient with a cold may use medication to relieve the symptoms but also may advise the patient on how to avoid colds in the future. Similarly, an optometrist may prescribe simple lenses for a symptom, as well as offer advice to the patient on how to avoid misusing his eyes in the future. For many patients, the drug that a practicing general physician prescribes is useful, but the advice and counsel given with it may be of equal or greater importance. In similar fashion, the lens prescribed by an optometrist may allay the symptoms, but advice and counsel may be of equal or greater importance.

While communication is highly important, it is also costly. It may take longer to *counsel* a patient than to *treat* one or more patients. For this reason, there is constant temptation to offer health care without this costly ingredient. In this way the cost can be lowered. Just as there are physicians who use assembly-line procedures in seeing patients, so some optometrists stress the therapeutic devices (lenses) and shirk the counseling aspect. The trend in medicine is definitely away from general practice; this may also be in store for optometry, a situation that would be most regrettable for the patient. As means have been sought to make health care available at reduced costs, this aspect has been the first to be sacrificed. Yet this much-discussed doctor-patient relationship may have more value to the patient than the drugs or spectacles he receives. Those who seek health care at reduced prices often fail to recognize the value of the counseling aspect of health services. This is a false economy that should be guarded against. In another section of the book, this phase of optometry is further treated. For the present, the reader should be well aware that a general practice service at its best includes genuine communication between patient and practitioner. This is one of the major characteristics, and perhaps offers the major value, of the general practitioner in health care.

We have dealt at some length with the marked similarity between the general practitioner in medicine and the optometrist. Some optometrists have complained of the limitations of the profession and of the limited horizons of optometric practice. Those who complain are frequently unaware of all the possibilities general practice offers and that the general practitioner in medicine has similar limitations. General practice, by definition, must be limited but it has its compensations. The personal relationship between doctor and patient, and the complete confidence of the patient in his family doctor are the chief rewards of general practice. High degrees of specialization, such as in surgery, are accompanied by much greater impersonality. Many physicians look with regret on what appears to be the passing of the general practitioner in medicine because they recognize that the patient has need for a family consultant. Optometry, in being a general-practice profession, is extremely fortunate, and its "limitations" are the price optometrists must pay for the privilege of being the general practitioners in the eye-care field.

Although the similarities between the general practice of medicine and of optometry are marked, there are differences. The most striking difference is the dispensing of the therapeutic agent. Drugs are to the physician what spectacles are to the optometrist, but the *prescription* for a drug and that for a pair of spectacles are very different. Optometrists insist on filling their own prescriptions and supplying the therapeutic device, while physicians write a drug prescription for another person to fabricate and supply. Because supplying the therapeutic device—the spectacles—is a basic part of optometry, it is advisable to explore this optometric concept, for supplying the device by the prescriber is a procedure contrary to medical concepts.

A pharmaceutical prescription calls either for a compound that has been prepared earlier by the manufacturing company and that the physician describes by name, or for a mixture of chemicals to be combined in prescribed amounts by the pharmacist. This latter method of prescribing is becoming increasingly rare. In either case, it is assumed that the prescription that the physician has written is sufficiently explicit so that any pharmacist who fills it will produce exactly the same compound as any other pharmacist following the same prescription. The variables of the pharmaceutical formula or prescription are the names of the chemical components and the amounts of each. The physician also specifies the form of the compound (liquid, tablet, capsule, and so on) and the recommended dosage.

An ophthalmic lens prescription, however, may have many unspecified variables in addition to those usually noted in the lens formula. The lens formula specifies the focusing power of the lens in two meridians and the orientation of the lens in the frame. It is customary also to state the distance separating the centers of the two lenses. However, beyond these vital characteristics of a pair of lenses, there are many variables, usually not specified, that are of great importance to the patient who will wear the spectacles.

The power of a lens differs according to its distance from the eye. Individual facial features differ, and a spectacle frame may place the lens anywhere from 7 to 19 millimeters from the eye. Were the optometrist to attempt to write a precise formula for lenses, he would have to specify the distance from the eye at which the frame would hold the lenses. The lens power used must differ according to the spectacle frame chosen and the distance from the patient's eye to the lens. The utility of the formula for the lens can depend on its carrier, the spectacle frame. In medical prescriptions, the characteristics of the chemical compound are not affected by the bottle or box it comes in.

Moreover, the choice of the front and rear curves of the lens, its thickness, and other physical characteristics may be important in certain lens combinations. For bifocals, the type of bifocal and the positioning of the bifocal component are very important variables that may affect the wearability of the lenses. However, one cannot specify the height of the bifocal segment until he knows the frame in which it will be worn.

Nor are all differences between an ophthalmic and a pharmaceutical prescription to be found in the descriptive aspects. The ophthalmic device must be fitted to the patient's face. No matter how skillfully written a lens formula is, if the lenses are not properly aligned for optical considerations, as well as for physical comfort, the patient will not derive maximal benefit. In pharmaceutical prescriptions, the patient is ordered to apply the therapy to himself at designated periods, but an ophthalmic device must be fitted and adjusted to the patient. One or more subsequent refinements in adjustment may be necessary. The difference even goes beyond this, for the ophthalmic prescription may be set one way at first and another way at a later time. Thus the optometrist may set bifocals in one orientation while the patient acclimatizes himself to them, and then by changing the adjustment, the optometrist may set them at a different position for use when the patient is accustomed to wearing the new bifocal unit.

For the reasons just enumerated and for many others of similar nature, optometrists, from their historic beginning on, considered examination of the patient's vision and supplying the spectacles as part of a unified service. Optometrists are trained to view the entire service as a single service and not to separate examining and prescribing from supplying, fitting, and adjusting the spectacles. Subsequent testing is often performed through the spectacles while they are on the patient. Occasionally, the effect on vision of altering the orientation of the spectacles is studied by the optometrist.

The unity of examination and supplying and adjusting the device is one of the unique aspects of optometry. As a result, patients receive optimal vision care service. It should be mentioned that there is an alternative to such a system. It is possible for an optometrist to write a lens formula, much as a physician writes a pharmaceutical formula. An optician can fill such a prescription just as a pharmacist fills a medical prescription. However, because of the nature of the two forms of therapy, the patient does not usually receive the best possible spectacle correction unless the system is a unified one. In the United States today, some people do receive their spectacles from someone other than the prescribing doctor. It is one of optometry's premises that such ophthalmic service is not optimal.

In a sense, the ophthalmic prescription resembles a dentist's choice of procedures more than it does a medical prescription. A dentist could examine a tooth and carefully design a filling or inlay. He could write a complex formula and submit a tridimensional design to another person who would perform the actual mechanical application of the restoration. However, such a procedure is unthinkable to dentists, whose training makes diagnosis and carrying out of the therapy part of a unified service. In this regard, optometric health care is much closer to dentistry than it is to medicine.

Therapy thus far has been discussed in terms of the importance of advice and consultation, and of spectacles designed, fitted, supplied, and adjusted for the patient by the optometrist. In addition to conventional spectacles, other forms of lens therapy are prescribed by optometrists. Special magnifying devices are designed for patients with low visual acuity. Contact lenses in the past decade or so have become used widely and are worn by millions in the United States.

Sometimes these procedures are considered to be specialties within optometry, but for the most part the optometrist who is practicing optimally also engages in them. Today most optometrists fit contact lenses. However, a few optometrists limit their practice to contact lens work only. These men become specialists in this regard and serve the useful role of consultant to other practitioners who have patients with special problems regarding contact lenses.

It is interesting to note again the comparison to medicine. Although the vast majority of practicing physicians of a few decades ago were general practitioners, today there are more specialty practitioners in the United States than general practitioners. In optometry, however, the vast majority of optometrists are general practitioners, while only a few specialize.

Another form of optometric therapy is vision training, or orthoptics. Several visual attributes, and particularly those that pertain to the use of the two eyes as a unified system, can be modified by training procedures. The patient, by repeating certain visual situations, is often able to change the operation of the visual system. For example, a patient who has difficulty in pointing both eyes at an object at the reading distance—that is, whose eyes tend not to converge on the object being viewed—may be trained to perform this necessary act more readily.

Several aspects of visual training as a therapeutic measure deserve discussion.

1. For the most part, vision training is considered a part of the

general practice of optometry. Certain anomalies are best alleviated through lenses, others through orthoptic exercises. The optometrist practicing his art to the fullest usually does orthoptic work for patients who require it. As in contact lenses, a few optometrists specialize in this area of optometry. For the most part, however, orthoptics is a part of the therapy provided by the optometrist in general practice. Most optometrists do not regard orthoptics as a specialty within the field.

2. Although some functions may be trained by orthoptic exercises, others cannot be changed. For example, many people have attempted to cure nearsightedness through exercises. Their failure has been clearly demonstrated. Nearsighted persons may be helped to see more clearly with lenses, but neither exercises nor lenses have any major effect on the consequences or progression of myopia. The competent practitioner recognizes the anomalies that respond and those that do not to each form of therapy.

As optometry has evolved, thanks to research in theoretical and applied physiological optics, optometrists have learned that some anomalies respond best to orthoptic training, others best to spectacles. The choice of overall procedure, as well as the specific choice of lens or form of exercises, is now part of the study of optometry. Through his understanding of the basic aspects of his field, the optometrist makes a prudent choice for each patient.

3. Many optometrists believe that orthoptic exercises are best administered by the optometrist himself. This belief is part of the premise of a total unified service. Just as optometrists believe that any division in the prescribing-fitting-adjusting aspects of spectacle procedures is artificial, they also believe that testing and actual administration of orthoptic training are best done by the general practicing optometrist. Some, however, believe this tedious and time-consuming task may be delegated to a technical assistant. There is no simple answer to this difference of opinion. (The role of assistants is discussed more fully in later chapters.)

In most optometric offices, the optometrist personally engages in the administration of the exercises and training procedures. Most optometrists practice this type of therapy as a part of their general optometric practice. The authors of this text tend to agree that the patient is best served by having as much of the total service as possible under the personal supervision of the optometrist.

4. Although optometrists think of orthoptic training as an in-office procedure, certain patients may be assigned exercises to perform at home. In these instances the optometrist, on completion of his examination, advises the patient. He teaches the patient to do home exercises, at frequent intervals he retests the aspects of vision that he

thinks the training should modify, he again teaches, and he again tests. There is no break in the total service; it is worked through as a unit. We may label one part "examination," one part "teaching," and the third part "rechecking," but in practice these are all parts of the unified service. The total procedure is designed to alleviate or neutralize original symptoms of the patient.

Exercises to do at home are not the only form of out-of-office training used optometrically. A patient may be given lenses on a temporary basis for the training effect they will have. A patient may be given special training lenses to wear while he watches television, a procedure designed to train certain functions while the patient is engaged in other pursuits. A patch may be used in front of one eye to force the patient to use the other eye. Any of these procedures, as well as subsequent office visits during which the optometrist reassesses and adjusts the homework, forms part of optometry's total service. This form of therapy emphasizes the artificiality of separating vision training from the general practice of optometry.

Sometimes it is necessary to have the patient follow certain procedures in order that more accurate testing may be performed on another day. In one anomaly, for example, in which one eye tends to point above its fellow, the patient may be requested to wear a patch for a day or two before returning for a retest. The tendency to turn is thus allowed to manifest itself when a patch is used. Again, testing and home procedures form part of a unified activity for optometrists.

THE OPTOMETRIC SERVICE—*Summary*

Through a description of what optometrists do on a day-to-day schedule with patients, the total service has been described. Of necessity, the description has not been complete but has involved major features only.

The optometric service is a unified service beginning with communication between optometrist and patient. It continues in the testing situation, those tests being administered that will throw light on the source of the patient's difficulties. If the patient's problem is non-optometric (disease, for example), the patient is referred to an appropriate practitioner. If it is optometric, the service continues with the fitting, supplying, and adjusting of spectacles, contact lenses, or special lens devices. It may also continue with the administration by the optometrist of vision training, either at the office or at home. Whatever therapy is used, the patient is informed of his problem. He is advised of hygienic measures or better ways to use his vision. The patient may make several additional visits to have the effect of lenses or orthoptic exercises reevaluated. The service is a total and unified one, and it does not end with examination or with the administration of therapy.

The total service is an excellent one for the patient. One aspect that the reader cannot have helped but note is that it is time consuming. This means that it will of necessity entail some cost. This part of the problem is explored in later chapters. The basic challenge, however, has been stated. Optimal service is time-consuming; it could be made less expensive by curtailing parts or by using assembly-line techniques (division of labor, employment of technicians, and so on). However, any separation, curtailment, or destruction of the unity and of the communicative aspects results in a less beneficial service. The challenge then is to find a way to make the service available to all who need it *without allowing it to become less than optimal.*

The practice of optometry described in this chapter is the classic form. However, the description here is by no means that of the complete scope of optometry. Some optometrists take special interest in the visual problems of motorists, aviators, or other occupations involving unique vision problems. Others take special interest in the vision of children or the aged. The scope of optometry is broad enough to include all aspects of human vision in addition to the services rendered in the classic form. A more complete listing of the various aspects of optometry is found in Appendix I. Although this list is quite broad, the vast majority of optometrists today practice the classic form of the profession described in this chapter. This they do in one-man, private-practice offices throughout the United States.

CHAPTER 3

PRE-OPTOMETRIC HISTORY

The optometric service has been described as one which amelio-rates vision defects. Man has had such defects for countless thousands of years; he has had a rational means for correcting them, spectacles, for only 700 years. Even though early man usually either tolerated his anomalous vision or sometimes perished because of it, sometimes he did make attempts to correct it. This chapter is a review of his efforts to correct vision defects in the period before the invention of specta-cles.

Optical defects of the eye were poorly understood during this period. Dimness of vision was attributed to causes other than the lack of focus of the eye. When man did have pain or dimness of vision that was intolerable, he sought the help of the priests and physi-cians—if he could afford to do so. Since the beginning of recorded history, the relief from pain or affliction has cost money. One of the earliest recorded laws provides for the compensation of those relieving affliction. The Code of Hammurabi, a collection of the laws of Baby-lonia in the period about 1700–1800 B.C., states that:

> If a physician opens an abscess of a man with a bronze lancet and saves that man's eye, he shall receive ten shekels of silver.

This same code, incidentally, contains provisions that are the earliest references to malpractice. If the lancing of an abscess resulted in the loss of an eye, the physician could be fined heavily if the pa-tient was a slave or have his fingers cut off if the patient was a freeman.*

IN THE BEGINNING—*Demons and Incantations*

Man's efforts to treat vision defects in the earliest days of re-corded history were not impressive by modern standards. A rational

* Unless otherwise noted, the material in this and the subsequent chapter was derived from Shastid (1917), Cox (1947), Hofstetter (1948), Gregg (1965), and the Encyclopaedia Britannica.

explanation for disease or for defects was not known. Most ills that befell men were believed to be due to demons, unfriendly gods, or other supernatural beings. Disease was believed to be caused by demons inhabiting the body; therefore, cure lay in driving the demons out by appealing to the good gods (incantations) or by using distasteful and disgusting remedies. The more horrible the remedy, the more likely it was to be efficacious in driving out evil spirits. Hence, purgatives were used for a multitude of diseases, and surgical incisions or blood-letting was also used to rid the body of the demons. The idea that various diseases were caused by demons and the practices of the day were part of the same lack of knowledge.

Surgery for certain eye afflictions was practiced 4000 years ago. Most afflictions of the eye, however, were treated by magic, incantations, and astrology. An early reference (cited by Shastid, 1917) to the treatment of anomalies of vision is found in an incantation used by Babylonian physicians about 2000 B.C.

> Disease of the bowels, the disease of the heart, the palpitation of the diseased heart,
> *disease of the vision,** disease of the head, malignant dysentery,
> the tumor which swells,
> ulceration of the reins,† the micturition which wastes,
> cruel agony which never ceases, nightmare,
> Spirit of the Heavens, conjure it! Spirit of the heavens, conjure it!

Thus, one of the earliest treatments for defects of vision that we encounter is the act of beseeching the heavens to help and ordering the defects to go away. Modern optometrists still see an occasional patient who relies heavily on this method.

In the records of Egyptian medicine of the period about 1500 B.C., there are references to several defects that today would fall within the province of optometry and that would be treated by lenses or orthoptics. In the Ebers Papyrus, which lists the diseases and remedies known to the Egyptians of this period, there are several prescriptions for "dimness of sight," which probably included large refractive errors, as well as various eye diseases. Swamp water was one; a compress of antimony and honey was another. Honey mixed with the excrement of a child was also recommended for dimness of vision. For "pain in the eye," which could be due to refractive errors as well as disease, antimony and charcoal were recommended. For "turning of the eyes," a condition that today is often corrected by orthoptic exercises and lenses, a mixture of tortoise brain and oriental spices was used.

* Present authors' italics.

† Kidneys.

Remedies like those described in the Ebers Papyrus were used for hundreds of years. During this period, the lot of an individual with defective vision was not a happy one. If he could pay for professional help, he might be prayed over or exorcised; he might be given one of several distinctly unpalatable nostrums. He was undoubtedly charged well, but he received little help other than the psychological impact of the treatments. Most patients ultimately must have decided to live and die with their defects of vision.

In Greece during the fifth century B.C., general medical practice became more rational. Magic and demonology were replaced by accurate descriptions of disease. The humoral theory, which attributed disease to the various fluids of the body, was accepted by most physicians. Disease was treated first by drugs designed to restore the balance of the humors of the body, then by surgery to drain off the ill humors, and finally by "fire," or cauterization.

The father of modern medicine, Hippocrates, lived between 460 and 377 B.C. Although his descriptions of general disease are excellent, Hippocrates made little contribution to the field of the eye and vision. For "nyctalopia" Hippocrates recommended liver of an ox and honey along with general purgatives. If this failed, surgery was recommended consisting of incisions and cauterization in the area of the occiput and neck. Nyctalopia probably meant photophobia or undue sensitivity to light, a condition treated today by tinted lenses. It sometimes meant dimmed vision at night, and thus could have included some patients with myopia.

For amblyopia, by which was meant reduced vision from any cause, surgery of the skull was used. To be sure, man was getting closer to a rational basis for healing. No longer was disease caused by demons, but rather by a physical cause—the body humors. Insofar as man's thinking was concerned, a tremendous step forward had been taken. But for the afflicted individual, surgery (before anesthesia, of course) or a different set of nostrums was hardly an improvement over the incantations and nostrums of a millenium earlier.

Some of the treatments of this period, if no more efficacious, were at least more humane. Demosthenes, the Athenian who lived from 384 to 322 B.C., mentioned eyestrain resulting from looking at brightness and particularly from reading. Among other symptoms, he mentioned watering of the eyes and a tendency of the lids to close. He recommended walking, running, holding the breath, and general gymnastic exercises. In lieu of the simple lens prescription for reading that the modern optometrist would use or of orthoptic vision exercises, this regimen leaves much to be desired. It does, however, mark a step forward. Progress was being made, but it was very slow and painful. Nor was there any marked improvement in treatment of the pa-

tient with vision defects for almost another two millennia. Some 900
years after Demosthenes, his treatment for eyestrain was still recommended by Aëtius, a Greek physician, born at Amida in Mesopo-
tamia.

THE SCIENTIFIC BASES OF OPTOMETRY

The applied sciences, particularly those in the health professions,
are based on knowledge in several basic science areas. Modern medicine, for example, depends on anatomy, bacteriology, biochemistry,
physiology, chemistry, and physics for fundamental knowledge. Three
broad areas represent the bases for modern optometry: (1) the life
sciences, especially anatomy and physiology of the eye and nervous
system; (2) the physical sciences, including particularly physics, optics, and the mathematics necessary to understand and work with optical problems; and (3) the psychology of sensation and perception, or
more precisely the psychophysical and psychophysiological visual
studies.

Developments in the basic sciences supply the knowledge on
which rational practice is based. This situation is true in medicine to
a great extent. Many of the great discoveries attributed to modern
medicine were actually made by basic scientists in other fields. Usually it was the chemists, the anatomists, the bacteriologists, or the
biologists who made the great breakthroughs in knowledge that were
incorporated into daily medical practice. This situation also applies
to optometry. In considering its history, it is advisable to look from
time to time at the progress being made in the basic sciences.

There is a myth, not only in optometry but in many other fields,
that a wide divergence exists between theory or basic knowledge and
the applied aspects of the problem. Misinformed people, even today,
speak of theory and practice as though these were two widely diver-
gent areas. This myth is nowhere better refuted than in a historical
review. The ineffective, almost barbaric, methods of treating eye
defects used for several thousand years went hand in hand with igno-
rance of a suitable theory of vision. Enlightened methods of treatment
depend very closely on advances in basic learning and knowledge
of the field as a whole. One does not encounter in history examples of theory and practice being anything but intimately bound together.

There are, to be sure, time lags. Often a discovery in a basic science is not recognized and does not find its way into the practice of
the applied branch for many years. However, ultimately knowledge
does triumph. One pressing problem of science today is the improve-

ment in communications among men of learning so that these time lags will be reduced. An even greater time lag is that between the discovery of information that will be of use to mankind and the time the discovery is actually put to use for man's well-being. This is the problem of sociology with which modern society is concerning itself more and more. In this historical review, we shall from time to time point to these time lags.

How Man Sees

Civilization reached a high point in many fields in Greece in the period 500 to 200 B.C. Philosophy reached a peak rarely achieved. Rational explanations for many phenomena were sought. Man sought suitable methods for governing himself. Among the many other inquiries that interested the Greeks were those in natural science, one aspect of which was an explanation of human vision. Among the natural scientists, or *physiologi,* there were differences of opinions as to how men see, but two concepts prevailed. The first was that the eye sent out an emanation that intercepted the object. Weakness in vision was due to a lack of this substance, and treatment by purgatives, by anointing, and by general gymnastics was designed to alter or increase the substance.

The second concept which some of the Greek philosophers espoused in differing forms was the notion that the object being viewed gave off tiny images of the object that passed into the eye, were fixed in the pupil, and became perceived by the soul. The proof was simple. When we gaze into the eyes of another, do we not see the tiny image of ourselves fixed in his pupil? Alcmaeon of Crotona, who lived during the sixth century B.C., was one who held this view. He was one of the first men to practice and learn from dissection. In seeking the seat of intelligence in animals, he noted that the eyes were connected to the brain by the optic nerves, indicating to him that the brain was the seat of intelligence. He described the optic nerve as a hollow tube, through which humors could pass.

These two concepts, alone or in combination, were utilized by most of the Greek scientists to explain vision. Some stressed one aspect more than the other, but the two elements appeared in most theories. The first theory, that rays are emitted from the eye and travel to the object of visual perception, played a strong part in the later theories of Euclid and Galen. The second concept, that tiny images were cast off by the object being observed and that these images entered the pupil of the eye, was held by Anaxagoras and Democritus, and other atomists in the fifth century B.C. This idea was further developed in the third century B.C. and was followed for many years by the Epicureans. This concept envisioned small images or hollow films of exceedingly fine texture being continually discharged from all objects and being exact replicas of the object. Some of these entered the soul through the various organs of sense. In the case of vision, they entered the pupil of the eye. For Democritus, the images consisted of subtle atoms that penetrated the body through its many pores.

A theory that combined both concepts is usually associated with Plato, who lived in the fourth century B.C., and Empedocles, who had lived 100 years earlier. It held that images proceeded from the object *and* that rays went from the eyes. These met at some point between the eye and the object and were combined to form a third type of ray, or picture ray, that ultimately was received by the pupil and perceived by the soul. The impact of this Platonic theory was great. It enabled dimness of vision to be described as a lack of power of the eye to send forth its emanation, and treatment was directed to correcting this condition. Although not impressive in comparison to modern knowledge, this concept was a vast improvement over the notion that visual malfunction was caused by demons.

This theory was predominant for almost 1500 years after Plato, a fact not in itself amazing, for advances in knowledge come slowly and with difficulty. What is surprising is that one philosopher of this age, Aristotle, had an opposing view that was much closer to the modern view, and his view was not accepted for 1500 years. It is interesting to speculate on how much sooner man would solve his problems if human thought proceeded in a straight line instead of being subject to time lags of 1500 years such as this one.

Aristotle was born in 384 B.C., and to this day mankind is indebted to the teachings of this great philosopher and teacher, who has been called the father of natural science. Aristotle believed that sense organs were acted on not by tiny images of the object (in the case of vision) but by motion. An object's color creates motion that produces light; this light acts on the sense organ and yields a perception. Light, according to the Aristotelian view, is not a body, and it is not emitted by a body; it does not occur by itself. It is a product of motion produced by the color of the object looked at. Hearing and smell, according to Aristotle, also were mediated by the objects causing the sensations setting into motion a medium that in turn impinged on the sense organs. Clearly, this concept approximates the modern view of sensation, and, except for the absence of a concept of waves of light or sound, it is consonant with the modern view of energy in the form of waves that excite the sense organs.

Aristotle was a teacher, philosopher, and advisor to the rulers of Greece of that period; he was not a physician. He did not describe or discuss diseases of the eye, but he did discuss errors of refraction as deviations from the normal. He offered two theories for the weak-sightedness of the elderly. One explanation was that ocular tissue, like the body as a whole, becomes dried out, no longer permitting light to pass through as readily as it formerly did. This is not too far from the modern explanation of senile cataract.

Aristotle's other explanation of presbyopia was that rays from the eye come together at a greater distance from the eye than they do in youth; thus the older person must hold objects farther from him in order to see clearly. Although this is of course not the case, and although Aristotle is guilty here of forsaking his own more nearly accurate theory of vision for the older view of something emanating from the eyes, the explanation is nonetheless important as an early optical explanation. The concept of rays coming together at an object bears great similarity to the modern one of light coming to a focus.

Aristotle described both nearsightedness and farsightedness. He seems to have understood these two varieties of visual anomaly quite well. For nearsightedness, for example, he describes the prominence of the eyeballs, the squinting of the lids together to obtain clearer vision, and the tendency of myopes to write small letters. He recommends that the nearsighted person look through a narrow tube to see distant objects more clearly! Here for the first time, a rudimentary optical device (a form of pinhole disk) is suggested for the correction of weak sight. Philosophically, this is a vast step from incantations and salves of children's excrement! Although a hollow tube was hardly a practical device for nearsightedness, it was the first rational remedy.

This observation of Aristotle, that nearsightedness is accompanied by protrusion of the globe, squinting of the lids, and a tendency to write small, is of interest because it supports a speculative statement that we offered earlier. We noted that early man with small amounts of myopia probably did not realize that he had a refractive error and probably did not seek help. Aristotle's description of nearsightedness would hold true only for those with marked degrees of myopia. The individual with smaller degrees of myopia does not manifest these symptoms. Thus, nearsightedness to Aristotle included only eyes that we would describe today as being *very* nearsighted. The many persons with lesser degrees of myopia probably were not recognized as having the same anomaly to a lesser degree.

Aristotle was an experimental biologist who observed and described more than he speculated. He differentiated nearsighted animals from farsighted animals. He described man as the only animal that has a variety of eye colors, and he noted (erroneously) that eyes the color of goat's eyes were possessed by people with the best dispositions and the most acute vision. He wrote that: "The eyes of some people are large, others small, and others of a moderate size—the last mentioned are the best." Surely, we cannot attribute to Aristotle, on the basis of this statement, a knowledge of the current biological theory for the genesis of refractive errors. However, he should be credited with taking the biologist's view of individual differences, a view he expressed throughout his writings.

Aristotle described the similarities and differences in the eyes of various animals, based on his keen and accurate observations. Many of his conclusions were erroneous (he held, for example, that the brain was not the seat of sensation and perception), but his methods were those of a modern biologist, and his accurate and astute observations on the eyes of various animals far outnumbered his false notions.

Thus, more than 1500 years before the invention of spectacles, one man at least had described the eyes of various animals with considerable accuracy, had differentiated and described nearsightedness and farsightedness, had described an elementary optical device for the correction of one error of refraction, had proposed a nearly modern theory of vision, had described the process of vision in modern terms vastly different from those used in theories then current, and had described presbyopia and offered two possible explanations for it, both wrong, but each incorporating ideas more like current ones than like those of the times. Truly, Aristotle should be adopted by optometrists as the patron saint of modern optometry.

Unhappily, the ideas of Aristotle were not readily accepted. Physicians did not accept the Aristotelian view. On into the Middle Ages, vision defects continued to be treated much as they had been before. The interesting phase of the history of sciences that deals with the long time lag between the time a correct and useful concept is first enunciated and the time it is put to use in alleviating man's suffering is nowhere better illustrated than here. The stage was set by Aristotle for an understanding of vision and of its errors and their correction. Yet, more than 1500 years were to pass before these ideas would again appear—this time to gain acceptance and to remain. For 1500 years more, vision would be thought of as due to rays coming from the eye, and weak vision would be treated by salves, surgery, and purgatives. Nothing new or startling would happen for another millennium and a half.

OPTICS

It is easy enough now-a-days to scoff at the Epicurean theory that objects emit images which are projected into the eye to be perceived by the sensorium; yet a more sophisticated theory of vision requires a greater knowledge of optics than the ancients had.

Edwin G. Boring (1942)

The ancients, it is true, had only rudimentary knowledge of optics. A great step forward was the work on optics of Euclid, the Greek mathematician who lived about 300 B.C. Little is known of Euclid's life other than through his writings. He was a teacher, and he founded a school at Alexandria. His *Elements*, the basis for Euclidean geometry known to every high school student presently and for many generations past, was a compilation of the work of his predecessors. The whole design of the work, however, was clearly his own.

Another book by Euclid that has been handed down is his *Optics*. So clearly does this text establish many of the basic principles of this field that Euclid has been undisputedly called the father of optics. An interesting anecdote about Euclid as a teacher has survived. Someone who had begun to read geometry with Euclid, after learning the first theorem asked, "What advantage shall I get by learning these things?" Euclid instructed his slave, "Give him three-pence, since he must make profit out of what he learns." Present-day optometric teachers of geometric optics are probably often tempted to offer similar compensation to their students.

In *Optics*, Euclid described the ray connecting the eye and a point on the perceived object as a straight line (Hofstetter, 1948).

> We must accept that the visual rays which pass out from the eyes proceed in straight lines, leaving between them certain intervening spaces. The figure formed by the visual rays is a cone, whose point lies at the eye, its base, however, upon the edges of the visual objects. We see only those things on which fall these visual rays; we do not see those things on which these rays do not fall. No visual object is seen as a whole simultaneously. We seem, however, to see the whole object because the visual rays are rapidly moved from one side to another.

Euclid thought of the direction of visual rays as emanating from the eye and proceeding to the object, rather than from object to eye, as we now know light travels. The concept of linearity, highly useful in later studies of optics, is nonetheless enunciated. Also, the concept of the visual cone is stated here. To Euclid the science of optics is indebted for the first mention of what we call today the "minimum visual angle," a concept that is the basis for the test type card so widely used in vision testing. He also demonstrated that the angle of incidence is equal to the angle of reflection, a natural law basic to much of the science of optics. In *Optics* is also a discussion of the geometry of binocular fixation of an object, and of parallax. Euclid developed a reasonably complete system of the basic science of optics; optometry was thus advanced by this mathematician and astronomer.

The science of optics was further advanced 450 years after Euclid by the writings of Claudius Ptolemy, who lived in Alexandria about 150 A.D. Ptolemy, best remembered as an astronomer and mathematician, left thirteen volumes on general physical sciences. Optics was one of the subjects treated by him. He is credited with the first discussion of the phenomenon of refraction, the action of light passing through media of various densities. He described the measurement of the angles of incidence and refraction from air to water, and explained astronomical refraction in terms of the density of air.

The traditional interest of astronomers in optics is worthy of mention here, for throughout the ages, discoveries by those primarily interested in astronomy have been important contributions to the basic science of optics, on which optometry is based. In passing, we might also note that the work of Ptolemy, like that of Euclid before him, was still based on the notion that rays travel from the eye to the object. Thus, although a more sophisticated theory of vision had to wait for more knowledge in optics, for many years optics developed without any change in the Platonic view of vision.

ANATOMY OF THE EYE

The only truly great ocular anatomist and physiologist of antiquity was Galen, who lived between 130 and 200 A.D. Born in Pergamum in Asia Minor, Galen studied at Alexandria, among other places, and at the age of 34 he went to Rome. A remarkable man, Galen wrote 125 treatises on philosophy, grammar, mathematics, and law; he wrote more than this on medicine and life sciences.

Our major interest in Galen is due to his book on *Anatomy and Physiology of the Eye,* the first of its kind. In this text of fifteen chapters, Galen discussed optics. However, it is for his work in anatomy and physiology that he must be remembered. For some 1500 years after his death, little in the field of ocular anatomy was forthcoming. This phenomenon, incidentally, typifies Galen; his writings on medicine were used and revered throughout the 1000 years of the Middle Ages. During this period, anything that was not mentioned in Galen simply was not accepted, and in medicine his teachings were rigidly adhered to longer than those of any other writer.

Galen's anatomy of the eye is complete and is based both on his own observations and on the writings of the period before him. From the past, however, he did not have much on which to draw. We have already noted that Alcmaeon of Crotona about 500 B.C. had written on the eye, and his work is cited by Galen. Herophilus about 300 B.C. is credited with describing the sclera, choroid, retina, and vitreous humor in his treatise *Concerning the Eyes.* The major contribution, however, was from Galen's own descriptions.

While the anatomical descriptions offered by Galen were excellent and were to serve as a basis for the ophthalmic sciences for so many years, his discussion of optics left much to be desired. Rays, of course, traveled from the eye out to the observed body. Of some interest are Galen's remarks (cited in Shastid, 1917) introductory to the subject of optics and the geometry used therein:

> We have spoken of almost everything concerning the eye, except one single matter, which indeed I had rather not describe at all, so that neither the difficulty of the explanation nor its length might cause me to be hated. For inasmuch as I, in connection with this matter, must touch upon mathematical theory—an unknown subject to the majority of educated persons, and one which makes even adepts therein hated and unacceptable—I had therefore rather not begin a discussion of any sort or kind about this ocular point. As however, a dream came to me and complained that I had badly conducted myself toward the most divine of organs, and had even committed an outrage against the Creator by omitting a work which so plainly exhibited his highest wisdom and providence for living things, I was obliged to take up a subject which, until then, I had completely neglected, and give it some attention.

In a later section, Galen again refers to his reticence at mentioning mathematics, geometry, and optics lest he be hated by "the majority of my readers, who would rather stand anything than betake themselves to geometry." This aversion to mathematical thinking and to optics by Galen's readers is not a phenomenon reserved to them. There is some reason to believe that, throughout the ages, those trained in the biological and life sciences and in their practical application in such fields as medicine encounter difficulty with mathematical subjects.

Galen's physiology of the eye, although complete, is not impressive. The crystalline lens is described as the seat of sensation (and will remain so for a thousand years until the Arabian scientists identify its true function). Galen espoused the humoral theory, and great stress is placed on the balance of the body fluids. Visual power proceeds from the brain to the eye, and much of disease is explained on the basis of the body fluids.

Because man sometimes adheres too long to dogma of an early writer, it is difficult to assess contributions as having an overall beneficial or detrimental effect. The Platonic and Epicurean view of vision was a marked advance over what preceded it, but its dogmatic acceptance because "Plato had said it" held back scientific inquiry for many years. So it was with Galen; his systematic anatomy was a vast step forward. That his anatomy, however, became the only word, dogmatically accepted by so many succeeding generations, is a phenomenon on which we might ponder.

We have just discussed the contributions of scientists in three different basic areas—psychology, optics, and life sciences—who contributed to knowledge about the eye. We now return to our pursuit of an answer to the question of how our ancestors were treated for defects of vision before there was an optometry and before there were spectacles.

VISION SERVICES DURING THE ROMAN ERA

The physicians of ancient Rome were usually of Greek origin. We have already seen that Galen was trained at Alexandria and later came to Rome. Many physicians trained in Greece did the same.

During the period of the Roman Republic and earlier, the practice of medicine was considered a trade and held in contempt by the higher classes. It was practiced by slaves and Greeks. With Julius Caesar, who died in 44 B.C., citizenship was granted to physicians who resided in Rome, and freedmen entered the profession. In the Rome of this period, medicine was practiced in offices that opened onto the streets. When not engaged in treating patients, the proprietor of a medical shop would stand at the door of the office and cry his merits to passersby. Rare and expensive drugs, impressive instruments, and pathological specimens were exhibited on counters for all to see.

The physicians of this period dispensed their own drugs, and there were many specialists. Some specialized according to the curative procedure used, such as herb doctors, wine doctors, or milk doctors. Others specialized according to the body part treated, and there were dentists, obstetricians, urologists, orthopedists, and in the greatest number, *ocularii*, or eye doctors, who, history reports, received excellent fees. The *ocularii* practiced in open shops just as the other doctors of that time did, and on occasion they made house calls.

We can best determine what the *ocularii* did for their patients from the writings of Galen and of Aurelius Cornelius Celsus, who lived from 25 B.C. to 50 A.D. The *ocularii* treated diseases of the eye with the medicines and surgery of the time. In the literature of the field that today is optometry, there are only a few references to the works of these ancients.

Writing about dimness of the eyes, Celsus (cited by Shastid, 1917) said:

> A dimness comes upon the eyes, sometimes from a lippitude [inflammation], at other times even without that, from old age, or weakness. [If due to inflammation, Celsus recommends medications composed of pepper, saffron, poppy tears, ceruss, psoricum, gum,

etc.] . . . if it arises from old age or weakness, it may be proper to anoint with the best honey, and cyprine and old oil.

Whoever is troubled with a dimness must walk much, use exercise, frequent bathing, at which time the whole body must be rubbed but principally the head, with iris ointment until it sweats; after that it must be veiled and not uncovered, till after he has got home, and the sweat and heat have ceased. Then he must keep to an acrid and extenuating diet; and after the interval of some days use a gargarism of mustard.

Celsus also discusses weakness of the eyes in which the patient sees well enough in the daytime but not at night. It is difficult to determine whether he is describing night blindness, an affliction caused by lack of vitamin A and possibly prevalent in those times, or myopia, which is worse at night than during the day. Probably both anomalies were sometimes considered in this category. Celsus notes that the disorder never happens to a woman when her menstrual discharge is regular. He recommends, among other things, anointing with the blood of a liver (preferably from a he-goat, but a she-goat would do), and "they ought to eat the liver itself." Liver, being rich in vitamin A, probably worked wonders for those with night blindness uncomplicated by refractive error. Exercises, bathing, and massage were also to be used.

Finally, Celsus describes nystagamus, "a palsy of the eyes," and states that it cannot be cured. (How true!) He also observes that patients so afflicted cannot see distinctly.

Celsus described many diseases of the eyes and the treatments for them but said little about dimness of vision. Probably, patients of this era either could not afford to have something as minor as moderate vision impairment attended to by an *ocularus,* or they did not notice small imperfections of vision. It is interesting that patients today take refractive errors as a matter of course while standing in awe of eye surgery. Yet surgery for lid afflictions, cataract, and growths on the eye was highly developed thousands of years before refraction was understood.

Galen, in addition to his contributions in anatomy, physiology, and optics, was also a practicing physician. In his writings on medicine, there are some references to the eye. Galen (cited by Shastid, 1917) was probably describing refractive errors when he wrote:

Finally, the patient may be affected by disturbances of the innervational pneuma. If the pneuma be abundant and clear, like ether, then the subject sees into the farthest distance and also very exactly. If it is only scantily present but pure, he sees nearby exactly, but distant objects not at all. If it be abundant but moist, he sees far but not exactly. If moist and scanty, he sees neither clearly nor far.

Because the various errors of vision depended on the "innervational pneuma," treatment was accordingly directed at the appropriate humor.

In 476 A.D., with the fall of the Western Roman Empire, the Middle Ages, which lasted 1000 years, began. It is thus appropriate to conclude this discussion of antiquity with a consideration of the status of optometric service at this time. The writings of Aëtius of Amida, who lived from 502 to 574 A.D., were available to later scholars and serve to describe the sum total of knowledge about vision defects at that time.

Aëtius, a resident of Byzantium, was trained at the University of Alexandria and was a devout Christian. He wrote a complete encyclopedia of healing in sixteen books, rare copies of which have been translated. Aëtius recommended, for making salves, that the following incantation be continually repeated:

> The God of Abraham, the God of Isaac, the God of Jacob, give virtue to this medicament.

Thus, by these particular words and the particular arrangement, a special magic would be transmitted to the salve being prepared. The only thing that had changed in 2500 years was the appearance of a new cast of characters!

Aëtius, whose encyclopedia of diseases was very long and complete, seems to have mentioned most of the defects of vision that the modern optometrist would correct. He describes atony, or atonicity, of the eyes, just as Demosthenes had done 900 years earlier, giving credit to Demosthenes for the treatment. This condition—probably discomfort caused by uncorrected farsightedness, astigmatism or errors of coordination of the eye—Aëtius (cited by Shastid, 1917) describes as follows:

> Those eyes are called weak which do not bear to look at white objects, or shining ones, or those which are fiery, but, when this is attempted, close the pupil and lacrymate: these things they do especially after much reading. They are to be distinguished from cases of epiphora in this way: that the latter produce tears without external cause, the former, however, only when such a cause is present. Weak eyes should be treated by the promenade, by protracted running, with gymnastics of the upper extremities, with massage and holding of the breath, with shearing of the head and light massage of the eyes after the gymnastics and with affusions of cold water to the head. Also to be prescribed is water-drinking and a temperate manner of living. It is also useful to read with a loud voice, and to write. In case we are obliged to resort to local eye-remedies, we shall use the astringent, the cooling, and the obstructive.

The description of nearsightedness, or myopia, is terse and to the point. It is also a most accurate statement for the times:

> Those are called shortsighted who, from birth onward, see small and near objects, but are not able to see those which are large and distant, and who, when reading, bring the script up close to the eyes. A few of them have irregular, bulbous eyes, others, however, normal eyeballs. The condition is incurable.

This quotation from Aëtius tends to bear out the idea that ancient man probably did not attempt to treat smaller degrees of refractive error because he includes only severe congenital myopia. Moderate myopia developing at later ages was probably thought to be a different defect.

This same observation also holds true for the definition of nearsightedness by Aristotle. The three characteristics of myopia he described were protruding eyes, the tendency to squint, and the tendency to see objects as small, and these are characteristics primarily of high degrees of myopia. The quotations from Aëtius and Aristotle support the view that only major degrees of myopia were of concern to the ancients; lesser degrees were not recognized as similar defects.

The discussion of amblyopia, a dimming of vision from many causes, is attributed by Aëtius to Galen. Aëtius (cited by Shastid, 1917) wrote:

> Amblyopia is a dimming of the vision and arises from various causes: either because the optic pneuma inspissates, or the membranes condense and thicken, or the ocular fluids become thick and tough. Visual weakness also occurs in those afflicted with tedious bodily diseases, and in consequence of heavy grief. In extreme old age there is generally added to the inspissation of the ocular fluids and of the membranes of the optic nerve, also relaxation of the optic pneuma and decided diminution in its quantity. Also collapse and a kind of rumpling of the optic nerve and of the condensed and thickened ocular membranes. For as the ocular fluids diminish in the aged, and less pneuma streams down from above to the pupil, the cornea waxes rumply to such a degree that, of the aged, some do not see at all, while others see indeed but badly and with great effort. For the folds lay themselves one upon another, and the membrane doubles itself to a certain extent and assumes a newly acquired thickness. The remedies for persons with amblyopia are made of the same materials as for those who have incipient cataract (hypochyma), some of which are used in the form of collyria; others (which are also good for inflammations of the ocular membranes accompanied by thickening) are moist; still others are dry.

The section on nyctalopia by Aëtius is lengthy but is included here because it illustrates the gamut of treatment used by the an-

cients who followed the humoral theory. Of the great number of procedures used concomitantly, probably only the eating of goat's liver
had any value to the patient. The lesson to be learned from this
example could be of inestimable value in assessing the efficacy of
modern multifaceted treatments.

On nyctalopia, Aëtius (cited by Shastid, 1917) wrote:

> One speaks of nyctalopia, when anyone can see by day, but sees
> more badly after sundown, finally, when the night has come, sees
> not at all. The cause of the disease may be a weakness in the head,
> and especially thickening of the optical pneuma and of the other
> humors and membranes of the eye.
>
> Other persons, however, see better by night and worse by day,
> while if, at night, the moon shines, they do not see at all. But this
> disease is rare, the former frequent.
>
> Nyctalopic persons should be treated, if robust, with venesec-
> tion at the elbow, and at the corners of the eyes, but, when the
> humors are corrupt, by purification with a proper purgative. Then,
> after the general evacuation of the body, gargles should be em-
> ployed, and purification should be practiced through the nose, and
> sneezing excited. As a nasal remedy the following is proper: pepper,
> lousewort, each 2 scruples; mustard, 1 scruple; pulverize, sift, add as
> much juice of the white-beet root as is needful to bring to the con-
> sistency of liquid honey; rub it together, instill it into the nose and
> let it draw the nose open. This do for from five to seven days. Also
> use the other nasal remedies which have already been communi-
> cated in the chapter on nasal diseases. The patient should take
> before meals, hyssop, organy, and rue. The manner of living should
> have for its object the reduction of bodily weight. When, however,
> all this fails one should give again a purgative, for example this:
> scammony, 3 oboli; beaver gall, 2 oboli; salt, 3 oboli. In case of
> great physical weakness, only 2 oboli of scammony should be used.
> This purgative has often freed the patient quickly from his disease,
> or at all events, produced a decided improvement.
>
> A few days later a different purgative should be given—one
> which brings away mucus and gall, for example this: bitter apple, 2
> oboli; scammony, 4 oboli; aloes, 4 oboli; make of this 6 pills and to
> those who are moderately constipated give 3, to those more strongly
> affected, all 6.
>
> Boiled honey should be rubbed in the eye, and the eyes held
> closed in order to retain the fluids. Very old oil may be used in this
> same way, or indeed fibrous alum roasted on a potsherd, 2 drachms;
> ammoniated rock-salt, or the Cappadocian, 1 drachm, rubbed up
> with honey and woman's milk. Or hyena gall with honey. The con-
> tinued use of acrid remedies should be avoided, but old oil should
> be persistently used. Goat's liver appears to be of use to these
> patients, with salt, but roasted without oil and eaten very hot.
> Others, however, are accustomed to anoint the eye with the broth
> which exudes from the liver during the roasting; others, during the
> roasting have the eyes held open in the uprising steam and so
> foment them.

The wild cucumber is also of service, rubbed in the eye from time to time with honey, and the gall of a partridge, or the wild she-goat, or of the he-goat. Then, too, the gall of the sole-fish, rubbed in, proves of great service. But, as stated, the entire way of life should be such as to make the humors thin. In the beginning one should refrain from wine, and avoid everything of a thickening nature (i.e., which thickens the bodily humors). In those who see better by night and worse by day, I take it that the pneuma is very thin or the membranes leaky, and that the dispersion of the pneuma which occurs by day, makes the pupil blind, while by night, a gathering together and thickening of the pneuma occurs, so that it then is in a condition to arouse the sense-perception. Therefore, one ought to provide for these day-blind persons a greater firmness in the eye. Herophilus, on the other hand, says in his work on ophthalmology; "For dayblindness take of gum, the dung of land-crocodile, vitriolic ore, and hyena gall, rubbed up with honey, and rub this into the eye twice daily; and give the patient to eat nothing but he-goat liver." I suspect, however, that this works better for nightblindness.

AND THEN THERE WAS DARKNESS

With the fall of the Western Roman Empire, western civilization entered the Middle Ages, a period of 1000 years of relative decline from which it did not emerge until the Renaissance. In previous sections, we have traced the knowledge of vision and its application to patients with defective vision from the earliest records some 4000 years ago up to the time of the fall of the Western Roman Empire. Certain general observations may be offered on this period of 2500 years.

The span of time we are discussing is but a fragment of man's time on earth. Man probably existed one million years ago. We can only guess that earliest man had defects of vision. Certainly, he had no effective means of correcting defective vision. Highly speculative theories on the evolutionary aspects of defects of vision exist and are of some interest in obtaining a better understanding of vision. For example, Gordon L. Walls, the greatest authority in the twentieth century on the vertebrate eye, in his lectures to students, stated that such anomalies as myopia probably came with domesticity. We know that myopia seems to be characteristic of domestic rather than wild animals. Although consideration of man's vision defects half a million years ago contributes little to the present discussion, it is advisable to remember how brief the period we are discussing is.

The first treatment of vision defects that we have encountered was based on magic, superstition, and a belief in demons as the cause of most of man's physical ills. The revolution in man's thinking that characterized the Greek and Greco-Roman eras was greatly significant. The shift from demons and supernatural agents to malfunction of the humors was a gigantic step forward in man's conception of his physical ills. Insofar as defects of vision were concerned, however, and particularly from the viewpoint of the patient, the change was minimal. It made no significant difference to the patient with poor vision whether a hole was cut in his head or neck or elbow to allow the demons to leave or whether the same surgical procedure was performed to allow the ill humors to escape. He was still cut, pained, and charged, and he still retained his vision defects. It made little difference whether he was given child's excrement and honey to drive out evil spirits or land-crocodile dung and honey to bring his humors to balance. Nor did the advice to engage in gymnastic exercises come much closer to relieving eyestrain than did the incantations of an earlier age.

Most significant, however, in considering this period of history, is the realization that many people throughout the world are today not in a very different situation from that of man several thousand years ago. We have offered the observation earlier that modern man corrects defects that ancient man tolerated. It must also be noted that modern man in an affluent and highly complex society corrects defects that modern man in a primitive or poverty-ridden society still tolerates.

The full impact of the history we have been considering is felt only when we realize that a large segment of the world's population today receives care for its defects of vision not too different from that found among the ancients. Here is a different time lag from that discussed earlier.

The lag between the time that scientific advances are made and the time that these are incorporated into the practice of healing is exemplified by Aristotle's theory of vision. The way to reduce this time lag is through better communication among educated people. The lag we are now discussing is the time between the improvement in practical procedure and its application to *all* people. It is the worldwide problem of making advances useful to people and is a problem for sociological study.

This immense time lag was the subject of a classic oration by Frank W. Weymouth (1961) on the occasion of his receiving life membership in the American Academy of Optometry. He complimented the Academy for reducing the lag between the time when knowledge was gained and the time it was applied to "all men and women whose vision is less useful than it might be." Weymouth coined a phrase that might well be optometry's slogan: ". . . any man or woman deprived of health or incapacitated for lack of application of known facts is a rebuke to mankind."

An interesting subject that illustrates the time lag between knowledge and its acceptance and utilization by man is that of the "evil eye" (Gifford, 1958). The superstition of the evil eye is the old belief that certain persons can do harm to others by looking at them. One who possesses the evil eye is said to be a sorcerer or witch and is to be feared. Countless remedies for overcoming the effect of the evil eye have been used by man. Another form of the evil-eye myth is that a person who looks at what he should not (for example, peeping Tom, who looked at Lady Godiva when she rode through the streets of Coventry) will receive an eye affliction—even blindness.

How closely the treatment of disease or defects of the eye has been bound to superstition is found in the dual role many substances have played through much of history. Human spittle has been used to avoid the evil eye and also as a curative agent. History also shows human urine to have held this dual role for many centuries. The herb rue has been used since antiquity as a curative agent (it is one of the substances recommended by Aëtius for nyctalopia) and also to break the spell of the evil eye.

Another form of the evil eye superstition is that of visual prenatal influence; a child may be born with stigmata associated with the mother's viewing of objects during her pregnancy. This myth was believed as early as the time of Hippocrates and undoubtedly long before. Illustrative of the tremendous time lags to which freedom from superstition are subject are the following relatively recent accounts of prenatal influence, all cited by Gifford (1958) : *

> A rabbit, with eyes glaring, had jumped at a pregnant woman and frightened her badly. The child was born with an enlarged head; the mouth and face were small and rabbit-shaped, and the skin was covered with short, dark hair (*British Medical Journal, 1868*).

> . . . an expectant mother, frightened by the gaze of a rattlesnake, whose child when born had an arm in shape and movements remarkably snakelike (*British Medical and Surgical Journal, 1839*).

> . . . a child with deformed arms and legs, whose mother was frightened in pregnancy by a large turtle (*International Medical Magazine,* Philadelphia, 1892).

> . . . a mother, terrified by a bull, whose child was stillborn with a cow's head; a mother, frightened by a black and white collie

---

* These four quotations are in Gifford's words and are not direct citations from the respective journals.

dog, whose child was born with a black mole studded with white hairs on the right thigh; and a mother, shocked by the sight of a crippled beggar, whose child was similarly crippled at birth (*Lancet,* 1890).

Impressive, and depressing, is the slowness with which superstition disappears. The recency of these quotations and their sources gives one an idea of the inordinately long time lags in intellectual development. The realization of the vast number of people who live in societies in which eye defects are still treated by methods used to avert the evil eye must serve as a challenge to all who are educated. The superstitions of antiquity described here still influence most of the world's population. Here is a problem the solution of which is worthy of any profession, for as each ray of light is thrown in dark corners, the time lag between knowledge and its utilization for man's betterment is slowly shortened.

One last cure for defective vision must be mentioned. Defects of vision during the early Christian era were often treated by various of the saints. There are records of saints who cured blindness by touching the eyes of the afflicted or by making the sign of the cross.

The discarded bath water used by certain of the saints was used as an eyewash, and cures of blindness by touching were recorded. The most exceptional cure, however, was that of St. Symeon Salos, who lived in the sixth century A.D. and was a most pious man. Having by accident cured a man's chronic eye inflammation, St. Symeon offered to kiss the eyes of young and pretty girls afflicted with crossed eyes. So successful was this method that girls with any eye affliction ran after him to be kissed.

With knowledge of the eye and its defects at this high point, man entered the dark ages!

CHAPTER 4

OPTOMETRIC SERVICE ON
A RATIONAL BASIS

The 1000 years after the fall of the Western Roman Empire in the fifth century is called the medieval period, or the Middle Ages; the first 600 years of this period have been called the Dark Ages. To regard this as an era when intellectual advancement was at a standstill is to oversimplify greatly. Western civilization was at a dark period compared to that which preceded or would follow, but for the Arabs or Saracens this was the period when their culture reached a high point.

During this long period, the people of Western Europe lived in cities—walled for more ready defense, but filthy, undrained, and disease-ridden. Sanitation and sewage disposal, necessary for man to live in healthy proximity to his fellows, were primitive and inadequate. Cities of Western Europe were plagued by frightful epidemics that threatened to wipe them out and left the survivors beaten in body and spirit. Infant mortality was exceedingly high; the lifespan of man was shorter than it would be subsequently or than it had been before the Dark Ages. When man took to the cities, he created problems he has not yet corrected. Improving living conditions in cities continues to be a necessity; slums and water pollution did not disappear when the Dark Ages ended.

The mere act of surviving in the walled cities of Western Europe was so difficult that very few had time for cultural pursuits. In Arabian and Eastern countries, however, the pursuit of culture was not as limited. The Arabs, settled in their newly won lands and pursuing their new religious belief with aggressive fervor, devoted greater efforts to learning. They became particularly interested in and kindly disposed toward the sciences.

As military victories were won by the Saracens, they tried at first to wipe out every trace of the learning of antiquity.* If a book of the Greco-Roman period agreed with the word of Mohammed, it was

---

* Such attempts to rid society of the thinking of the past are a recurring phenomenon in history. Large scale destruction of the written word began as soon as men learned to fear whatever ideas might be written. Such attempts to obliterate opposing ideas occurred during the middle of the present century in Germany and following the death of Ikhnaton (Amenhotep IV) in Egypt, about 1362 B.C.

deemed unnecessary; if it disagreed, it was considered pernicious. In either case, it was destroyed by the Saracens. When the library at Alexandria was destroyed, its many books were used to heat the 4000 public baths of that city. So vast was the Alexandrian collection that the volumes supplied heat for this purpose for six months!

The Arabs, having destroyed so much early literature, then had a change of mind. Almost as if to make amends, they leaned over backwards to accumulate and preserve as much ancient learning as they could. For several hundred years, the learning of antiquity was preserved and passed on by the Arabs. Among the works that survived and were carefully handed down from generation to generation were those of Galen and Aëtius. These works prevailed as the accepted learning in general and in eye medicine respectively into the middle of the eighteenth century in Saracen countries—and later in Western European countries. As late as the eighteenth century the anatomy and physiology followed by physicians were those of Galen; the pathology, surgery, materia medica, and therapeutics were those catalogued by Galen, Celsus, or Aëtius.

Insofar as the history of optometric service is concerned, it made little difference whether the works of antiquity were saved or destroyed, because the correction of defects of the eye had not been understood in antiquity. The discoveries that were to place optometry on a sound scientific basis were yet to be made. In fact, the rapid development of the optometric service after about 1300 A.D. may be due partly to the fact that so much of it developed without a false basis of misinformation.

Two scientific achievements toward the end of the Middle Ages served to place the optometric service on a rational basis. The first of these, Alhazen's two treatises on optics, served as the basis for modern optical science. Later mathematicians and scientists elaborated on Alhazen's optics. By the middle of the seventeenth century, optics was progressing on a sound scientific basis.

The invention of spectacles sometime in the last quarter of the thirteenth century was the other great contribution of this period to the optometric service. Within a short time thereafter, spectacles were fabricated and supplied in sufficient quantities as to be fairly common. These early spectaclemakers were the first optometrists, although they were not called by that name. They supplied the optometric "service" as a matter of daily routine on a more or less rational basis.

ALHAZEN—*Desert Mathematician and Opticist*

The first major contribution during recorded history in the field of optics was that of Euclid, the father of optics, in the third century B.C. Four hundred years after Euclid, Ptolemy recorded what was then known about optics. Almost another millenium passed before Alhazen made the significant contributions that finally placed optics on a sound footing.

Alhazen is the generally accepted and Latinized transcription for Abu Ali Al-Hasan ibn Alhasan, although his name also appears as Alhasan, al-Haitham, or al-Haitam.

Little is known of the life of Alhazen. He was born in 965 A.D. at Basra and became a practical or applied mathematician. He boasted that he could build a device to control the inundations of the Nile River, and the caliph, Hakim, summoned him to Egypt to make good this claim. Whether Alhazen began the project and failed, or whether he immediately realized the impracticability of the undertaking is not clear. Whatever the answer, Alhazen was aware that Hakim would be angered, so he hid himself (according to one source) or feigned madness (according to another) until Hakim's death in 1021. Alhazen spent the remainder of his life in Egypt and died in 1038 in Cairo.

Alhazen is credited with writing about 200 works, most of which were abstracts of earlier writings, commentaries, and miscellaneous minor papers. The two works for which we remember him are his treatise on optics and his treatise on light. These had a marked effect on the modern science of optics.

In his book on optics, Alhazen solved several optical problems, including the "problem of Alhazen." In this particular problem, the location of the eye and the location of the object being viewed in a mirror are known; the point of reflection must be located. He possessed a knowledge of, and described the principles of the camera obscura, to which he compared the eye. He showed that the angle of incidence is related to the angle of refraction.

In the treatise on light and in the treatise on optics, Alhazen stated clearly that light from a luminous body travels in transparent media in straight lines; it proceeds from every point of the luminous body and in the direction of every straight line that can be drawn from each point. He explained that light traveling from one medium to another changes its direction.

The field of optics is indebted to Alhazen for these and many similar contributions. But by far the most important contribution of this desert philosopher was his clear denunciation of the earlier theories of vision that had the eye giving off a substance or emanation that traveled to or toward the object. Alhazen completely disagreed with this concept. He believed, as do modern theorists, that vision depends on light from the object reaching the receptor organ—the eye.

Thus, Alhazen's great contribution was to free man's mind from the Platonic-Epicurean view, which had enslaved it for some 1400 years. Because Euclid has been accepted as the father of optics, we cannot, as some authors have, also give Alhazen this appellation. A better term would be liberator of optics, for with the two treatises of Alhazen, the groundwork was laid for optics to move forward, free from the myth that had held it back.

Aristotle had come closer to the truth than any other ancient philosopher, but his views were generally not accepted. Alhazen, through his discussions, examples, and proofs, gave man a basis for the modern concept of vision, but many more years passed before his ideas prevailed. Both Aristotle and Alhazen lived before the time man was to be ready for their particular truths, but Alhazen was 1400 years closer to that time.

Old myths die hard, and there was no sudden realization of the truth of Alhazen's concept of vision. For hundreds of years after Alhazen, authors still said that vision was due to emanations from the eye. In other areas, however, the truth as recounted by Alhazen was recognized earlier. His work was preserved and used by later scientists.

The ideas of Alhazen certainly were not all correct. For example, he believed that the crystalline lens was the receptive element of the eye. It was many years before man would learn how the eye focuses the image of distant objects on the retina.

Alhazen's treatises were transcribed by his son-in-law in 1083 A.D. About 1270, a fairly complete book on optics was written by Vitello, a Pole. Whether he translated Alhazen, as some authorities claim, has not been proven, but his manuscript clearly shows that he was familiar with Alhazen's work. We do know that Alhazen's treatise was translated into Latin about the time Vitello lived. By the middle of the fourteenth century, Alhazen's treatise on optics had been translated into Italian. A Latin translation was published by F. Risner of Basel in 1572. Arabian copies of the treatise on optics have survived to the present. Thus, there were copies and translations available to later scientists. Between 1400 and 1650, many significant contributions to the field of optics were made by workers to whom Alhazen's thinking was available. The liberation of man's thinking by Alhazen from the earlier ideas of vision made possible to a great extent the many contributions in optics of the fifteenth to seventeenth centuries.

Knoll (1965), writing on the thousandth anniversary of the birth of Alhazen, notes that this great thinker was centuries ahead of his time. Practical applications of, and advances beyond his optical theories did not appear until the seventeenth century. During that century, Galileo demonstrated the telescope (1609), Snell expounded the law of refraction (1621), van Leeuwenhoek made his microscope and discovered bacteria (1675), and Huygens and Newton expounded more sophisticated theories of the nature of light. That the foundation of all of these and many other advances was present in Alhazen's work is another example of a time lag in scientific thought.

Alhazen truly deserves the description Knoll (1965) offered when he called Alhazen "a lone voice crying in the wilderness."

THE INVENTION OF SPECTACLES

The importance of spectacles to man is perhaps nowhere better described than in a paragraph by Clendening (1927):

> It is doubtful whether any one thing which man has accomplished has raised him further above the level of the beasts than the wearing of spectacles. As Clarence Day said some time ago, this being a simian civilization, and the outstanding characteristic of simians being chatter, we are likely to attach a disproportionate amount of importance to those inventions which in some way increase our ability to talk—to the telephone, the radio, the phonograph. Humbler inventions are, however, really of much greater usefulness, and none more than spectacles. Suppose a wild animal has myopia, or shortsightedness; it cannot see the approach of its enemy, nor the exact location of its prey, and dies by violence and starvation. A modern woman with the same optical defect and intellectual purpose is fitted with glasses, and in consequence spears her prey and defends herself gallantly.

More eloquent and in the style of his time are the words of William Molyneux of Dublin. In 1692 he published *Dioptrica Nova,* a text on optics that was used and quoted well into the nineteenth century. His description (cited by Barnett, 1943) of the importance of spectacles appeared in the third chapter of his treatise:

> Were there no farther use of *Dioptrics* than the invention of *Spectacles,* for the help of the defective eye; whether they be those of *Old Men;* or those of *pur-blind* * *Men;* I should think that the advantage that mankind received thereby, inferior to no other benefit

* *Pur-blind.* Used here to mean shortsighted or myopic.

whatsoever, not absolutely requisite to the support of life. For as
the *Sight* is the most noble and extensive of all our senses; as we
make the most frequent and constant use of our eyes in all the
actions and concerns of human life; surely that instrument that re-
lieves the eyes when decay'd, and supplies their defects, rendering
them useful when otherwise useless, must needs, of all others, be
esteemed of the greatest advantage. In what a miserable condition,
do we most count those, in whom it has pleased the *Great Con-
triver of Eyes and Sight,* to shut those two little windows of the
Soul? And we may imagine that they, in whom these lights are but
partly obscured, do in some measure partake of the misery of the
blind. How melancholy is the condition of him who only enjoys the
Sight of what is immediately about him? With what disadvantages
is he engaged in most of the concerns of human life? Reading is to
him troublesome, War more than ordinary dangerous, Trade and
commerce toilsome and unpleasant, and so likewise on the other
hand, how forlorn would the latter part of men's lives prove, unless
Spectacles were to hand to help our eyes, and a little form'd glass
supplied the decays of nature? The curious engaged in any minute
works could no longer follow his trade than till the *fiftyth* or
sixtyth year of his age. The scholar no longer converse with books,
or with an absent friend in a letter. All after would be melancholy
idleness, or he must content himself to use another man's eyes for
every line. Thus forlorn was the state of most *old men,* and many
young before this admirable invention, which on this account can
never be prized too highly.

Knowledge about the invention of spectacles is sketchy. The
exact date of the invention is not known, although the last quarter of
the thirteenth century seems the most probable period. The area of
the world in which spectacles were first used to correct defective
vision is also not known, although the most probable area is Western
Europe.* The identity of the inventor to whom subsequent generations must be indebted is also not known, but evidence supporting
three individuals, Roger Bacon, Salvino d'Armati, and Alessandro
della Spina, has been suggested.

The first spectacles had convex lenses and were used by presbyopic individuals to improve vision at close range. It was at least 100
years after the invention of spectacles that concave lenses for myopia
were used. Cylindrical lenses for the correction of astigmatism were
not used until the nineteenth century. From all the evidence, we may
reconstruct the most probable sequence of events in the invention of
spectacles:

* Claims that spectacles originated in China seem to be based on the finding
of tortoise-shell spectacle rims (but no lenses) dating from before the fourteenth
century. The tortoise was an animal associated with good luck, and these devices
were probably used in accordance with this superstition rather than as holders of
lenses.

1. Convex spherical lenses were used as burning glasses many hundreds of years before spectacles were invented.

2. The most primitive lens aid to vision was a convex spherical lens (half a sphere, for example) placed directly on the object to be viewed, such as on a written page. This device aided vision solely through its magnification properties.

3. Someone who knew of such magnifiers discovered that the lens could be lifted from the page and held before the eye. Whoever first performed this simple act and recognized its value was the inventor of spectacles.

4. The lens was mounted in a holder that had a handle. This primitive device was used monocularly.

5. For use with both eyes, two such monocular devices were joined by a pin at the handle of each. The user held the pinned handles of this device over his forehead while reading, or the device was perched on the nose and the two elements were pinched together to hold the device on the nose.

6. The monoculars, paired together by riveting, were replaced by a solid bar with two convex lenses suspended from it. The user of this device held it before his eyes or allowed it to perch on his nose, where its hold was precarious.

7. Temples that pressed against the head were added to the solid bar to steady the device before the eyes.

From this brief overview, it is apparent that there was no one inventor of modern spectacles. Many years probably elapsed between each step in the sequence. Some time after 1250, someone lifted a magnifying lens from the page he was reading and noticed its effect while it was held closer to the eye. By 1300 the convex lens that had been used for centuries as a burning glass and for many years as a magnifier evolved into spectacles, with all the major features of the modern corrective device for presbyopia.

BEFORE SPECTACLES—GLASS, BURNING LENSES, AND MAGNIFIERS

Glass was probably made as long as 4500 years ago. A good deal of the ancient glass found is not transparent, but Barnett (1943) notes that a glass bead dated 3500–4000 B.C. and now in the Berlin Museum is perhaps the oldest piece of *clear* glass. It is certain that clear glass was known long before the birth of Christ.

Several ancient small bottles have been unearthed, and they bear testimony to the antiquity of glass. Such a spherical bottle, when filled with water, would have served as a convex lens, and Taylor (1924) notes that such an observation by some ancient man may have led to the discovery of lenses. Some early man holding such a bottle filled with water probably observed how it focused an image of the sun; another may have noted its magnifying properties.

Convex lenses made of glass or crystal were known at least 1000 years before the invention of spectacles. Many such lenses have been unearthed and are now in museums around the world. Some of these finds are:

1. Two crystal lenses found in Crete. One is ⅘ inch in diameter with a focal length of one inch and has been dated 1200–1600 B.C. These are probably the oldest of the lenses (Barnett, 1943).

2. A plano-convex lens from the ruins of Nineveh and now located in the British Museum has been given a construction date of 700 B.C.

3. Lenses of +5.50 D power and 1½ inches in diameter were found in a fourth century B.C. sarcophagus in Tunis, close to ancient Carthage (Taylor, 1924). Barnett (1943) describes a series of six lenses in the Lavigeril Museum, Carthage. They are catalogued as burning glasses and are dated between the sixth and fourth centuries B.C.

4. A crystal 2⅝ inches in diameter and dated second century A.D. is now in the British Museum (Barnett, 1943).

Whether these ancient lenses were used as burning glasses, as lenses to aid vision, or both is not clear. The evidence that they were used as burning glasses is good; that they were used as vision aids is less convincing. Aristophanes, in *The Clouds* (423 B.C.), clearly describes a "burning glass." Pliny, in the first century A.D., described hollowed spheres of glass filled with water used by physicians to focus the sun's rays on an area to be cauterized.

The evidence for the use of convex lenses to magnify is less clear, although it is difficult to believe that many years elapsed during which burning glasses were used without anyone noting and putting to use their magnifying properties. One early reference in literature is the frequently quoted observation of Pliny that the Emperor Nero watched gladiatorial contests in a *smaragdus,* the generic term for all green stones. This has led to speculation of later historians that Nero used a concave lens made of an emerald to correct his myopia, that he used a concave mirror for a similar purpose, or that he merely used a green mirror as a toy to avoid looking directly at the arena. Some of the earliest spectacle lenses were made of beryl, a green, transparent stone. Most historians agree that Nero's *smaragdus* was not an early concave lens. More likely he was influenced by the still current myth that "green is such a restful color"!

Barnett (1943) offers somewhat better evidence than the Nero story for the early use of devices to aid vision. Iamblichus, who wrote a biography of Pythagoras several centuries after the latter's death, states that the famous Greek mathematician sought an aid for deafness that would do for the sense of hearing what *dioptra* did for vision. This statement would indicate that Pythagoras knew of a device (*dioptra*) that aided vision. What, however, was a *dioptra?* If Pythagoras did in fact understand spectacle lenses in the fifth century B.C., this invention was lost and not rediscovered until much later.

In summary, glass was known for well over 5000 years before spectacles were invented; clear glass was known for almost as long a time. Convex spheres used as burning glasses were known at least at the time of Christ and probably long before. Convex lenses, probably used for burning, have been found; these date as long as 2000 years before the invention of spectacles. The discovery that a convex lens magnifies was probably made by many people during a period of some 2000 years. The discovery cannot be attributed to any one person. A possible explanation for the discovery having been made and lost over so long a period is that few people read or used their eyes for close work before the thirteenth or fourteenth century. Surely, if a large number of ancients had been literate presbyopes, the use of convex lenses as a vision aid would not have been forgotten once it had been discovered.

THE INVENTOR OF SPECTACLES

Alhazen knew about planoconvex lenses with thickness greater than the radius. Because translations of Alhazen's work were known in many monasteries, it is possible that such clumsy magnifiers were used on written manuscripts by weak-eyed monks. Roger Bacon, Franciscan monk, scientist, and philosopher, in his *Opus Majus* of 1266, advised the use of such lenses placed on the page to help old or weaksighted persons (von Rohr, 1923–1924). In this he was restating what Alhazen had said.

Barnett (1943) has reviewed the evidence favoring and refuting the claim for Bacon as the inventor of spectacles. The date of the invention of spectacles has been narrowed to the last quarter of the thirteenth century. According to a book of sermons preached about 1305 by Jordan di Rivalto, a Florentine monk, it was not yet 20 years since the art of spectaclemaking had been discovered. He described this invention as one of the best and most necessary in the world. According to this statement, the date would be some time close to 1285 A.D., the year in which Bacon was 61 years old. Bacon lived another nine years and thus was alive and presbyopic at the proper period. Moreover, it is known that Bacon described and made drawings of biconvex lenses (Hill, 1915). The kind of lenses drawn would much more appropriately be held before the eye than placed on a page.

Two others, both Italians, have frequently been considered as the inventors of spectacles. An inscription on a tombstone in a Florence church states: "Here lies Salvino d'Armati of Florence, the inventor of spectacles. God forgive him his sins. Died in the year of our Lord, 1317." This memorial is often cited as evidence for this Italian being the inventor; the date usually given is 1285.

According to a chronicle of the Convent of St. Catherine at Pisa of the period between 1280 and 1311, one of the monks, Brother Alessandro della Spina, first communicated the secret of spectacles that was his own invention (Barnett, 1943). According to another and conflicting manuscript, Brother Alessandro, a good and humble man with the ability to copy anything that he saw or that was described to him, made spectacles for himself and his friends when the inventor would not show him how to do so.

The real inventor of spectacles may have therefore been (1) the English monk, Roger Bacon, whose writings indicate that he understood biconvex lenses and who wrote of lenses as an aid to those with old or weak sight; (2) the Italian Salvino d'Armati, named on a tombstone as the inventor; or (3) the Italian Brother Alessandro della Spina, listed in the chronicles of a convent as maker and/or originator of spectacles. Despite the conflicting evidence, two facts stand out. First, the date is pinpointed very close to the year 1285; second, there is a close association between the church and spectacle-making, a relationship readily understood when one realizes that most of the reading and writing of that period was done in monasteries. A short time later, with the advent of printing, books moved outside the monasteries and, as one might predict, so did spectacles.

In addition to being the places where most reading and writing were done, the monasteries in Europe served another useful function, that of communication. The monks traveled and spread knowledge to other parts of the continent. This aspect of monastic life led Casemaker, a Belgian optician who studied the history of spectacles diligently in an effort to unravel the mystery of their origin, to offer an interesting theory connecting Bacon to della Spina (Barnett, 1943). Casemaker found in the histories of various monasteries and convents that Bacon had spent some time at the Convent of Cordeliers at Lille where he met Henri Goethals, who is also known as Dr. Solemnel. Goethals was a great traveler. In 1286 he journeyed to Rome to visit Pope Martin IV. While Goethals was en route, the pope died, and the traveler ended his journey at Pisa and Florence. It is possible that Bacon could have told Goethals about his invention of spectacles; perhaps he gave a pair to his friend. It is possible that Goethals showed such spectacles to della Spina at Pisa, affording that talented man an opportunity to copy them for his own friends.

This theory nicely accounts for the time difference. Strengthening this theory further, Hill (1915) speculated as to why Bacon might have invented spectacles but kept the information to himself and to a few friends. Bacon had suffered the same fate as many scientists of that period of history. By 1285 he had already been imprisoned for "black magic." Spectacles might well have been regarded as impertinent human efforts to defeat what was accepted as divine purpose, the infliction of disabilities on the aged. Bacon may have wished to avoid further notoriety.

The inventor of spectacles will probably never be known with certainty; perhaps none of the three candidates mentioned was the actual inventor. We shall probably never know who first discovered that a convex lens could magnify objects viewed through it and, hence, could aid vision. We may safely assume, however, that spectacles came into being at the end of the thirteenth century in Western Europe.

The invention of spectacles, like most great inventions, is a relatively simple concept. Agriculture, the wheel, the zero, domestication of animals—the great inventions of man—are all simple concepts. The invention of spectacles was little more than the concept of lifting a lens off the page. Clear glass was long known; convex lenses were long available. The great invention was the simple idea—*place the lens before the eye instead of on the page.* As is true of so many other great inventions, the name of the individual who first had the idea remains hidden in the past.

THE DEVELOPMENT OF SPECTACLES

The invention of spectacles is a further example of the long time lags between man's major accomplishments. Clear glass was probably known for some 2000 years before a lens was made of it; convex lenses existed for perhaps 1000 years before they were used as an aid to vision; lenses were used as magnifiers for some time before their value in focusing light was recognized and before they were placed in front of the eyes. In sharp contrast to these long time lags is the rapidity with which spectacles, once invented, came into widespread use.

Shortly after their invention, spectacles appeared in paintings and in the literature of the time. Chaucer, before 1400, wrote in the "Tale of the Wife of Bath" (*Canterbury Tales*):

". . . . a spectakel . . . thurgh which he may his verrey frends see."

Another poet, Thomas Hoccleve, in 1415 wrote:

"Right as a spectacle helpeth feeble sighte."

Thus, within the 100 or so years after spectacles were invented, they were sufficiently familiar to find their way into the poetry of the day.

Unquestionably, spectacles caught on as rapidly as they did because the time was ripe for them. The need created by increased literacy had reached a point where a significant number of people required visual improvement in order to read. The invention of spectacles, the manufacture of paper, and the invention of printing all occurred within 200 years in Western Europe. The interrelations of the three events have been noted by historians. Without paper there could be no meaningful printing process; without spectacles, those past middle age could not read the printed word. Printing and increased literacy made the use of spectacles imperative once they were invented.

By the middle of the fourteenth century, paper was being used for all literary purposes in Europe. Prior to this, vellum was used and manuscripts (as their name implies) were handwritten. By the middle of the fifteenth century, Gutenberg had invented movable type; by the last quarter of that century, Caxton had introduced printing to England. There were no long time lags in the spread of printing. It caught on very rapidly. The steady increase in literacy and in the annual output of printed material was closely paralleled by the increased use of spectacles. Optometric service was more than just a health service. Its history is intimately tied in with man's literacy and his intellectual development.

The close association between the church and the invention of spectacles has been noted. For several hundred years, the clerical community continued to make contributions to the art of spectacle-making and to the science of optics. When we recall that before Gutenberg most manuscripts were produced in monasteries, where the brothers copied books by hand, the association between church and spectaclemaking is not surprising.

Cox (1947) described the contributions to optics during a period of several hundred years by churchmen in general and members of the Jesuit order in particular. Jesuits who contributed to optics were: Francis Maria Grimaldi, born in 1613, who experimented with prisms; Balthasar Conrad, born in 1599, who wrote on optics; Dechales, who described late in the seventeenth century his own observations of entoptic phenomena and muscae volitantes, as seen by a high myope (cited by Donders, 1864).

Father (Christoph) Scheiner, born in 1575, was one of the great early contributors to optometry. Scheiner made and recorded numerous observations. These included measurements of the indices of refraction of the eye, the first measurements of the corneal curvature, the location of the optic nerve in the eyeball, and the observation that pupillary contraction results from the action of light on the eye. He probably demonstrated the inversion of the retinal image. He is best known for the famous Scheiner experiment, a simple demonstration in physiological optics that is the basis of most optometers.

Many other monks and priests, during the 400-year period between the thirteenth and seventeenth centuries, ground and adapted lenses, made observations on the eye and optics, and left their manuscripts for others to read and learn. As might be expected, there was a short period when the new invention was condemned by the church or segments of it. We have already noted that Bacon, aware of the possible reaction of the church to any device which seemed contrary to God's design, may have preferred not to claim the invention of spectacles as his own.

For a short period, women were forbidden to wear spectacles, lest they become vain. Objections, however, rapidly died away.

More lasting objections to the use of spectacles came from another source. Physicians, both general and those practicing eye medicine, did not readily accept spectacles; some of their objections lasted well into the nineteenth century.

The first medical reference to spectacles of which we have a record is, in fact, a negative statement. Bernard de Gordon, the French physician who taught at the medical school at Montpelier from 1285 to 1307, mentioned in his book on medicine that he knew of a collyrium which would make spectacles unnecessary. Guy de Chauliac, born in 1300, also a member of the school at Montpelier and physician to several popes as well, wrote that he recommended spectacles only if his own eye lotions were incapable of effecting a cure.

Thus, within a very few years after the invention of spectacles, some physicians were discouraging their use and offering medications instead.

The first European to be considered a scientific oculist was Georg Bartisch, born in 1535. He began as a barber-surgeon and is remembered most for several advances in cataract surgery and for his writings on the eye in the German language. Bartisch, sometimes called the father of modern ophthalmology, was in 1588 appointed court oculist to the Elector of Saxony. Bartisch was bitterly opposed to the use of spectacles (Shastid, 1917), noting that he had known of many eyes to be destroyed by them. People see better, he claimed, with nothing at all in front of the eyes; one should use the correct eye powders or eye waters rather than spectacles. Thus, the practice of discouraging the use of spectacles began almost as soon as they were

invented and was continued by the father of ophthalmology several
hundred years later. Nor did the practice end in the seventeenth
century.

Duke-Elder (1949) notes that on into the nineteenth century
oculists "universally discouraged the use of spectacles." Having cited
Bartisch as having written in 1583 on "protecting oneself from the
need of glasses" and on "ridding oneself of the habit of wearing
them," Duke-Elder goes on to cite Mackenzie, who, in 1840, held that
concave lenses aggravated myopia; Sichel, who, in 1848, forbade
convex lenses for distance use by hypermetropes; and Jaeger, who, in
1855, wrote that he could not warn too insistently against "the mad
fashion of wearing glasses."

This consistent discouragement by physicians over a period of
500 to 600 years against the wearing of spectacles played a major role
in the development of the optometric service outside the realm of the
medical profession. Not only did physicians discourage and warn
against the use of spectacles, but they referred prospective wearers to
an optician to have them fitted, or they suggested that the patient
select the lenses himself. This long tradition of deprecating the use
and fitting of spectacles continues, in part, at least, to this day as a
difference in the optometric and ophthalmologic evaluation of the
importance of testing for spectacles.

In the sequence of events of the invention and development of
spectacles cited earlier, the monocular form was said to have preceded
the binocular. The sequence cited follows von Rohr (1923–1924);
however, Greef (cited by Hill, 1915) held the opposite view—that
binocular spectacles were used first and that the monocular device followed as an affectation. It is difficult to tell which form was used first,
since both forms were in use within a short time after the invention
of spectacles at the end of the thirteenth century. By the middle of
the fourteenth century, both forms were in use. In a painting originating at Treviso in 1352, one subject is using a monocular on a
handle, while another is using a pair of monoculars riveted together
and pressed against the nose to hold the device in place.

Further evidence that the monocular form was used first and that
the binocular form originally was merely two monoculars hinged together comes from the fact that in all modern languages the plural
form "eyeglasses" or "spectacles" is used. This fact has suggested to
historians that the initial device was monocular.* Whatever the case,

* In the poetic quotations from Chaucer and Hoccleve, the singular form of the
word "spectacle" is used. This is cited by Barnett (1943) as indicating that the monocular form was in use in England at that time. However, a poet and contemporary
of Hoccleve, Lydgate, used the plural form, an indication that both forms were already in use.

two monoculars riveted together came into being almost contemporarily with the monocular eyeglass. Most of the paintings during the fourteenth and early fifteenth century that portray a subject wearing a vision aid show two monoculars hinged at the bridge and used for reading.

Concave lenses came into use in the latter half of the fifteenth century. A painting from 1480 shows a subject, who is not reading, with a pair of lenses perched on his nose and his head thrown back to hold them in place. A portrait of Pope Leo X by Raphael dated 1517 shows the Pope wearing spectacles the reflections of which clearly identify them as concave. Furthermore, Leo is known to have boasted that despite his visual affliction he could do better as a huntsman with his spectacles than his normally sighted companions.

Concave lenses were frequently called "young glasses." They were worn by young, nearsighted people to enable them to see at great distances. Convex glasses were called "old glasses." They enabled presbyopic wearers to see things close.

Concave lenses worn during the Renaissance in most European countries were mostly monocular in form. Binocular convex lenses mounted in a leather or shell frame with a rigid bridge could be held before the eyes for reading or could be perched loosely on the nose. This form, however, was not used with concave lenses in the viewing of distant objects.

Myopes, particularly those in the "refined classes," preferred the monocular form and carried the monocular concealed, bringing it out stealthily only to view a distant object and then returning it to hiding. This custom prevailed in most of Europe except Spain, where even concave lenses were worn binocularly and were held in place by loops of thread attached to the frame at the outer edges and fitted behind the ears. The monocular lorgnette so characteristic of French and English refined society during the Renaissance was not an affectation at that time. It was simply the accepted way to use a prosthetic lens for a myopic eye.

The earliest spectacle frames were made of bone; horn was used shortly thereafter. Court and von Rohr (1928–1929) describe the earliest lens carrier as one made of bone, holding a single lens and with an eye wire which was split, to enable the lens to be mounted, and then tied together by thread.

Leather, which has the advantage of being less breakable than bone or shell, was used for spectacle mountings in the sixteenth and seventeenth centuries; metal frames of gold, silver, and tin came into common usage later. Frames with a combination of leather and metal have also been found. Binocular devices with rigid bars were used, particularly for reading, and various modifications were used to hold them onto the bridge of the nose. One form (Court and von Rohr, 1928–1929) was made of horn or bone and had a bridge in which slits were cut to make it more pliable. In seventeenth century England, the numbers of slits in the bridge determined the price. A frame with a rigid bridge was cheapest, while a bridge with four slits (five thin pieces of material) was the most pliable and the most expensive.

Spectacles were used for over 400 years before temples were added. Although the Spanish, about the end of the sixteenth century, began fastening spectacles to the ears by thread loops, throughout the rest of Europe spectacles were hand-held or balanced solely by means of the nose bridge. In 1728 in England, E. Scarlett (Court and von Rohr, 1928–1929) published a description of his invention of spectacles with temples. Early side-pieces, unlike modern ones which fit behind the ear, extended only three or four inches back and pressed against the side of the head of the wearer at his own temples. The upperclass people of this period wore wigs. Hence, the temples of the spectacles were flat bars between the wig and the head. With advances in metallurgy, pince-nez glasses became popular. It is only quite recently that side-pieces which fit behind the ears (and hence probably should not be called temples) have come into use.

We have noted that convex spherical lenses for presbyopia were known by 1300; concave spherical lenses for the alleviation of the symptoms of myopia were in use about 200 years later. We can no more name the inventor of the concave lens form than we can name the inventor of spectacles. Cylindrical lenses for the correction of astigmatism did not appear for another 300 years (approximately 1825) ; bifocal lenses were first used about 1785.

In the preceding history of spectacles, we have not discussed optometric service. For the 600 years from 1300 to 1900, spectacles were known and were used. For all of this period, convex lenses were used; during the last 400 years of this period, concave lenses were used; and for approximately the last century of this period, cylindrical and bifocal lenses were used. Who fitted and supplied the spectacles during this rather long period? Medicine as a profession advised against their use or advised patients to obtain them from someone other than a physician. Optometry as a profession did not emerge until the turn of the present century. Each year more and more people found aid and comfort from spectacles—but who supplied them? Who, in short, were the suppliers of the optometric service before there was an optometric profession? The answer to this question is to be found in the history of the guilds of Europe.

THE GUILD SYSTEM

In modern society, there is a scale of social acceptance of the various skills involved in supplying vision care. If, for example, we were to ask a modern layman to place the various vision service tasks on a scale of social importance, he would probably place eye surgery at the top of the scale; somewhat below this would be the examination of the eyes for glasses, a service which, however, he would rank markedly higher than the manufacturing of spectacles. The one who determines which spectacles shall be worn and who writes a formula (prescription) is entitled to be called "doctor," while the artisan who fabricates the spectacles is considered distinctly lower in the social scale.

This same order, however, did not always exist. One of the most striking aspects of the early days of the optometric service is that the social scale was almost the reverse of today's. The spectaclemaker was the one who formed a professional organization; only certain people could make spectacles; one had to prove, through a system of apprenticeship and examinations and association membership, that he was worthy of being allowed (licensed in the modern sense) to make spectacles. But anyone was allowed to fit spectacles to a patient and to make them available to the patient. Today, the examinations, schooling, and association restrictions are required of the vision examiner. The maker of spectacles does not have to demonstrate special knowledge or skills to anywhere near the same extent. Accordingly, he finds himself lower in the social scale.

The earliest spectaclemakers were churchmen, often monks who manufactured spectacles. Soon, however, lay organizations of spectaclemakers were formed. These organizations of spectaclemakers were typical guilds with all of the characteristics of other guilds of the time. A guild in Europe during this period was an organization of artisans in a single branch of industry in a single town.

Most guilds were formed in the twelfth to fourteenth centuries, although there are records from an earlier date of a few guilds in some industries and in some communities. By the fourteenth century, the system was flourishing, and most branches of industry in most major cities had guilds. The peak of the guild system for industries as a whole occurred in the fifteenth and sixteenth centuries; by the eighteenth century, the guilds were on the decline, and most of them had disappeared before the nineteenth century.

A major function of the guild was to secure good and honest

workmanship. The officers of the guild inspected the workmanship of apprentices and set standards by which an apprentice could become a master craftsman and a member of the guild. The product which the applicant prepared for his master's examination, his *masterpiece,* was passed upon by his seniors. The regulation of the industry was the major aim of the guild. Although there were common funds and religious and social aspects, the guild mainly controlled the monopoly of working within a specific branch of industry. Laws were passed by the various cities which protected the home industry and forbade the import of goods made outside the city. The laws allowed the officers of the guild to levy fines against local members who did not comply with local work regulations. They could confiscate products made outside the city, by non-guild members within the city, and by guild members whose procedures did not conform with the local rules.

The guild system had aspects characteristic of a number of modern institutions. Guilds were similar to present-day trade unions in that they set standards for working conditions and pay scales. But they were more than unions. They assumed some of the functions of the modern state boards of examiners in that they tested applicants for the occupation. They also controlled the quality of workmanship and materials. Unlike modern state boards, which forbid advertising of superiority, the guilds permitted it. For example, Marshall, an Englishman, advertised in 1694 that he had grinding tools made of brass superior to those of all other spectaclemakers.

The guilds had a monopoly of a given trade within a city, a fact which makes them different from either state boards or trade unions. They were a part of the city system of government and were designed to protect local artisanship. This monopolistic control often had harmful effects. The guilds, for example, fought the introduction of many advances. Leather frames were bitterly opposed by those already geared to work with other materials. Court and von Rohr (1928–1929) tell of another advance which was fought by the Worshipful Company of Spectaclemakers in London:

> About the end of the 17th Century some of the more advanced London opticians tried to introduce plano-convex instead of bi-convex spectacles, but they encountered the very energetic opposition of the Company and its officers. Judging from our modern standpoint, the plano-convex form is decidedly to be preferred as the astigmatism of oblique pencils in looking through the glasses with the natural movement of the eye is diminished in comparison with that produced by any bi-convex form. The freemen of the guild, however, objected to this form because the old rules were against any advantage that one of the brethren might obtain by making a form of glass which was more easily finished than the bi-convex glasses ordinarily in use.

Guilds, then, were a part of municipal government in Europe which served some of the functions of modern examining boards, professional associations, and trade unions. First and foremost, however, their purpose was the protection of local industry and the establishment of local standards.

The earliest spectaclemakers' guild was formed in Antwerp, Belgium, in the mid-fourteenth century (von Rohr, 1923–1924). In the neighborhood of Antwerp, a spectaclemaking center grew, and spectacles were made and exported to nearby countries. This guild was probably the model for those in the German (Bavarian) cities of Nürnberg and Regensburg. Here two famous spectaclemaker guilds were formed some time in the latter half of the fifteenth century. A spectaclemakers' guild was organized in Paris during the latter half of the fifteenth century. Guilds also were in existence in Frankfurt-am-Main and in Strasbourg. Guilds also existed in other European cities during this period, some as far away from their point of origin as Spain and Italy. All are believed to have spread from the original Antwerp guild (Court and von Rohr, 1928–1929).

What was perhaps the most famous guild, patterned after those at Antwerp, Nürnberg, and Regensburg, was not founded until about 180 years after these continental guilds. The Worshipful Company of Spectaclemakers was chartered in London in 1629 by King Charles I "for the better order, rule and government of those using the Art and Mistry of Spectaclemaking." The books of this company were destroyed in the great fire in London in 1666, but the charter and bylaws were saved by the devotion of its clerk. These, together with the books since that date, are still in existence.

Thus, in Europe shortly after spectacles were invented, guilds of spectaclemakers were founded in the various cities. These groups policed the quality of the spectacles and the working conditions under which they were made. The spectacles themselves, however, were sold in haberdashery stores and by itinerant peddlers, who often also sold toys and notions. These men made no attempt to help the recipient choose the spectacles. Thus, optometric service was supplied by the patient to himself. Later, however, the retailers of spectacles began to help the buyer make his selection. As time went on, spectaclemakers began to have their own shops for retail supplying of spectacles as well as other optical devices, such as telescopes or microscopes. The spectaclemakers who owned such shops and who purveyed the spectacles they fabricated directly to their customers were unquestionably forerunners of modern optometrists. Many of these men were well versed in optics and were skilled and learned artisans as well as merchants. Many made distinct contributions to the field of optics.

For the most part, the European guilds died out and were replaced by another economic and governmental pattern. The spectaclemakers company of London, however, evolved in a very interesting fashion into modern optometry in England. Because of its complete records and because of its extreme importance as a direct forebear of the profession in England, this guild will be discussed in greater detail.

THE WORSHIPFUL COMPANY OF SPECTACLEMAKERS *

Although originally limited to the city of London, the Worshipful Company of Spectaclemakers came to include all of England. It was granted the right to regulate the conduct of those engaged in spectaclemaking by its charter, granted and signed by King Charles I and countersigned by Wolseley in 1629. The resemblance between it and the guilds at Antwerp, Nürnberg, and Regensburg is sufficient for the conclusion that it was patterned after these city guilds, which had been created 130 years earlier.

The spectaclemakers were fortunate in that there was no overlap between their field and that of other guilds. The clockmakers, for example, fought the lockmakers for jurisdiction over parts of their trade. No existing company, however, was injured by the formation of the guild of spectaclemakers. This advantage, however, was also a disadvantage. The craft of lens grinding was sufficiently simple that it was not considered as skilled as some other crafts; hence, its members enjoyed only modest social standing.

By the beginning of the seventeenth century, there were 69 craft guilds in London, but no spectaclemakers' guild. However, according to Champness (1952), unless tradesmen and craftsmen were members of a guild, they labored under many handicaps. Those spectaclemakers who did practice in London at this time were usually members of some guild the major area of which was not spectaclemaking. Of the 16 spectaclemakers who initially applied for a charter, 13 were members of the brewers' guild.† In addition to the 16 men (including 13 brewers) who applied for a charter, there were 15 other

---

* A history of the Company has been written by Court and von Rohr (1929–1930) who had the opportunity to examine the books of record of the Company. Their treatise and an earlier paper by the same two authors (Court and von Rohr, 1928–1929), and an address by Sir John F. L. Rolleston in 1917 while he was Master of the Company, form the basis for information in the present section.

† The 13 members of the Brewers Company who petitioned to have the Spectaclemakers Company chartered, and who then transferred from the Brewers to the Spectaclemakers are listed by Champness (1952) as follows: John Turlington, Robert Clifford, Thomas Dumblebee, Robert Allt, Thomas Peale, William Peale, John Baylis, John Jenkinson, John Allt, John Boote, Robert Dumblebee, John Allt the Younger, and Thomas Copeland.

spectaclemakers in London, ten of whom were members of other companies and did not transfer to the newly formed guild. Thus, the total number of opticians or spectaclemakers in London at the time of the founding of the guild was 31 (Champness, 1952).

The period of apprenticeship was seven years, the applicant being bound to a master at the age of 16 and completing his term at 23. Two more years were spent as a journeyman before the spectaclemaker could advance to master. To achieve this advancement, a candidate presented spectacles made by himself to the court of the Company. These *masterpieces* were examined; if they were satisfactory, the applicant became a master in the Company and was allowed to take on apprentices.

In the early years of the Company, most apprentices attained their ultimate freedom by serving seven years. However, it was also possible to obtain freedom either by patrimony or by redemption, that is, by making a payment without previous instruction. Toward the middle of the eighteenth century, many sons and daughters of master opticians took up their freedom without complete training; some became members through redemption without full training. As a result, the Spectaclemakers Company underwent a considerable downward change of status; the Company was not as highly regarded by journeymen during the latter half of the eighteenth century as it had been in earlier times. Court and von Rohr (1929–1930) note that the same deterioration took place in Germany. They state: "The decay of the Nürnberg factories in the 17th Century is largely to be attributed to the undue influence of family relations which prevented the selection of the fittest."

Members of the Company paid quarterly dues. They also paid a modest fee each time they advanced, as from apprentice to journeyman. A fee was levied if they refused to take an office (master or warden) to which they had been elected. Masters who took on apprentices paid a fee for each apprentice, the fee becoming higher for each succeeding one. The books of the Company during the eighteenth century show fees of two pounds paid for a first apprentice, three pounds for a second, and four pounds for a third apprentice. If a master changed apprentices, or if he employed a "youth before his time" (under age, such as 15 instead of 16 years), or if he employed an apprentice not bound to him, he was fined varying amounts. The books of record show that there was wide latitude in assessing these fines; they were often reduced for extenuating circumstances or for hardship. In employing a second apprentice to replace one who had run away, for example, one master had the fee waived; another master's fine was reduced, the member "not being in good circumstances."

The Company was responsible for the quality of optical goods within the city of London; its wardens had the right to search for and confiscate inferior materials. Foreign-made spectacles were forbidden and were confiscated and destroyed. The fines were often of sufficient magnitude to be ruinous. They were levied with greater regularity during the seventeenth than during the eighteenth century. At the latter time, there was considerable laxity in enforcing the rules. Examples of penalties given for violations during the last half of the seventeenth century, drawn from the Company's records, are:

1. J. Clark was arrested in 1667 and fined for selling 16 pairs of spectacles which were "looking glass," being ground on one side only. He was referred by the Lord Mayor to the Company. The latter mitigated the fine. In 1669 he was fined for many bad pairs of spectacles, and in 1670 he was fined three pounds for selling three pairs of looking glass spectacles. Despite these infractions, Clark became a full-fledged member of the Company in 1672 and took on apprentices. His own child, Lucretia, was apprenticed to him in 1692 and freed by patrimony in 1699.

2. J. Penny was fined in 1670 for making and selling a dozen pairs of bad spectacles. Six pairs of his spectacles were also found at a haberdasher's shop, were judged to be poor in quality, and were scratched with a diamond to make them unsalable.

3. J. Hackett, apprenticed in 1658 and freed in 1666, was fined in 1671 for making bad spectacles. Later in that decade he took on an apprentice. In 1682 he became a master of the Company.

4. Several members were fined for selling spectacles to nonmember spectaclemakers or for selling frames without glasses. One member was expelled for this infraction.

Some members of the Company had their own optical shops, while others sold the spectacles they had manufactured to retail outlets, usually haberdashers. The Company controlled not only its members. It had complete control of the sale of spectacles by anyone within the city. The spectacles sold by a haberdasher were subject to scrutiny by the wardens of the Company. The records of the Company show that in 1671 ten dozen pairs of spectacles made in France and with tin frames were found in the haberdashery shop of J. Whitehead. The Company had them broken. Twenty-two dozen pairs of bad English spectacles were seized from the haberdashery shop of E. Bagnall in 1671. They were taken to Mayors Court, adjudged to be of poor quality by a jury, and condemned to be broken, "both lenses and frames." The judgment was carried out in public, the spectacles being placed on the street and "with a hammer broken all in pieces."

The major output of spectacles was not sold directly to customers by the spectaclemakers, at least in the earlier years of the Spectacle-makers Company. Thus, the optometric service, an important part of which is the prescribing of appropriate spectacles, was not nearly as closely controlled as was the making of the spectacles. The purveyor of the device, often a haberdasher, had to pass no tests of competence. Anyone could supply spectacles to the public, provided the spectacles themselves were of good quality and had been made by a member of the city Company. What criteria the haberdasher may have used to help the customer select the spectacles is obscure. Probably for convex lenses ("old spectacles" for presbyopic wearers), the age of the intended user was suggested by the manufacturer. Concave spectacles ("young spectacles") were probably selected by the intended user by trial and error from a series of pairs of differing power.

Many people in the United States today receive no better service than that offered in seventeenth century England. Despite the tremendous scientific advances in this richest of countries, "ready made" convex spectacles known as "glazed goods" can still be purchased in many states in stores not greatly unlike the English haberdashery shop of the 1600's. Millions of Americans still receive no vision service other than the purchase of a self-selected pair of inexpensively fabricated convex lens spectacles from a drug or variety store counter. Some states have outlawed the practice, but many have not. This is another example of a time lag between the development of knowledge and its universal application. For millions of people in the richest country of the world, the scientific advances of 300 years of optometric service are still not being used.

Not all spectacles were sold by haberdashers and novelty sales persons, however. Some spectaclemakers, even in 1629, when the Company was chartered, had their own shops. In these shops, the optical goods were fabricated and supplied to the buyer. Microscopes, telescopes, and other optical instruments were manufactured and supplied in addition to spectacles. The proprietor of such a shop, usually a free member of the Company, advised the client of the type of spectacles (or telescope or microscope) to purchase. These men often had considerable knowledge of optics and were in a better position than anyone else at the time to offer an optometric service.

For several hundred years, this was the only optometric service available. Physicians did not examine the eyes for spectacles, nor did they recommend them. Physicians preferred to use medication—solutions and salves. Members of the Spectaclemakers Company or their equivalent, the opticians of the day, fabricated spectacles that were either supplied to clients by them or were sold to haberdashers who, for the most part, allowed the client to select his spectacles for himself. Little by little, the optician who supplied spectacles became interested in the function of aiding the client in his selection. This slow evolution, lasting several hundred years, gave rise to modern optometry. The first modern optometrists were the best educated and most advanced of the opticians.

OPTICIANS—*1700 to 1900*

From 1700 to approximately 1900, spectacles were supplied in England in one of three ways: (1) by a member of the Company who owned his own shop; (2) by a peddler who bought his supply of spectacles at wholesale in the city and then traveled from farm to farm selling spectacles along with other small items such as needles, thread, toys, and buttons; or (3) by a store, such as a haberdashery, which purchased spectacles at wholesale and allowed the purchaser to select the most appropriate pair. During this 200-year period, the trend was more toward individual shops, and fewer spectacles were sold by peddlers or by general merchandisers. A trend also developed for the optician and even for the peddler to do some sight testing. Thus evolved the proto-optometrist who tested for, as well as supplied, spectacles.

In the British colonies in America, the optician shop, along with many other traditions from the parent country, was retained. Spectacle peddlers supplied the sparsely populated areas in the United States. Some spectacles were sold in general merchandise stores. The only marked difference between British and American opticians was the absence of the formal guilds in the new country. Learning was by apprenticeship. By the time the colonies were well populated, the guild system was on the decline in Europe. It never flourished in the United States. The British optician of that period, however, was the pattern for the American optician.

The British optician of that period and his American counterpart were direct ancestors of the present-day optometrist. Many of these men were well-educated in the field of optics. Numerous contributions in lens systems for telescopes, microscopes, and spectacle lenses and frames were made by these opticians.

During the seventeenth and early eighteenth centuries there were no house numbers on the streets of London; a sign was the method for identifying a place. The early opticians in London had signs which were in keeping with the custom of the times. Thus, when John Yarwell opened his optical shop called "Archimedes and the Crown," his sign showed Archimedes looking through a refracting telescope of considerable length. In the four corners of this sign were four pairs of split spectacles in tortoise-shell rims. Most opticians' signs had Archimedes, Bacon, or Sir Isaac Newton on them. Signs disappeared in London toward the end of the eighteenth century, for their creaking noise in the wind became an intolerable nuisance. At that time, street numbers were introduced to identify houses; and the opticians, along with others, took down their signs.

Each shop also had what was known as a "shop print," an advertising sheet with the sign and a list of the goods sold at the shop. The shop prints were usually given away and have become valuable documents today for the insight they give us into the trade of that time. From them we have learned what materials were sold and the prices that were charged.*

Court and von Rohr (1929–1930) attribute the decline of the Nürnberg Company to educational weakness and to economic factors. The instruction of apprentices from the beginning was poor; with members entering the trade through patrimony or through purchase, even poor instruction became absent. The old rules and methods, which were vigorously preserved, became inefficient compared to the new methods developed elsewhere. Thus, lack of adequate education and failure to keep up with advanced methods contributed to the decline.

Equally important was the economic problem. Since the members of the Company were allowed to deal only in spectacles and since the amount of retail trade in a medium-sized town like Nürnberg was limited, the members were compelled to develop a wholesale trade of some size, manufacturing spectacles in quantity through division of labor, and supplying them to other towns. Other factories sprang up, and competition became great. In the south German free towns, the optical industry developed mass production means; it managed to put on the market eyeglasses "of indifferent quality but at a marvelously

---

* We encounter here a time lag of a different sort from the ones previously discussed—the time lag in the behavior of individuals. Optometry today, recognized legally and academically as a health profession, is practiced by the vast majority of its members in conformity with the patterns of health profession members. A few optometrists, however, in spite of modern educational advances, sometimes adhere to earlier patterns. Thus we occasionally encounter an optometrist in a metropolitan area who uses advertising signs reminiscent of eighteenth century London. An occasional optometrist utilizes a public display of his wares reminiscent of the *ocularii* of third century Rome. Even the shop prints survive for some few optometrists in the form of newspaper or mailing advertisements. The association of spectacles and the London haberdashery store has its modern counterpart in the minority of present-day optometrists who have offices in mercantile establishments.

There are today individuals who either do not recognize or reject the evolutionary process toward professionalism which has occurred over several centuries. These recalcitrant members of the optometric profession sometimes trouble their more professionally-minded colleagues. In any evolutionary process throwbacks are to be expected. The main evolutionary trend is in the direction of advancement; the throwback emphasizes the progress which is being made by the group as a whole.

low price." Finally, the German guilds "came to an ignominious end as the makers neglected quality in the attempt to reduce costs to the lowest possible."

A similar decline was noted in England, but the results were not fatal in England as they were in Nürnberg, according to Court and von Rohr. After some decline in the seventeenth century, the British spectaclemaker of the eighteenth century stressed high quality and pride in workmanship; he would not impress his stamp on materials unless he felt they were of the best quality. This, plus the retention of rigid instructional standards, enabled the British spectaclemaker to survive.

The decline of the Nürnberg Company offers valuable insight into present optometric problems; this will be discussed again in later sections. Optometry today in the United States has developed perhaps the finest vision service of all time. But this service, because of its completeness and high quality, is not within the financial means of all people. We again face the problem of making it available to all. One suggestion has been to reduce the total service to simple component parts that could be performed by persons with far less education than the optometrist has. But this may lead to complete disintegration of the overall service, judging from the experience of the south German guilds. Another temptation is to reduce quality to make for greater availability. This, too, was tried at Nürnberg and failed. Consequently, when in a later chapter we discuss the sociological problems of the present, we will reject the suggestions for increasing availability by reduction in education or in quality. The sociological problem will be to *retain* excellence and yet increase availability.

Mass production of spectacles did ultimately contribute to the evolution of the optometric service. Court and von Rohr note that, when large factories, such as that of the Dunckers in Rathenow, grew rapidly, the former "professional men" were induced to purchase ready-made spectacle lenses, if not complete spectacles, from them. As a result, the spectaclemakers became spectacle vendors and later, spectacle fitters. This same trend developed later in both England and the United States. Interestingly, the new profession developed far more healthily in these countries, where quality and educational excellence were retained for a longer period. To this day the quality of optometric service is highest in the English-speaking countries.

From 1700 to 1900, then, spectaclemakers evolved slowly into spectacle vendors and finally into spectacle fitters. Spectaclemaking became a function of large factories using the methods of the newer industries. The present development of the optometric profession evolved in a different manner in various countries. In most of Europe today, optometry has not reached the degree of professionalization or independence that it has in the United States or England. In England, the Worshipful Company of Spectaclemakers played a role in the changes which occurred at the turn of the present century. In 1895, the British Optical Association was formed and was the first body in that country to set up an examination for refracting opticians. In 1898, there was a revival of the Worshipful Company of Spectaclemakers, which gave examinations. Those who passed these examinations were granted diplomas entitling them to practice opticianry. In 1904, sight-testing was included as one of the subjects in the examination. Thus, the same guild which was once restricted to spectaclemaking became a testing and accrediting body for sight-testers (optometrists).

In the United States, there was no equivalent to the Spectaclemakers Company. At the turn of the century, sight-testers (optometrists) gained recognition. But it happened in a different way than in England; the story of how the optometric profession emerged in the United States is discussed fully in Chapter 6.

CHAPTER 5

SCIENTIFIC CONTRIBUTIONS

Sometimes in the history of scientific disciplines, distinctly different groups have branched from a common stock. Initially, healing and religion were bound together intimately. Physician and priest in the earliest days of recorded history were almost indistinguishable; hospital and temple, incantation and therapy were practically inseparable. Often the individual who drove *out* evil spirits with white magic was also believed able to drive *in* evil spirits with black magic. The evil eye tradition was a part of such beliefs. Then, from the common stock of priest-medicine man two branches formed. With Hippocrates, a group began to practice healing primarily. Eventually, in parts of the world there were two distinct fields: professional healing and the professional priesthood. Several hundred years passed before this separation took place. In some areas of the world, it still has not occurred. However, in the period of Hippocrates, the die was cast; after that, it was only a matter of time for the separation to be accepted among civilized people.

Another separation took place toward the end of the Middle Ages. Early in history, vision was so poorly understood that diseases of the eye were not recognized as different from defects of vision, and they were treated similarly (Chapter 3). When vision anomalies were attributed to a lack of humors of the eye or to a deficiency of the spirit that emanated from the eye, errors of refraction and diseases of the eye were treated by the same healer and with the same therapy. With advances in optics, however, came the realization that defects of vision were not due to disease. When this was understood, two separate disciplines dealing with eye abnormalities could and did develop.

Treatment of diseases of the eye remained within the field of medicine, but a new group evolved to care for treatment of eye defects. This new group was composed of men who applied their knowledge of optics and their special skills to the making and fitting of spectacles for correcting vision defects. It was not made up of physicians, nor did it evolve from the physician group. Although these newcomers were a far cry from the modern optometrist, they were his ancestors and contributed their knowledge of optics, of spectacles, and of defects of vision to their heirs.

Since modern optometry evolved not from those whose province was the treatment of eye disease but from those who learned to correct for eye defects, this text will now no longer concern itself with the former group. We shall limit ourselves for the remainder of the text to the development of optometry as a separate service.

For the 600 years between 1300 and 1900, "optometric" service was provided by spectaclemakers, spectacle vendors, and opticians. These men, particularly the better educated opticians, made many contributions to optometric scientific knowledge. But no health art or science is self-sufficient. Just as medicine has been indebted to anatomists, physiologists, bacteriologists, biologists, and other general scientists, so optometry has been indebted to physicists, astronomers, mathematicians, and other physical scientists. Moreover, the human eye is part of the living biological system, and so optometric science has depended upon the same biologists, anatomists, physiologists, and psychologists for basic knowledge, as has medicine.

Finally, optometry is indebted for some discoveries to medicine, just as medicine is indebted for some of its knowledge to men of optics. No field of science is isolated; all are dependent on other fields.

The present chapter is a summary of the many contributions to the body of knowledge which comprises modern optometry—contributions from physical scientists, from life scientists and biologists in the broad sense of the word, from the men who practiced medicine, and from the men who practiced primitive optometry itself, the opticians and spectaclemakers.

THE THEORY OF VISION

Many men helped discover the means by which the eye mediates vision. Philosophers, artists, natural scientists, mathematicians, and physicists have contributed. For 1400 years, it had been thought that the eye sent forth an emanation to the object. Then Alhazen identified light as the stimulus that traveled from object to eye. But the problem was not solved *in toto* with the work of the Arabian mathematician.

Alhazen, for example, did not understand the nature of the crystalline lens or the retina. He believed that an image of the object was brought to a focus on the front surface of the crystalline lens and that this structure functioned as a receptor rather than as a refracting body.

For many years, different authors held to the Epicurean theory even after the work of Alhazen disputed it. Abelard of Bath (about

1130), a teacher at monastic schools in Gaul, had traveled among Moslems and greatly admired their work. Nonetheless, he held a theory of vision similar to Plato's rather than Alhazen's. In postulating that the "visible spirit" passed from the brain to the eyes through hollow nerves and thence to the object and back again with great speed, he demonstrated that he was not acquainted with the optical research and treatise of Alhazen, who lived 100 years earlier. Robert Grosseteste, Roger Bacon's teacher at Oxford University, and Bartholomew of England also postulated theories of vision in the mid-thirteenth century in which an emanation from the eye plays a part.

Vitello, whose book written about 1270 may have been a translation of Alhazen, and Peter of Albano, born in 1250, both maintained that the theory of vision by extramission of rays was impossible. Yet, as late as the latter half of the fourteenth century, at least 350 years after Alhazen and 100 years after Vitello and Peter of Albano, the Arabian author As-Sadili explained vision as being dependent on the emission of something from the eye.

Leonardo da Vinci, born in 1452, is usually credited with identifying the crystalline lens as a refracting body rather than a receptor. Da Vinci, famous as sculptor, architect, painter, musician, mechanic, engineer, and physiologist, was one of the greatest scientists of all time; certainly he was one of the most versatile intellects who ever lived. He correctly identified the cornea and the crystalline lens as the two major refracting elements in the eye. However, he located the lens toward the center of the eye and thought of the image as erect and formed upon either the posterior surface of the lens or upon the optic nerve head. To this Italian genius, then, goes credit for moving the image back from the lens itself toward the retina—but not to the retina itself. This latter concept was not postulated for another 100 years.

The identification of the retina as the receptive layer and of the crystalline lens solely as a refractive element was the work of Felix Plater, born in 1536, a professor of anatomy at the University of Basel in Switzerland. Before Plater, it was believed that impulses from the crystalline lens passed over the suspensory ligaments. Plater cut the suspensory ligaments, which disconnected the lens, and demonstrated that vision persisted in spite of this procedure. He therefore reasoned that the crystalline lens and suspensory ligaments are not essential to reception of the visual stimulus.

Very shortly afterward, the German mathematician and astronomer, Johannes Kepler, born in 1571, not only placed the image upon the retina, but also differentiated the function of the central and peripheral retina. In his writings on vision, Kepler correctly identified the crystalline lens as a refracting body and the retina as a receptor, although he did not offer the experimental proof that Plater did. His evidence was theoretical and based on mathematical computations.

In 1619, the Jesuit opticist, Father Scheiner, demonstrated that an inverted image was formed on the retina. He cut a window through the sclera and choroid in the back of sheep and ox eyes and demonstrated the existence of the inverted image in this region. This demonstration is still repeated annually in optometric laboratory courses by student optometrists. Thus, the two simple experiments of Plater and Scheiner and the optical and mathematical reasoning of Kepler demonstrated conclusively that the image utilized in vision is formed on the retina. This is now the accepted theory.

Kepler's treatise on optics (1611) explained scientifically the process by which the eye received and formed an image. Light from an object entered the eye, was refracted by cornea and lens, and formed an inverted image on the retina. The eye was no longer an organ which sent forth spirits, rays, atoms, or substances to interpret the object. It was an optical instrument, an image-forming device the retina of which was the true receptor.

But once again there were time lags. Duke-Elder (1940, p. 731), for example, notes that as late as 1813 Horn believed that the image was received in the vitreous; in 1817 Reade believed it was received by the corneal nerves; in 1825 Lehot held that a tri-dimensional image formed in the vitreous was the essential image in vision; and in 1830 Plagge held that the image used in vision was that reflected from the cornea. Thus, even within the recent past, a time lag of over 200 years was to exist between the time knowledge was clearly available and the time it was accepted and utilized universally. And this lag occurred after Scheiner's irrefutable demonstration, after Plater's experimental proof, and after Kepler's complete optical treatises. More than discovery is required before new knowledge is assimilated and put to use. Examples of time lag indicate how necessary it is for those in scientific pursuits to keep an open mind and be willing to examine evidence. Today's student and scientist should ponder this problem. There have been so many examples of time lag, periods when better facts were at hand but were not adopted. It is always possible that some important point or points of information have already been discovered that today are neglected. Someone 100 or 200 years from now may point to our period and note with derision that certain information was already at hand and was not generally accepted.

This fact might suggest that one accept all new ideas. This is anything but the lesson we should learn. Rather, time lags can be avoided or cut down by examining all new ideas *critically* and accepting or rejecting them on the basis of their conformity with facts.

Truth does not come pre-labeled; it often appears not greatly different from untruth. Thus, scientists need two attributes: an open mind and a willingness to examine evidence critically. The key word in modern experimental science is *evidence*. Time lags can be cut and knowledge can advance more rapidly if all new ideas are considered on the basis of the evidence for and against their being true. Time lags are reduced by acceptance of the true *and* by rejection of the untrue. Even with the best scientific methods, time lags will undoubtedly plague man for years to come. But they can be reduced, and this is a major aim of modern science.

CONTRIBUTIONS OF THE PHYSICAL SCIENTISTS

The science of optics is an important base for modern optometry. The first major contributions were made by Euclid and Ptolemy. About 1000 years later, toward the end of the tenth century, Alhazen made his notable advances. Then a long period elapsed before another major breakthrough was made, involving many men. During the seventeenth century, a great deal of modern optical theory and practice was formulated. The publication in 1611 of *Dioptrice* by Kepler may be said to be the beginning of the modern period. Today's optometry student is often surprised at the number of references to this seventeenth century publication. Through the three great works of Euclid, Alhazen, and Kepler the history of optics is traced; however, Kepler's period is particularly significant because it is one of many discoveries and one in which many men made significant contributions to optics.

The period between Alhazen and Kepler was not without some contributions. The first European treatise on optics was by Vitello (about 1270); his *Ten Books of Optics* played a dominant role until Kepler's time. Vitello's work, however, contained little original material. It was mainly a restatement of earlier Greek and Arabian works. The optical writings of Roger Bacon, the English friar, born in 1214, had some significance in that they spoke of lenses as an aid to vision; but, as Polyak (1943) notes, these writings, too, showed little originality of optical thought.

During the seventeenth century, physical science reached a higher degree of sophistication than did biological sciences. There were several reasons for this development. For one thing, other sciences depended on advances in physical instrumentation, the lack of which delayed their further development. Electrophysiology had to await a knowledge of electricity; histology had to await the invention of the microscope.

Reluctance to allow study of the human body, whether dead or alive, slowed development of life science. Complacency in the belief that Galen's system was both complete and correct was another contributing factor.

Astronomy, in which such marked advances were made during the seventeenth century, was particularly fortunate among the physical sciences. Astrology was allied to astronomy and, therefore, the latter was considered practical. This made it a subject in which rulers had considerable interest; consequently, it was subsidized by the government even in early times. Astronomy is the science which deals with the bodies of the universe and with their positions, motions, constitution, and origin. Astrology is the ancient art, science, or pseudo-science of predicting the future of human beings on the basis of the positions of the stars and planets. Astrology has an ancient history, and as late as the fourteenth and fifteenth centuries, astrologers played a dominant role in the courts of Europe; even in the seventeenth century the interest of western rulers in astrology continued.

The development of optics early in the Renaissance was in part the result of the belief in astrology, since kings and rulers subsidized students of this lore. To study the heavenly bodies, better optical systems were required. The science of optics which developed was far more scientific than the purpose for which it was originally used.

The leading figure of this golden period in optics was the German astronomer, mathematician, and, in his early years, theologian, Johannes Kepler. Born in 1576, the eldest child of a reckless soldier of fortune and an undisciplined, poorly-educated mother, Johannes suffered from smallpox in his fourth year. This left him with poor vision and crippled hands. At first, he studied for the ministry. He turned from this pursuit in 1594 to accept a post in science at Gratz; in 1601 he replaced Tycho Brahe at the observatory at Prague.

Kepler found that a good many of his duties were of an astrological nature. Emperor Rudolph II believed in astrology and paid Kepler's salary; Kepler drew the emperor's horoscope. He seems to have believed that astrology was not completely invalid and stated that he hoped to preserve the grain of truth contained in that field. Although he used necessity as his excuse for this compromise, he did keep careful records of his own life to determine what planetary influences might have occurred.

In 1604 in his *Supplements to Vitello's Optics,* Kepler presented his theory of vision, which was a great advance over that of Alhazen and was so close to modern thinking. Crombie (1964) points out that all of the necessary knowledge was available to Kepler. For example, Kepler was acquainted with Plater's work on the retina. However, he succeeded in seeing the problem in a new way. Earlier scientists such as da Vinci and Porta had thought of the eye as a form of camera obscura but had encountered a stumbling block in supposing that the image had to be right side up. Kepler compared the eye to a camera obscura *and* accepted the fact that the image is inverted.

Kepler also recognized (Crombie, 1964) that the explanation of how the eye forms an image was only a part of the explanation of vision. He recognized that the way the physical occurrences in the eye were transformed into sensation (the psychophysiological portion of the visual process) lay outside his mathematical solution. Of this he said, "I leave it to natural philosophers."

In 1611 Kepler's *Dioptrice* was published. For its time, it was a complete system of optics. The mathematical relationships of lenses, prisms, and mirrors were presented, as well as further description of the process of vision. With the publication of *Dioptrice* and of *Supplements to Vitello's Optics,* the visual process was described accurately insofar as the image-forming aspect of the eye is concerned. From then on, a systemized knowledge of optics was available. For these contributions Kepler has been recognized as the founder of modern optics. Although he made contributions to astronomy and mathematics, Kepler's great contribution was his original and systematic treatment of optics.

Another outstanding scientist of the same period was the Dutch mathematician and astronomer, Christian Huygens. His father was a statesman and an author often described as the most brilliant figure in Dutch literary history. In 1666 the younger Huygens accepted an offer by King Louis XIV to become a resident of France and pursue his work in that country. He remained in France until 1681. Then he returned to Holland. His contributions to the physical sciences were numerous. Optics, in particular, is indebted to him for the wave theory of light. The concept that light travels as waves, all points on a wave front serving as the origin for secondary waves, became one of the foundations on which modern optical science is built. Huygens also did work on polarized light. This resulted from his experiments with double refraction in Iceland spar crystals.

Another scientist, usually classified as a mathematician and physicist, who made a great contribution to optics about this time is Sir Isaac Newton. His father died before Isaac was born in 1642, and the boy's early scholastic record was unimpressive. He worked on his mother's farm for a short period and then matriculated at Trinity College in 1661, remaining at Cambridge University for most of his life. In 1689 he was elected a member of parliament as a representative of the university. In 1701 after 40 years at Cambridge as student and faculty member, he resigned his professorship to become warden of the mint in London, a position he held until his death. He became president of the Royal Society in 1703 and was knighted in 1705. His great scientific contributions were made during his earlier period at Cambridge.

Newton's contributions to the general field of physics are well known. He was an astronomer. His interest in optics stemmed from his desire, to perfect telescopic lens systems. An attempt to remove defects from lenses probably led to his study of color. His experiments led to the discovery that white light is composed of different colors, each refracted to a different degree. He did a great deal of work on lenses and optical systems, all in order to aid his astronomical endeavors, but all serving as contributions to the general field of optics.

Although Kepler, Huygens, and Newton were the major figures during the seventeenth century, other physical scientists made contributions. Unlike the three major contributors, each of whom produced a treatise on the broad subject of optics, these others made lesser but worthwhile contributions to human thought, even though they did not produce major systematic works.

Willebrord Snell, born in 1591, succeeded his father as professor of mathematics and natural philosophy at the University of Leyden. To this mathematician we are indebted for the sine law which describes the relationship between angle of incidence and angle of re fraction. Although he imparted this discovery to his students, he did not publish it. After Snell's death, Descartes published the sine law in *La Dioptrique,* 1637.

F. Maurolycus, an older contemporary of Kepler, studied the properties of lenses; some of his contributions to the science of optics were incorporated in Kepler's work. His explanation for the basis of vision was similar to Kepler's, but it was not published until after his death and after Kepler's work had appeared (Crombie, 1964).

Another contemporary of Kepler, Giambattista della Porta, described by Polyak (1943) as "the great Neapolitan dilettante," also made some studies of the properties of lenses and added a convex lens to the camera obscura.

The English physicist, Robert Hooke, born in 1635, was a contemporary of Newton. Often described as one who originated much but perfected little, Hooke conceived in incomplete form the undulatory theory of light wave propagation; this work was perfected several years later by Huygens.

These and other mathematicians, astronomers, and physical scientists during the sixteenth and seventeenth centuries developed optics to a point close to its present state. Throughout the next 350 years, new single discoveries would be made, and new problems solved. But the groundwork was well laid during this era. To describe the contributions of each opticist in the next years (and there have been many) is beyond the scope of this volume. The period from Kepler to the present was certainly not sterile in the field of optics.

In the seventeenth century, there was a large number of contributors in optics. Unlike Alhazen, who worked without colleagues, the men of the seventeenth century knew each other and discussed problems in common. In seventeenth century physical sciences, we see a beginning of organized science. Other physical scientists and natural philosophers, such as Descartes, Bernoulli, and Leibnitz, knew and communicated with the men we have discussed. When in 1694 Newton was ill, Huygens wrote to Leibnitz inquiring if he had heard about the illness of the "good Mr. Newton."

More important, these men were members of an organization which offered them the opportunity to meet with each other, to discuss their work, and to be challenged. The organization was the Royal Society, of which Newton was president from 1703 until his death in 1727.

The Royal Society of London for Improving Natural Knowledge was founded in 1660 and is one of the oldest scientific societies in Europe. It is an outgrowth of a group that had been meeting weekly for some years at Oxford. In 1661, the society granted the king of England membership and adopted its present name. At Royal Society meetings, members and scientists presented papers and performed experiments for the edification of their fellows. Of those already mentioned, Newton, Hooke, and Huygens were all members. Reports of the meetings were published in the *Philosophical Transactions,* a scientific journal of world renown. The performance and discussion of experiments were the major functions of the society. Many of the great discoveries were first presented to the Royal Society.

More recently, the Royal Society has served as consultant to government, has awarded medals, has provided honorary lectureships, and has disbursed a sizeable fund for research grants. At present, 25 new members are elected annually. Although primarily devoted to the physical and mathematical sciences in its early years, the Royal Society in 1887 divided the *Philosophical Transactions* into two sections: one for physical and mathematical sciences, the other for biological sciences. Unquestionably, this society contributed greatly to the advance of knowledge.

Although the physical scientists of the seventeenth century displayed little academic interest in spectacles and did not envisage their work as a cornerstone of what would one day be a profession called optometry, their work nonetheless became just this. But of deeper significance than their overall contributions regarding the laws of optics and theories of light was their encouragement of and adherence to scientific methodology, a heritage which has been adopted by scientific specialties, including optometry.*

CONTRIBUTIONS OF THE LIFE SCIENTISTS

The work of physical scientists contributed to optometric knowledge of lenses and light. However, optometrists deal not only with spectacles, but also with the human organism, which is a biological system. The life scientists contributed knowledge about the structure (anatomy) and functioning (physiology) of the eye. When psychology and physiological optics came into being during the nineteenth century, workers in these disciplines also made significant contributions to the science of optometry.

ANATOMY

In the second century A.D., Galen produced a system of anatomy and general medicine so encompassing that it was followed almost without deviation for nearly 1400 years. The descriptions of structures listed by Galen were accepted as unqualified truths. Yet there were many errors in Galen's work. He had performed no human dissections, although he had done some work on Barbary apes. The dogmatic acceptance of Galen's work held anatomy and medical research back many centuries. Yet, as Atkinson (1956) notes, the fault was not Galen's. Nowhere in his writings did Galen insist on unreasoned acceptance of his every word. He did perform dissections; he was an experimentalist. It was only the blind acceptance of his work by later generations which made it possible for Haggard (1933) to comment: "Hippocrates opened the wide road of medical advancement; Galen closed it, and it remained so closed for nearly 14 centuries."

Because of this lack of questioning of Galen's interpretation of the structure of the eye and of all other body parts, Galen's beliefs were adhered to exactly as he had stated them until the middle of the sixteenth century. Then in 1543, Andreas Vesalius (born in Brussels, 1514), a teacher of surgery and anatomy at the University of Padua, presented his great book, *De Fabrica Humani Corporis*. Vesalius had performed many systematic human dissections. He obtained the bodies by bribing deadhouse keepers, robbing graves, and using cadavers of criminals. His plates were made as woodcuts and were prepared by several artists; the volume was printed in Basel. Saunders

---

* The biographies in the present section were derived from many sources. Particularly worthy of note, however, are Polyak (1943) ; Southall (1933) ; Boring (1942) ; Bausch & Lomb (1936) ; and, above all, the *Encyclopaedia Britannica* (1958 edition) .

and O'Malley (1950), in their introduction to a modern reproduction of Vesalius' volume, report that it is not only a scientific work of sufficient importance to make its author one of the great medical scientists of all time, but it is also one of the "most noble and magnificent volumes in the history of printing." The last plate of the volume showed a series of dissections of the eye.

Thus, from Vesalius and those who came after him, man obtained an accurate knowledge of the structure of the human eye. But an understanding of the minute structure had to await technological improvements. Histology, the branch of anatomy which deals with microscopic studies of tissue, did not develop until technological advances permitted it.

Some idea of the recency of man's understanding of the minute structure of the tissues of the eye may be obtained from Table 1. Several tissues and structures of the eye are named after those who described them. These structures include the Meibomian glands, the Zonule of Zinn, and Descemet's membrane. Table 1 lists the names used today for several tissues and the name, nationality, and period in history of the discoverer. From inspection of the table, we note that most of the anatomists who gave their names to parts of the eye lived in the eighteenth and nineteenth centuries. Half of the anatomists were German, a quarter French. An understanding of the histological structure of the eye, as can be seen from the table, was obtained only within the past hundred or so years.

Galen began the investigations on the structure of the eye in the second century A.D. For 1400 years, until Vesalius' work was published, no new contributions to anatomy reached the public. Following Vesalius, many other anatomists contributed to the information which we have today on the structure of the eye. It is to all of these anatomists that modern optometric science is indebted for such knowledge.

PHYSIOLOGY

The eye is living tissue, and many physiological discoveries from the seventeenth to the nineteenth century also applied to ocular function. William Harvey, in 1628, described the mechanism for circulation of blood. His contribution to general knowledge about blood circulation helped in the understanding of the physiology of the eye, since blood courses through arteries and veins in the eye just as it does throughout the body. When Lavoisier, born in 1743, explained how oxygen in the air (previously described by Priestley and others) is taken into the organism and utilized in the metabolism of foodstuff, this knowledge, too, had application to the eye; most eye tissues, just as those elsewhere in the body, utilize oxygen.

TABLE 1

STRUCTURE	NAMED AFTER	NATIONALITY	LIFE SPAN	DISCOVERY OR DESCRIPTION DATE
Glands in the Lid	Meibom (1)	German	1638–1700	1666
Suspensory Ligament of the Lens	Zinn	German	1727–1759	1755
Membrane of Cornea	Descemet	French	1732–1810	1758
Spaces in Iris	Fontana	Italian	1720–1805	1781
Capsule Surrounding Eye	Tenon	French	1724–1816	1806
Muscle (Lid)	Horner	U.S.A.	1793–1853	1822
Canal in Vitreous where Fetal (Hyaloid) Artery Passed	Cloquet	French	1790–1882	1821–1831
Canal in Sclera	Schlemm (2)	German	1795–1858	1831
Layer of Retina	Henle	German	1809–1885	1839
Membrane of Choroid	Bruch	Swiss	1819–1884	1844
Muscle (Meridional Fibers of Ciliary)	Brücke (3)	German	1819–1892	1846
Membrane of Cornea	Bowman	English	1816–1892	1847
Muscle (Radial Fibers of Ciliary)	Müller (3)	German	1820–1864	1855

(1) Galen first discovered these glands in the lids; but Meibom, having made the first exact description, has been honored by the use of his name.

(2) Schlemm made his first observation of the canal which bears his name on the eye of a criminal who had been hanged. He observed and described blood in the canal, a phenomenon which occurs in strangulation. For many years the function and contents of the canal in a living being were disputed vigorously by various authorities.

(3) The ciliary muscle, so very important to optometrists because of its role in accommodation, was described by Eustachius in his anatomical plates in 1552–1574. His work was seemingly forgotten, and so Kepler in 1611 and Descartes in 1637 in describing accomodation merely assumed the presence of such a body as the ciliary. Although it was studied and described by the English anatomist, Knox, in 1823, and the American Waller in 1835, its discovery is usually attributed to Brücke in 1846. The meridional fibers are named after Brücke; the radial fibers after Heinrich Müller, who described them in 1855, although Waller had also described them some twenty years earlier. The ciliary was also described almost simultaneously with Brücke's work by Bowman (1847). (Text of this footnote, after Duke-Elder, 1940, p. 61.)

Thus, advances in general physiology provided a physiological base for those who studied the eye and vision. Some physiological advances were more prominent and pertinent to vision scientists than others.

Albrecht von Haller founded modern physiology with the publication, between 1757 and 1766, of his *Elements of Physiology*. This text includes a full discussion of the senses. Haller was an experimentalist; he rejected the concept that nerves are hollow tubes through which a liquid flows. He did this by a simple experiment which demonstrated that ligatured nerves do not swell up on the side toward the brain (Hulin, 1933).

Charles Bell, a British anatomist and physiologist, described in his *New Idea of the Anatomy of the Brain* (1811) the different functions of nerves from different parts of the brain. In *The Nervous System of the Human Body* (1830), Bell clearly differentiated the functions of sensory nerves and motor nerves. Independently, in 1822, the French physiologist François Magendie demonstrated the difference in the function of the sensory and motor nerves. Boring (1942) explains this discrepancy in dates; he states that Bell made the observation first; however, his text was distributed almost exclusively to friends and was not seen by Magendie. The latter, working without benefit of Bell's earlier paper, performed the more conclusive experiment. The law which describes the function of the sensory and motor nerves' emerging from the spinal roots has been named the Bell-Magendie law in tribute to the contributions of both men.*

Work on both the nervous system and the visual system was performed by Johannes Müller, the German physiologist and anatomist who is often referred to as the father of experimental physiology. His *Handbuch der Physiologie des Menschen* was published in several volumes between 1833 and 1840, and an important part of the work was that on the nervous system and the special senses. His theory of

* While his work in neurophysiology was brilliant and his experiments excellent, Magendie's work in other areas of visual physiology was notably poor. He held, for example, that there was no mechanism of accommodation, the eye having universal focus like a pinhole camera. He believed that the crystalline had some function other than that of a lens. He based his conclusion on his repetition of Scheiner's experiment of observing the image formed in the back of an enucleated eye. Magendie used the eye of a white rabbit; he changed the object distance and found little change in the scleral image. Helmholtz later pointed out the flaw in the experiment: namely, the unsuitability of the sclera to act as the screen. Descartes a hundred years earlier had pointed out the value of using a thin screen (paper) in place of the sclera in performing Scheiner's experiment, but Magendie had not read Descartes. In this instance, in his duplication of Bell's work, and in several other efforts, Magendie appears to have experimented brilliantly but failed to keep up on his reading. This tale is often told to novice scientists to stress the importance of "keeping up with the literature."

"specific nerve energy" (1838) became a base for an understanding of the sensory processes. We have already noted that by the time of Kepler (1611) and his *Dioptrice,* there was a comprehension of the formation of an image on the retina of the eye. But the steps between the formation of the retinal image and the perception of the object in space were still not understood. Müller's theory led to the understanding that impulses in the optic nerve and those in the auditory nerve, for example, do not differ from each other. What is different is the action of the receptors *and* the area of the brain to which the respective nerves lead.

This phase of physiology that deals with the nervous system was further advanced by many investigators in the present century. Details of the nervous system continue to be a fruitful subject of study. Neurophysiology has been important to optometry even when it has not dealt with the visual process itself. Its overall significance is emphasized by the fact that three workers in this field have received Nobel prizes: the Russian Ivan Pavlov, born in 1849, the Englishmen Charles Sherrington, born in 1857, and Edgar D. Adrian, born in 1889. Although only Adrian * and his co-workers at Cambridge University devoted any considerable effort to the visual system specifically, the work of all greatly abetted the understanding of the visual process.

The optometric base in the life sciences was developed before the middle of the nineteenth century by those anatomists and physiologists who were advancing knowledge of the total living organism. In addition to these general advances, a great deal of experimental work in visual sensation and perception was being carried out in various German physiological laboratories by the middle of the nineteenth century.

The functioning of the eye from its cornea to its retina was understood. The time was approaching for a systematic exploration of such problems as how man sees color, how he perceives depth, what determines the sensitivity of vision, and how form is perceived by the organism. In Johannes Müller's laboratory, many physiological experiments were conducted on the senses. Then, during the middle of the nineteenth century, two new disciplines were founded, each incorporating within its scope the sort of problems which had been worked on in experimental physiology. With the publication of his work on *Physiological Optics* (1866), Hermann von Helmholtz, a physiologist who was influenced in his student years by Müller, founded physiologi-

* At the time this volume is being written, Horace B. Barlow, a former student of Adrian, is studying the processes of neurophysiology of the visual system as part of the research program of the School of Optometry, University of California.

cal optics. In 1874 Wilhelm Wundt, a student of both Müller and Helmholtz, founded modern psychology. The time was ripe for both of these disciplines to emerge. The peculiar problems involved with vision required more knowledge of optics than was possessed by most physiologists and more knowledge of physiology than was possessed by those working in optics; processes such as learning and perception required special approaches.

Physiological optics is perhaps the most important body of knowledge in the present optometric curriculum. It is, in fact, the science of which optometry is the applied branch. Yet its founder, Helmholtz, was a physicist and a physiologist and remained so throughout his life.

Hermann von Helmholtz was born at Potsdam, Germany, in 1821. His father was a military officer and later a teacher of classical languages; his mother was a descendant of William Penn, founder of the state of Pennsylvania. Helmholtz was a sickly child who had trouble in school with subjects requiring memory. However, he excelled in mathematics, physics and, later, optics. He had wanted to become a physicist, but his father prevailed upon him to study medicine because of the family's need for money. Nonetheless, he never conducted a private practice of medicine; after serving as a military physician, he became professor of physiology at Königsberg (1849), professor of anatomy and physiology at Bonn (1855), professor of physiology at Heidelberg (1858), and professor of physics and director of the Physical Institute at Berlin (1871). He died in 1894.

Throughout his professional life, he was a teacher, a researcher, and, most of all, one who organized knowledge. As a teacher, he could claim many great scientists as his pupils, including Wundt, the founder of psychology, and the great physicist Hertz. As a researcher, Helmholtz made contributions to physiology and to physics. He measured the speed at which the impulse travels within a nerve. Primarily, he utilized the inspiration of others and fitted the pieces together into a unified whole.

The great discoveries associated with the name of Helmholtz were usually made by predecessors. Helmholtz recognized discoveries and evaluated their importance. The ophthalmoscope, said to be invented by Helmholtz in 1851, had actually been described four years earlier by the English lensmaker Charles Babbage. Babbage had presented it to a leading physician; the latter had failed to recognize its usefulness. The ophthalmometer, which Helmholtz used in his work, had been described earlier (1796) by the English lensmaker Jesse Ramsden. The theories of accommodation and of color vision associated with the name of Helmholtz had both been suggested half a

century earlier by the great British scientist Sir Thomas Young.*
Helmholtz's contributions were refinement, careful investigation of
all the intricacies, utilization of learning, and synthesis.

His great work was the three volume textbook, *Physiological
Optics*. The first volume appeared in 1856, the last in 1866. A second
edition appeared during Helmholtz's lifetime in 1885; a third edition
was published in 1909–1910 with added notes and corrections by
Gullstrand, von Knies, and Nagel. The additions and comments by
the physiologist and physicist, Alvar Gullstrand of Sweden, 1911
Nobel prize winner, are particularly valuable; they extended the usefulness of the treatise to the present period. In 1924, the third edition
of Helmholtz was translated into English by Southall, and its publication was underwritten by the Optical Society of America.

From the time of Helmholtz, the discipline of physiological optics
has made tremendous strides. During Helmholtz's life and shortly
thereafter, the science of physiological optics also developed in
France. Louis Emile Javal, born in 1839, initially an engineer, became interested in the strabismus of one of his relatives; he studied
medicine because of this interest and was the first to translate Helmholtz's work. In 1876, a laboratory was created for him at the Sorbonne. In 1881, he developed a clinical model of the ophthalmometer. He became blind from chronic glaucoma shortly afterward and
devoted the remainder of his life to studying the problems of blindness.

In 1884, M. Tscherning became director of the Sorbonne laboratory. Tscherning, born and educated in Copenhagen, produced a text
on physiological optics, conducted experimental work in the subject,
and advanced the science in France. Some of his theories differed
from those of Helmholtz regarding aspects of physiological optics.
The "how" of eye accommodation was one point of disagreement.

Before Helmholtz, physiological optics had been part of physiology. Why did it emerge as a new discipline? Why was vision a function which required a separate discipline, yet such equally complex
phenomena as respiration or metabolism remained within the main
body of physiology? The answer to these questions is of great significance to modern optometrists, inasmuch as optometry is the applied

---

* Tscherning has named Thomas Young, who lived between 1773 and 1829, the
founder of physiological optics, although that title is usually bestowed on Helmholtz.
A versatile genius, Young read fluently at the age of two and spoke a dozen or more
foreign languages while still in his early 'teens. Both a practicing physician and a
professor of natural science, he made contributions to optics, physiology, and physics,
and translated the hieroglyphic inscription of the famous Rosetta Stone. Helmholtz
described him as ". . . one of the most clear-sighted men who have ever lived." (This
biography is based on Duke-Elder, 1940.)

branch of a body of knowledge of which physiological optics is the academic aspect. The rationale for optometry as a separate applied art and science is the same as that for physiological optics as a separate discipline.

The main reason for the separation is to be found in the nature of the problem and the types of solution. An understanding of vision requires a knowledge of *both* the biological sciences, such as physiology and anatomy, *and* the physical sciences, such as mathematics and optics. Physiological optics is the academic science which synthesizes both physics and biology in the understanding of vision; optometry is the applied art and science which utilizes both disciplines to solve vision problems on a day-to-day basis. The early developers of physiological optics were well versed in *both* physical *and* biological science. Young was both physician and physicist; Helmholtz was both physicist and physiologist; Javal was first an engineer, then an ophthalmologist. In recent times, however, most workers in physiological optics have been trained from the outset in *both* of these branches of science. They are not physicists who later learned physiology, nor physiologists who later learned mathematics. The premise for optometry's existence as a separate discipline is based on the same circumstances as physiological optics, because optometrists, too, are trained at the outset in *both* approaches—the physical as well as the biological. The discipline of physiological optics is basic in their training.

Physiological optics has remained an active and fruitful discipline throughout the century since Helmholtz delineated its scope. A better understanding of the visual process has resulted from research within this field during its hundred year history. Almost to the day of its hundreth anniversary as a separate discipline, physiological optics received worldwide public recognition. The 1967 Nobel Prize in Physiology was awarded to three researchers in physiological optics: Ragnar Granit who worked on the electrical potential of retinal nerve cells at the Caroline Institute in Sweden; Halden Keffer Hartline of Rockefeller University who also worked on the electro-physiology of receptor cells of the visual system; and George Wald of Harvard University who studied the biochemical nature of the pigments of the retina which mediate vision.

CONTRIBUTIONS OF PSYCHOLOGISTS

Like the biological and physical sciences, psychology also contributes to the basic knowledge on which optometry is dependent. Unlike biology and physics, however, psychology is a new science. It is less than 100 years old. It was established as a separate science by Wilhelm Wundt in 1874; experimental psychology was founded by Wundt in 1879.

The history of psychology is analogous to that of optometry in that both histories are short. However, men thought about psychological phenomena long before psychology emerged as a separate discipline. Just as "optometric service" was offered by spectaclemakers and opticians for hundreds of years before optometry as a modern discipline came into being, so natural scientists and philosophers concerned themselves with areas of thought which would now be considered part of psychology. Sensation and perception did not suddenly spring into being in 1874, the date usually given for Wundt's founding of psychology.

In science, the lines between disciplines have been and still are indistinctly drawn; overlap is the rule rather than the exception. Knowledge is indivisible. Knowledge about the eye and vision has come from many different disciplines. Correspondingly, the field in which an individual works is not always clearly demarcated. Helmholtz, as has been pointed out, was a physician, a physicist, a physiologist, and the founder of physiological optics as a separate discipline. In addition, his work was important to psychology. Boring (1942) dedicated his *Sensation and Perception in the History of Experimental Psychology* to Helmholtz.*

Although many different disciplines may contribute to academic knowledge of any particular subject and one individual may function within several academic disciplines, sharp lines are drawn between the practitioners of the various branches of applied science. Optometrists test vision, but psychologists do not; clinical psychologists do mental testing, but optometrists do not; physicians prescribe drugs, but optometrists and psychologists do not; surgeons operate on the human eye, but physiologists do not. This distinction between academic and applied branches of the various disciplines is important.†

* At the time that one of the authors was a student at Stanford University (MJH, 1943–1947), Professor of Psychology Farnsworth submitted a questionnaire to a group of psychologists asking them to rate all psychologists, living or dead, in the order of importance. Helmholtz was rated fourth highest; only Wundt, James, and Binet rated higher. Clearly, experimental psychologists consider Helmholtz a psychologist.

† In the 1950's an attempt was made to carry the distinctions of the applied sciences into the academic field. An organization of applied medicine passed a resolution declaring it unethical for physicians to teach or have discourse with optometrists. Although on the academic level contributions to the common body of knowledge continued to be made by physiologists, psychologists, optometrists, and physicians, the attempt was made to keep knowledge away from students of one discipline. Because the concept of exclusive ownership of knowledge is so foreign to the academic community, the attempt met with little success. Happily, as this is being written (1966), this restriction against dissemination of knowledge has been revoked.

A true history of psychological thought begins, as does Boring's (1942) history, with philosophers such as Aristotle, the Epicureans, and Plato; it also includes the later contributions of physiologists. Thus, until the middle of the nineteenth century, the history of psychology, like that of optometry, is closely intertwined with the history of many other disciplines. Much of the history of psychology has already been presented in this text in the discussions of other disciplines.

Crombie (1964) claims for Descartes the distinction of having recognized that vision entails an optical, biological, and psychological aspect. Before Descartes, students of vision never clearly recognized that there were three different kinds of questions: physical, physiological, and psychological. The problem had been dealt with as though a single question only was involved. Kepler separated out the physical, but noted that he left the remainder for the "natural philosophers." The mechanistic philosophy of Descartes, according to Crombie, set the stage for differentiating physiological or psychophysiological areas from psychology and the nature of perception.

René Descartes was born in 1596 into a learned French family. He was sickly through most of his life and appears to have done a considerable amount of work in bed.* He was trained at Jesuit schools. From 1618 to 1628, he traveled about Europe as a gentleman soldier and then settled in Holland. There he spent most of the remainder of his life. Having inherited wealth, he never held a regular job or university post but spent all of his later years writing, thinking, and experimenting. The impact of his writings in mathematics, philosophy, and optics created a major change in the thinking of mankind.

Through most of his life, Descartes had an interest in optics and in vision. Before settling in Holland, he carried on some optical research with the help of the optician Ferrier. He repeated the Scheiner experiment, noting the necessity for using a thin membrane over the window in the sclera.

Descartes' *La Dioptrique* is similar to Kepler's *Dioptrice,* published 25 years earlier. It may be considered a refinement of Kepler's treatise. One major improvement was the inclusion of the sine law, discovered but not published by Snell a few years earlier. Some authors believe that Descartes discovered this relationship independently of Snell.

Descartes' major contribution to human thought, however, was not his optics text, although it was read and utilized by visual scien-

---

* Biographical material on Descartes is based on *Encyclopaedia Britannica* (1958). Description of his scientific contributions follows Crombie (1964).

tists for many years. His mechanistic philosophy and his concept of man as a machine called attention to the body-mind problem. His thinking encouraged physiological advances for the next 200 years by removing the necessity of considering the mind in physiological problems. Then, in the middle of the nineteenth century, the new science of psychology appeared which dealt with the mind and, hence, with sensation and perception.

Wilhelm Wundt, who had performed physiological experiments in the laboratories of both Müller and Helmholtz, established the first laboratory of experimental psychology at Leipzig in 1879. He attracted students from all over the world (Hulin, 1934). With the establishment of his laboratory and the problems he proposed for it to solve, experimental psychology was founded. In Wundt's laboratory, all of the sense organs and their responses, including visual functions, were measured. Knowledge of other sciences was brought to bear on psychological problems. For example, the description of the photochemical action of the retina advanced in 1877 by Willy Kuhne was taken into account immediately by Wundt and his students in their work on vision.

Historians have classified many of those who worked on vision problems in the years just before Wundt as experimental psychologists. There is a tendency to place scientists within fields not only according to their academic posts but according to the nature of the work they did. Ewald Hering, born in 1834, held theories on color vision and on space perception that were at variance with those of Helmholtz; Hering did considerable work in physiological optics. He held the post of professor of physiology at Vienna from 1865 to 1870, at Prague from 1870 to 1895, and thereafter at Leipzig. He is listed in the *Encyclopaedia Britannica*, however, as a physiologist *and psychologist*.

Psychology in its short history as a separate discipline has grown markedly. Today, psychology includes not only the experimental subdivision but also abnormal, animal, child, clinical, individual, and many other subdivisions. Theories or approaches, such as behaviorism, Gestalt, and functionalism, have had their various advocates, many of whom have made significant contributions. Because psychology has become one of the sciences basic to optometric knowledge, the student of optometry becomes acquainted with the major individuals, theories, and schools of psychological thought. A history of psychology is, obviously, too broad to be included in this book.

One aspect of psychology, however, should be alluded to for its deep influence on vision training. Problems of the learning process and of reflex behavior have been widely studied. Optometrists, making practical use of this knowledge about learning and reflex behavior gained by psychologists, judge which visual functions are trainable and which are not. They are also indebted to psychologists for the methods used in vision training or orthoptics. Furthermore, there are many investigators working within departments of experimental psychology on vision problems, particularly the problems of perception.

CONTRIBUTIONS TO CLINICAL OPTOMETRY

The clinical aspects of optometry for a period of 200 or 300 years were advanced more by persons outside the clinical fields than by the opticians or physicians of the period.

The first major treatise on the fitting of spectacles was made by one who did not practice the clinical art. In 1623 in Seville, an essay on spectacles and vision was published by Diego Perez (Wood, 1921). The author was Benito Daca de Valdez, a notary (clerk) of the Holy Office (Inquisition) in the city of Seville. The manuscript was read by a censor who was an agent of the Vicar General; he found nothing in it contrary to the teachings of the church or state. Wood (1921) notes that: "Neither Church nor State took chances in the brave days of old."

The Valdez essay is a treatise on optics and ocular biology as well as a practical dissertation on the prescribing of spectacles. The sections on physiology, anatomy, and optics *per se* are of slight historical importance. The section on spectacles, however, is a distinct contribution—the first in literature. Valdez, after discussing the happy invention of spectacles, describes convex, concave, and plano lenses as well as protective (conservatio) spectacles. He discusses why convex lenses magnify and concave lenses minify objects viewed through them. A system for numbering lenses according to their power is included; this was a distinctly important clinical advance. In addition, a method is offered for determining the focal distance of each lens; according to this method, it is necessary that the one who is making the determination be a "person with perfect sight."

Valdez differentiated between congenital and acquired visual defects (Wood, 1921) and offered a system for determining which lens the patient required. He offered a table for determining the strength of convex lenses for presbyopia based on the age of the patient if the patient was not "at hand." From Wood's treatise we have converted the Valdez data to the modern dioptric notation, since Valdez expressed lens power in degrees or "vara," a measure equal to about 6/5 of a diopter:

Age of Patient	Presbyopic Lens Recommended Diopters
30–40	2.4 D
40–50	3.0
50–60	3.6
60–70	4.2
70–80	4.8
over 80	6.0 to 7.2

Women were said to require slightly stronger presbyopic lenses than men.*

Many other notes on the selection of properly fitted spectacles are offered by Valdez. The monocle will make the vision in the two eyes unequal and is, therefore, not to be used. A pair of stenopaic slits in metal discs mounted in a spectacle frame assists certain defects of vision. The lens fitted to a myope must not be so strong as to diminish the size of viewed objects. A somewhat weaker lens than that which gives clearest vision is superior because it is worn with greater comfort. Weak lenses should be planoconvex or planoconcave; stronger lenses should be biconcave or biconvex. Colored lenses are recommended to protect the eyes from the winds of winter and the bright lights of summer. Spectacles should be steadied by fastening to ear or temple as well as over the nose.

Many of the suggestions of Valdez are still valid even though written over 300 years ago. The most amazing feature of the essay is that it was written not by a clinician but by a clerk of the Inquisition. He justified his writing on the basis that God had created our eyes. Hence, a study of the eye and spectacles was a compelling duty.

Half a century after Valdez, a text was published in England that dealt with the prescribing of spectacles. This, too, was written by a non-clinician, one William Molyneux. This Irish philosopher, mathematician, astronomer, and politician wrote *Dioptrica Nova* in 1692. Molyneux was a friend of Locke and author of a book that dealt with the legislative freedom of Ireland.

In *Dioptrica Nova*, Molyneux pays tribute to the invention of spectacles.† He then describes the fitting of spectacles to both pres-

---

* The Valdez manuscript is over 300 years old. Today in many parts of the United States it is still possible to submit one's age and sex to a company which sells ready-made spectacles through the mail and to receive a pair of "reading glasses" not unlike what would have been supplied in seventeenth century Spain. The clients of such a company accept prosthetic devices little affected by 300 years of scientific achievement.

† Molyneux' statement on the importance of spectacles was cited earlier.

byopes and myopes. Like Valdez, he included a host of "practical tips," most of which are as valid and valuable today as when they were written over 250 years ago. Molyneux suggests that: the weakest lens that solves the problem is the one to be chosen; myopes may require more than one pair of spectacles for different viewing distances; and some eyes will not be helped by either convex or concave spectacles. His book served as a valuable guide to those who first practiced optometry, that is, the opticians who helped the client select spectacles.

The books by Valdez and Molyneux contain many suggestions with which modern optometrists would agree. The problem of fitting spectacles, however, was much simpler then than it is today. Spectacles were made up in spherical convex or concave lenses only, and lenses of equal power were used before both eyes. Such spectacles could be prefabricated. A dozen or so pairs of "old glasses" and perhaps twice that number of pairs of "young glasses" were sufficient to satisfy most presbyopes and myopes. Thus, the rules for spectacle fitting took into account a very small number of possible combinations. With the inventions of cylindrical lenses and bifocals, however, the number of possible combinations increased tremendously. With this increase in combinations, persons who had previously needed correction not available to them were able to wear helpful lenses. Most important, such lenses could not be prefabricated as ready-made spectacles, and such lenses could not be selected by the patient himself or fitted by a haberdasher or spectacle seller. Such lenses had to be prescribed, a process that demanded a knowledge of special sight-testing techniques.

Although there is evidence that some opticians and spectacle-makers had experimented with bifocals, their invention is usually attributed to Benjamin Franklin—publisher-printer, scientist, inventor, and American patriot-statesman. One of the true geniuses of all time, Franklin was respected by scientists for his pioneering experimental work in electricity, by physicians for his writings on the success of smallpox inoculation, and by political scientists both for his successful diplomatic missions to France and for his help in establishing the governmental foundations of the United States. With all his achievements, he was kind, generous, wise, humorous, and a great humanitarian.

Finding that he could see distant objects best through one pair of spectacles and near objects clearly through a different pair, Franklin, in 1784, made for himself a pair of what he called "double spectacles." He had the two pairs of lenses cut in half and placed within the same spectacle frame; the upper halves of the distant-viewing lenses were placed on top, and the lower halves of his near-seeing lenses were placed below them. He not only did this for himself, but he described to others what he had done.

The correction of astigmatism was undertaken by many men. Undoubtedly the English spectaclemakers had experimented with it. The famous scientist Thomas Young described astigmatism and measured the anomaly in his own eye about the year 1801. The English optician William Cary is credited with having called the defect to Young's attention. Cary suggested tilting a spherical lens in order to correct the defect. However, the actual description of cylindrical lenses was made by an English astronomer, George B. Airy.

Airy, who was graduated from Trinity College of Cambridge University in 1823, became a fellow of the college in 1824, professor of mathematics in 1826, and professor of astronomy and director of the Cambridge observatory in 1828. His long career thereafter in astronomy was characterized by many valuable achievements and honors, including his appointment as royal astronomer in 1835. Early in his career, he measured the astigmatism in his own eye and had James Fuller, an optician, construct for him a pair of spherocylindrical lenses. In 1825, when he was only 24 and barely past his student days, he presented a paper "On a Peculiar Defect in the Eye and Mode of Correcting It" (Gregg, 1965). This work by Airy with the aid of Fuller is usually cited as the beginning of the practical correction of astigmatism by spectacles. Airy's contributions in astronomy were so significant and numerous that the *Encyclopaedia Britannica* (1958) in a half page biography fails to mention his work on the correction of astigmatism.

Although Airy was the first to order a lens for the correction of astigmatism and Fuller was the first to make it, another layman-optician combination arrived at the same solution to the problem of astigmatism independently. Snyder (1965) reports that in 1825 or 1826, a clergyman, Rev. Goodrich, about whom very little is known, described his own visual anomaly in a letter to the Philadelphia opticians, the McAllisters. The Rev. Goodrich had obtained a pair of concave spherical spectacles. He observed that vertical lines appeared clearer with his naked eye, while with his concave spectacles, horizontal lines appeared clearer. He wrote this in a letter to the McAllisters, sending along his spectacles. He reasoned that the lens of his eye was probably cylindrical and that ". . . a glass whose shape resembles the crystalline lens of my eye, placed before my eye, so that its greatest length would be at right angles with the lens of the eye would produce a perfect image." The McAllisters ground a planoconcave cylindrical lens from this information and supplied it to the Rev. Goodrich. The entire transaction was carried on by mail. The Rev. Goodrich began wearing these spectacles in May, 1828. The Airy-

Fuller lens was made in 1825, at which time Airy reported his findings to the Cambridge Philosophical Society; his paper, however, was not published until 1827. Thus, Rev. Goodrich could not have known of the work of Airy and Fuller in 1826. He must have worked out the solution himself. Moreover, unless they had seen the Airy publication very shortly after it appeared, the McAllisters probably also should be credited with independently having figured out how to fabricate a lens for the correction of astigmatism.

By the middle of the nineteenth century, physiological optics had reached a golden age; Helmholtz and others had made significant contributions to visual science. Clinical optometry at that time was still poorly developed. Opticians and spectaclemakers had made advances in the fabricating and supplying of spectacles. John Dolland, for example, in 1757, had found a way to reduce chromatic aberration in lens systems. But the major developments—the two early books on spectacle fitting, the invention of bifocals, and the invention of a means of correcting astigmatism—came from non-clinical people. The closest the physicians or opticians of the age came to making a major contribution was the work of the opticians Fuller and McAllister in carrying out Airy's and Goodrich's requests.

Several opticians and spectaclemakers of the time did make a tremendous scientific contribution, but it was not to clinical optometry; rather, it was to medicine and biology. The microscope, so necessary for medical and biological advancement, was the invention of spectaclemakers. But conversely, a practicing physician made a contribution of inestimable value to the science which was to become clinical optometry.

The microscope and the telescope were invented by spectaclemakers Zacharias Janssen and Hans Lippershey in the town of Middleburg, Holland, some time between 1590 and 1608. Miller (1964) attributes the microscope to Janssen in 1590 and the telescope in 1608 to Lippershey, who knew of Janssen's invention of the microscope. Both inventions depend on a combination of lenses to produce magnification. Miller (1964), citing Ariel and Will Durant, states that Janssen was experimenting with lenses and hit upon a combination that acted as a microscope. The *Encyclopaedia Britannica* (1958) cites as a common story that Lippershey was holding a spectacle lens in each hand; he directed his gaze through both lenses toward a church steeple and noted that it appeared closer to him; from this experience came the invention of the telescope.

It is significant that both the microscope, described by Haggard (1933) as the instrument which is "one of the most valuable in all medical discovery," and the telescope that had such a profound influence on astronomy in particular and science in general were the inventions of spectaclemakers, the optometrists of the time.* Nor did the contribution of spectaclemakers to microscopy end with the *invention* of the microscope. High resolution required an achromatic lens, and this device was the invention of the English optician John Dolland. His lens was of greater significance to improved microscope design than it was to spectacle design.

During most of the three centuries following the invention of the microscope and telescope, the spectaclemakers in many European countries made and sold both of these instruments as well as spectacle lenses. In the history of the Worshipful Company of Spectaclemakers in England there are many evidences that the members of the Company dealt in all three devices.

With the invention of the microscope, *scientific* medicine had its beginning. Optometry, thanks to the invention of spectacles and scientific advances in optics, had arrived at a point of rational treatment of anomalies of the eye at a much earlier period. Convex lenses in a spectacle frame to neutralize the effects of presbyopia were used after the thirteenth century and are still the basic treatment of this anomaly. Cylindrical lenses, different lenses for each eye, and bifocals have all been improvements; but the basic principle, spectacles with convex lenses to correct presbyopia, has remained unchanged for 600 years. During this period it has been applied for the benefit of millions of people.

Medical therapy, on the other hand, well into the eighteenth century still used the types of medication which have been described in Chapter 3: the excrement of various animals, useless herbs, bits of moss, bone, and tortoise shell. These were the ingredients of medical prescriptions still in use long after convex lenses for presbyopia and concave lenses for myopia were in frequent use. Surgical blood-letting and the application of leeches to drain blood from a patient were common techniques in medicine long after optics was on an essentially modern basis.

The earliest users of the microscope during the seventeenth century are greatly responsible for the ultimate emergence of medical science. Anton van Leeuwenhoek was born in Delft, Holland, in 1632, and was a draper by trade and janitor at the city hall. He worked with a microscope for many years, placing under it "anything he could lay his hands upon" (Haggard, 1933). His description of the

---

* Miller (1964) notes that the term "optometrist" can be used to describe those who in earlier times were called "opticus, opticker, optician or spectaclemaker—just as the term 'physician' is used to encompass the earlier designated medicus, algebraist, leech, barber, physicker, or chirurgeon." In the present text we have considered the history of the earlier spectaclemakers, opticians, and opticists to be the history of optometry on the grounds that these men practiced the optometric service at the time.

"little animals" which were revealed under his microscope led to an understanding of protozoa and bacteria.

Robert Hooke also used the microscope and subjected vegetable matter to examination and observation of cellular structure. He observed tiny compartments which he called cells, from the Latin, *cella*, "little rooms." His book *Micrographia* described his findings; Pepys mentions his fascination upon reading this book. Both Hooke and Leeuwenhoek reported their several findings to the Royal Society in London.

Marcello Malpighi, an Italian physiologist born in 1628, made numerous observations of minute anatomical structure with the microscope. He is considered the founder of microscopic anatomy (Haggard, 1933). Jan Swammerdan, a Dutch naturalist born in 1637, also utilized the microscope in the study of the micro-anatomy of human beings and insects.

Athanasius Kircher, a Jesuit teacher, mathematician, professor of philosophy, linguist, and scientist, born in 1601, was the first to use the microscope in an attempt to discover the cause of disease. He proposed the theory that disease is spread by living infectious particles, described by him as tiny worms of contagion.

Thus, by the beginning of the eighteenth century in Europe, cellular structure had been described, microscopic anatomy or histology had been established, protozoa and bacteria had been seen, and a relationship between these tiny living organisms and diseases of mankind had been theorized by at least one author. Yet, more than a century was to pass before these findings would be incorporated into clinical medicine by Koch, Pasteur, and others.

Just as the founders of clinical optometry were not the clinicians of the time, so the founders of scientific clinical medicine were not the physicians of the time. Medicine was to be advanced with the help of spectaclemakers, academic biologists, philosophers, physicists, and naturalists—and even a haberdasher and janitor. Just as optometry was dependent on many disciplines, so too was medicine; just as there were long time lags in optometric development, so there were in medical development. Of the two disciplines, optometry attained an age of rational procedure and science several hundred years before medicine. However, scientific refraction had not yet been developed, and it did not develop until the middle of the nineteenth century. Its development is largely due to the great contributions of Frans Cornelis Donders, a physician. From his work developed the field which was to become clinical optometry.

Donders was born in Tilburg, Holland in 1818, the ninth child and first son of a simple burgher family (Flick, 1952). He was a good student, fluent linguist, and accomplished violinist; as a boy, he worked as a paymaster for a local employer, and was in charge of the accurate running of the village clock. At the age of 17, he entered the medical school at the University of Utrecht. After graduation at age 22, he spent two years as a military surgeon and then became a teacher of anatomy, physiology, and histology at the Military School of Medicine in Utrecht. In 1847, he became Professor Extraordinary at the University of Utrecht and lectured in biology, anthropology, forensic medicine, and ophthalmology. He was a handsome man, quick, refined, artistic, congenial, a good conversationalist, and intellectually inclined.

Donders' major contribution was his book published in 1864, *On the Anomalies of Accommodation and Refraction of the Eye, with a Preliminary Essay on Physiological Dioptrics*. The New Sydenham Society in London was the publisher. The original publication was in English, having been translated for the publisher by William D. Moore of Dublin from Donders' Dutch original. Later it was translated into many languages. The original English edition was reprinted in 1952 by the Hatton Press in England. Although he published over 200 papers and had a long and fruitful career, the importance of his classic on refraction far overshadowed Donders' other achievements.

On the 50th anniversary of the publication of Donders' book, one commentator noted that "Not a single one of Donders' essential teachings has been proved wrong; they have stood the test of half a century. Of how many men can this be said?" (Flick, 1952, citing Ernest Clarke). Now, 100 years after his book first appeared, essentially the same comment can still be made.

The modern optometrist finds within Donders' classic the basis for clinical optometry. Optics and physiological optics are utilized to justify the clinical procedures. Unlike most of the physicians of the time, Donders recognized the value of spectacles and made the prescription of them a scientific procedure. The symptoms of hypermetropia were shown by Donders to be amenable to relief by the use of convex lenses. Spectacles rather than lotions and eyewashes were the answer to refractive problems. The relationship between accommodation and convergence was noted by Donders and its significance was recognized. Today's optometry students read Donders' original text, amazed at how much of the modern clinical art and science was clearly presented by this author. Truly, as the founder of scientific refraction, Donders also founded modern clinical optometry.

THE OPTOMETRIC SERVICE—1900

The various disciplines and many of the individuals who contributed to the body of knowledge that constitutes the basis for modern optometry were discussed in the previous sections. After the invention of spectacles, the first basic science to achieve a relatively modern status was optics; by the end of the seventeenth century, this aspect of visual science was on a sound footing. At least two books on clinical optometry were also contributed during the seventeenth century, both by non-clinicians.

The eighteenth and nineteenth centuries brought marked advances in the biological sciences, particularly physiology, and an understanding of the biological aspect of vision. In the last half of the nineteenth century, physiological optics and psychology, dealing with the perceptual aspect of vision, came into being. To this day, optometric science is based on the disciplines of mathematics, physics (optics), anatomy, physiology, physiological optics, and psychology.

By the middle of the nineteenth century, several events had occurred that acted as immediate stimuli to the emergence of a new profession. When the need for cylindrical lenses, bifocals, and different lenses for each eye was understood, prefabricated spectacles could not satisfy this need; the patient could no longer choose his own spectacles if he was to be benefited by the new discoveries. For almost 500 years, spectaclemakers and opticians had supplied an optometric service as good as was available, but the new knowledge demanded greater clinical skills than these trades could offer.

With advances such as Helmholtz's in physiological optics and with the clinical studies of Donders, the knowledge was available to make spectacles that were fitted to the individual. As has been noted, the physicians who practiced eye medicine or ophthalmology had historically ignored the fitting of spectacles. Duke-Elder (1949) notes that ophthalmologists well into the nineteenth century advised those patients who might require spectacles to "try a series of them at an optician's shop." He cites Franz in 1839 of Leipzig, Mackenzie in 1840 of Glasgow, and Ruete in 1853 as authors during this period who held this view.

Several medical authors recognized the existence of a problem and exhorted their colleagues in ophthalmology to learn to fit spectacles. Frederick Ritter von Arlt was one such author. Born in 1812, the son of a Bohemian blacksmith, Arlt studied ophthalmology at the University of Prague, was a professor there from 1846 to 1856, and professor at the University of Vienna from 1856 until 1883, when he was retired. In a book he wrote in 1846, Arlt called upon members of the medical profession to fit spectacles, claiming that so important a matter should not be left to opticians.

Arlt's pleas, however, were not answered by any large number of physicians. Wood (1918) wrote:

> There can be no doubt but that if the medical profession as a whole does not in some effective manner provide for the needs (or demands) of that rather large percentage of the laity who continue to frequent the shops of the optician the so-called 'optometrist' will, sooner or later, under pressure of public opinion, receive legal recognition, either through legislative action or, as in the case of Columbia University, by the establishment of optical (or optician's) courses. For good or evil, that portion of the public that goes (or is sent by physicians) to the optician believes that much of the oculist's work is as well done by the 'optometrist' as by the ophthalmologist. They also learn, or are being taught, that doctors are pursuing a sort of dog-in-the-manger policy in that they are opposed to 'simple refracting' by a 'qualified' optometrist and still refuse to do the work themselves.

Wood then calls upon the medical profession to meet the demand for more effective refractive work "than the oculist is now able to furnish the public."

Thus, after a long history of non-participation in the optometric service, physicians began in the mid-nineteenth century to recognize a need, but did not act on it. From Arlt's plea in 1846 to Wood's comment in 1918, three-quarters of a century elapsed. Three reasons might be offered for the resistance of physicians to doing refracting themselves. First, of course, there was the tradition of deprecating spectacles and their use. So long-standing and deep-rooted an attitude was not to disappear overnight. Second, some ophthalmologists, engrossed with the new discoveries in the treatment of eye diseases and in surgery, must have felt that vision testing was not the work they wished to do. Third, and perhaps the most important, the skills and attributes that led an individual to study medicine were not those required in clinical optics. It was one thing for a Helmholtz, trained in physics as well as medicine, or a Javal, trained initially in engineering, to cope with the mathematics of optics; it was another matter for the average physician, trained in microscopic examination, observation of tissue change, biological sciences, bacteriology, anatomy, and other sciences basic to medicine to add mathematics and optics to his armamentarium.

During this same period—the last half of the nineteenth century and first few years of the twentieth century—events were occurring in another group. Among the opticians and spectaclemakers there were also a few men who recognized the need of the public for clinicians who could test vision and fit spectacles according to the new knowledge in physiological optics and in the science of refraction. During the late nineteenth century, these opticians had begun to perform vision tests and to urge their fellow opticians to do the same thing. Since they had a good grounding in optics, it appears that it was less difficult for these men to learn those aspects of biology that applied to their work than it was for the physicians to learn optics.

These few farsighted opticians began the phenomenal bootstrap operation that was to see a new profession born at the turn of the century and, within the very short period of 65 years, arrive at a point where the field was clearly defined and was recognized by legislative bodies and academic senates. Their story, the story of modern optometry, is told in the next few chapters.

CHAPTER 6

EMERGENCE OF A PROFESSION—
JURISDICTIONAL
& LEGISLATIVE PHASES

Of the thousands of occupations in the United States, only a few have attained the status of profession. The reasons why some occupations attained professional status and others did not have been subjected to careful study by the sociologist Wilensky (1964). He found that most of the favored occupations followed a distinct pattern. After careful analysis, he presented the typical process by which the established professions have arrived:

> . . . men begin doing the work full time and stake out a jurisdiction; the early masters of the technique or adherents of the movement become concerned about standards of training and practice and set up a training school, which, if not lodged in universities at the outset, makes academic connection within two or three decades; the teachers and activists then achieve success in promoting more effective organization, first local, then national—through either the transformation of an existing occupational association or the creation of a new one. Toward the end, legal protection of the monopoly of skill appears; at the end, a formal code of ethics is adopted.

The sequence of events for the process of professionalization which Wilensky gives, along with the dates at which optometry attained each step are:

Became a Full Time Occupation	*
First Training School	1892
First University School	1910
First Local Professional Association	1896
First National Professional Association	1897
First State License Law	1901
Formal Code of Ethics	about 1935

Wilensky noted that this sequence was followed in general by all occupations which attained professionalization. In each instance,

---

* Wilensky did not give a date here, but clearly the occupation had been practiced on a full time basis in America from Colonial times, the early opticians being trained in the tradition of the British spectaclemakers.

however, one or more dates are not in the listed order. In optometry, which was one of the 18 professions which Wilensky studied, the only item which is out of order is the establishment of the first university school. Law and medicine also were licensed by the first state before they established their first university-affiliated school. Aside from this one item, however, optometry followed the classical pattern for professionalization in the United States.

In discussing the professionalization process in optometry, we shall follow Wilensky's outline. In previous chapters, the development of the area and the scope of the optometric service have been described. In the present chapter, we shall discuss the status of the service in the United States at the time the professional emergence began, the legislative aspect, and the men who engaged in the legislative phase. In the following chapter, the educational, organizational, and ethical aspects—the other characteristics of professions—will be discussed.

OPTOMETRY IN THE UNITED STATES
IN THE LATE NINETEENTH CENTURY

Until the latter part of the nineteenth century, the optometric service was supplied by men who were engaged in a highly skilled trade. Then, in a remarkably short period of time, a profession emerged; thereafter, the service was rendered on a professional basis.

The professionalization of optometric service was primarily an American phenomenon. To a lesser degree, a similar professionalization occurred at about the same time in England and some of the British Commonwealth nations. But in most of the civilized world, an optometric profession did not develop; it is only in the very recent past, almost three-quarters of a century after optometry has emerged as a profession in the United States, that we begin to see signs of similar developments in several other countries. (See Chapter 8.)

The early stages through which the optometric profession passed in England have been described in Chapter 4. The Spectaclemakers' Company consisted initially of men who fabricated spectacles. These spectacles were sold in general merchandise shops, such as haberdashery shops in the cities and by peddlers in the country. Then the makers of spectacles opened their own retail shops as opticians and sold the products which they manufactured directly to the public. Finally, late in the nineteenth century, these opticians began to increase the advisory capacity of their work by actually testing sight.

The changes in England were gradual. It was not a big step for the optician who had formerly "advised" clients of what the various types of spectacles would achieve actually to begin to test the client's vision and fabricate spectacles specifically for that patient. To a great extent, the introduction of toric lenses for astigmatism and bifocals for presbyopia made such a change imperative; the number of possible lens prescriptions available with cylinders and bifocals made prefabrication impossible.

In England, all of the changes occurred within the framework of the Worshipful Company of Spectaclemakers. The British optometrist (called an ophthalmic optician in England) is still usually a member of the Spectaclemakers Company. In the United States, the changeover was more abrupt. To understand the phenomenon, it is necessary to understand a little bit about the sociology of the United States and about the men who were providing the optometric service at the turn of the century.

What was the environment in the United States in the last part of the nineteenth century and the beginning of the twentieth century? The industrial revolution had made its impact on all phases of American life. The United States, rich in natural resources and blessed by a government that allowed the development of new ideas, was going through a radical redistribution of jobs as well as the creation of hundreds of new ones. Farm jobs, which accounted for well over 60 percent of the work force in the 1860's, declined to less than ten percent in the next century. The great relative reduction in cost of most commodities brought a standard of living undreamed of 50 years previously. With this new emancipation came man's realization that increased education would further raise his standard of existence. He could now afford to take his children out of the work market and keep them in school. The new jobs, the high standard of living, and the increased education all tended to create demands for better vision unique in the history of civilization.

Hofstetter (1948) has stated that "on a day to day basis professions are costly luxuries and it is only on a long range basis that civilization profits in the maintenance of a given vocational group in a professional status." The United States in the early 1900's was a wealthy nation. It could afford the luxury of a profession if there were a need for that profession. Rapid technological advances and increased education had brought on the need.

The visual needs of the American people were not being met by any profession in existence at that time. If they had been, it would not have been necessary for a new profession to be formed. Credit must be given to the early optometrists who saw the need for establishing an independent profession to care for these needs, especially considering the conditions that existed.

Vision care was obtained by people in America in the late nineteenth century in one of a variety of methods. As in England, there were opticians, highly skilled men who practiced much in the same fashion as their British counterparts. John McAllister, Jr. is credited with opening the first optical shop in America in 1783. The next hundred years saw the rapid development of opticianry as a highly skilled trade. The guilds of England had developed a fine tradition of excellence in optics. This tradition was carried on in the new world. The invention of many unique optical instruments and the rapid development of optics in the 1800's were stepping stones in the emergence of the profession of optometry.

But the optical shop was not the only place in which optometric service was offered. In many areas, optometry was a side-line in the better jewelry stores of the day. Watchmaking and spectaclemaking were often practiced by the same individual in the jewelry store; instruction in these two trades was often offered in the same school with a short and restricted curriculum. In the outlying communities, itinerant peddlers distributed spectacles in much the same fashion as their antecedents had in western continental Europe several hundred years earlier.

The story of the American spectacle peddlers is a fascinating and often forgotten one. Many of these traveling spectacle purveyors were flamboyant charlatans who affected top hats, broad capes, and drove highly polished fancy carriages with high-stepping horses. Stories are told of how these men fleeced the farmers, for example, by discovering a cataract (where one did not exist). For a fee, they would go through motions of performing surgery (amazingly bloodless) and then produce a bit of onion skin which they had palmed earlier, informing the patient and his family that this was the cataract that had been removed. The myth still held by many laymen that a cataract is a skin removed from the front surface of the eye may have had its roots in this old bit of quackery. Lenses, of course, were then supplied, and behold the patient's vision improved. The peddler was well paid for the spectacles but better paid for the bit of onion skin he left behind.

All peddlers, however, were not of this nature. One of the authors (MJH) in his student days was fortunate enough to meet and have many friendly chats with Ephraim Weiss, then aged about 90, who was one of the last American spectacle peddlers. This remarkable man traveled the roads of rural California selling spectacles; he numbered among his clients such people as the noted scientist, Luther Burbank, who carried on his plant-breeding experiments in Santa Rosa, California, between 1875 and 1925. Burbank purchased his spectacles from Weiss, and in a letter expressed his great satisfaction and requested extra pairs the next time Weiss would pass through.

Weiss had learned many useful rules for prescribing lenses. Each quarter diopter of minus lens added to a prescription, he told us, should increase the acuity one line of Snellen type or else it was an overcorrection. Although we never understood how he determined muscle balance, he knew that one should "add a little plus if the eyes tend to turn in and a little minus if they tend to turn out." Self-taught, he practiced a most acceptable brand of sight-testing for the time, seemingly with great patient satisfaction. In later years, he became sufficiently wealthy to endow a room at the Stanford Library and to leave an apartment house the income from which was shared by the University of California and Stanford University.

For a further description of the early spectacle peddlers, many of whom ultimately "got religion" and settled down into opticianry or optometric practice, the reader is referred to Cox (1947).

In some areas, some members of the medical profession practiced optometry as a side-line during this era. There were many dedicated men—the forerunners of the present ophthalmologists—who contributed greatly to the care of vision during this time. The training and interest of these men, however, were not primarily in optics. No medical schools trained students in the optics needed to prescribe lenses. In fact, early ophthalmologists studied in the same short courses and correspondence schools used by the men in optometry at that time.

It was not uncommon during this period for an elderly physician to seek semi-retirement in a small community as an "eye, ear, nose and throat specialist." Tired of the arduous life of general medical practice or surgery, these doctors took a short course in optics, purchased a trial lens case and some spectacles, and set up practice.

Thus, at the turn of the century, there were opticians who supplied spectacles but did not test vision, opticians who supplied spectacles *and* tested vision, itinerant spectacle peddlers, and watchmaker-jewelers who offered some form of optical service. In addition, there were some physicians who tested vision and, depending on the community, either supplied spectacles or referred their clients to an optician to obtain spectacles.

Throughout the United States there seemed to arise spontaneously a dissatisfaction with the hodge-podge of people who were allowed to care for man's vision. The exact date when such a phenomenon occurred would be difficult to pinpoint. It most probably occurred sometime in the 1870's or 1880's.

Not only was the general public dissatisfied with the type of vision care in this period, but many of the sight-testing opticians themselves recognized the need for reform. Cox (1947) notes that ". . . it is a tribute to the honest purpose of the early optometrists that [spectacle] peddling was gradually eliminated [as was practice by all other unqualified persons] through regulatory legislation of their own seeking. In fact, in order to . . . outlaw such unwholesome practices, they had a generation of struggle, with medical opposition the greatest impediment that had to be surmounted."

Although the early optometrists who laid the groundwork for optometry as a profession were undoubtedly motivated by a concern for the visual welfare of the American public, they were certainly also cognizant of the personal advantages of a profession as opposed to a trade. The need of the early optometrist for esteem and prestige did much to stimulate him to adopt the standards which distinguish a profession from a trade.

Kahl (1964), writing on the American class structure, makes some important observations which help explain the emergence of optometry as a profession. Kahl says the activity that is most important to Americans is occupation. He feels that prestige in small groups is determined by an individual's behavior in living up to the standards of the group. This, of course, is a basic part of all professional behavior.

According to Kahl, the significance of work is best measured by those who understand it. The criteria used are the skill the job demands, the talent and training necessary to produce the skill, the responsibility, the pay, and the nature of the services. A professional man doing a good job at his work enjoys the esteem of his fellow workers as well as of his patients. Optometry attained most of these criteria early in its development; as in all professions, however, public acceptance came slowly.

Kahl says that the key to the solution is in the income level of the group involved. The American value system tends to match prestige with income. Most Americans believe that income is a fair measure of occupational success, and the less they know about the work the more likely they are to assume this to be true.

Kahl substantiates his views of the American class structure with surveys conducted by the National Opinion Research Center. In the survey which was conducted concerning the rating of certain jobs as having excellent standings, the characteristics giving such jobs these standings were listed as: (1) the jobs pay well; (2) they are a service to humanity (that is, they are essential jobs); (3) preparation requires much education, hard work, and money; (4) the jobs carry great social prestige; (5) they require high moral standards (honesty, responsibility); and (6) the jobs require intelligence and ability. Using these criteria, the optometrist of today practices a highly desirable profession.

Although there were many men who contributed to the founding of the optometric profession, most historians agree that Charles F.

Prentice and Andrew Jay Cross did the most to bring about the transition from trade to profession, particularly in the legislative phase. The work of these men as well as many of the other leaders would have gone for naught, however, if the environment just described had not been suitable. But the time was right—and their efforts led to the rapid establishment and growth of optometry as a profession.

CHARLES F. PRENTICE—*The Father of Optometry*

Charles F. Prentice stands out in optometric history as the inspiration to the refracting opticians to unite and form a new and separate profession with legal recognition. Prentice's personality comes through in his book, *Legalized Optometry and Memoirs of Its Founder.** It is necessary to know Prentice's background to understand his devotion to optometry.

Charles Prentice was raised as an only child—the only one of eight children to survive infancy. There was great attraction between father and son; Prentice frequently quotes from the philosophy of his father. James Prentice, the father, had opened a retail optical shop. It was his desire that his son Charles ultimately assist him in this venture.

Charles' early schooling, commencing at five years of age, was in a private German school. His later education was continued in Europe and was planned quite thoroughly by his father. There were no courses in optics available in the United States that Prentice, Senior, thought sufficiently good. Charles Prentice spent three years in the Royal Polytechnicum at Karlsruhe. His education was largely in engineering, physics, and mathematics. An observation that may be of interest to American students is that "lectures began at 7:00 A.M. hourly until noon and from 2:00 P.M. until 5:00 P.M. during the winter semester; every day of the week including Saturday. The lecture notes were required to be put in writing so that one rarely went to bed before midnight. Instruction in Germany is strenuously thorough, provided the student ardently applies himself. A collegian there is put on his honor and not treated as a school boy." Instructors addressed the students as "Mister."

When he returned to America in 1874, he was not particularly impressed with the occupation of selling and fitting spectacles. According to his memoirs, it seemed to be beneath his dignity.

His first engagement after college was with a mechanical engi-

* Some time during his student years, every optometrist-to-be should read this biography of the profession's founder. An understanding of Prentice and his aspirations will make a great many contemporary developments more understandable.

neer. He left this position after a few months because of his employer's mischievous monkey. Young Prentice apparently could not put up with the monkey's habit of stealing his drawing instruments!

After a short period in a steamship yard, at his father's request, Charles left this occupation and went to work for his father. At first, he did not work in the optical shop but supervised the installation of his father's exhibit of engineering instruments at the World's Fair. In addition, he did some drafting and worked with the patent office in Washington for private concerns.

About this time Prentice suffered an unfortunate marriage that lasted only a short time. During a fit of violent disapproval, his wife swept his writings from the table. He was writing his paper on *The Metric System of Numbering and Measuring Prisms*. Prentice then philosophized in his memoirs that it had always been a mystery to him why the well-meaning and helpful wife generally gets the worthless husband and the most beautiful and considerate husband is usually cursed with a frivolous woman of easy virtue or a shrew.*

Soon after he began working with his father, Prentice felt his shortcomings in optics and began a program of self-education in optometry. He devoted his evenings to reading the works of Donders, Helmholtz, and others. He noticed a serious omission in the writings of the so-called authorities in his time—none of them had written a description of the properties or construction of lenses used to correct defective vision. This observation resulted in his writing a short treatise on *Ophthalmic Lenses*. This 48-page book was favorably reviewed in several ophthalmological journals and brought about a feeling of mutual respect and friendship between Prentice and several ophthalmologists that was to last throughout his life.

Prentice found something lacking in the operation of the optical shops then in existence. He felt the need of a more "dignified attitude" toward the "clients." During this period, he visited John Ailman, a competent and successful optician in Boston. Prentice was particularly impressed by Ailman's dignified attitude toward his clients and the confidence they seemed to place in him. Ailman's name does not appear in any of the other early optometric historical literature. His interest apparently was not in the politics of his profession. Nevertheless, his willingness to impart his knowledge and office management procedures to young Prentice is an important part of the story of vision care. (Incidentally, this willingness and desire to assist fellow optometrists has characterized optometry throughout its existence.) In Ailman's office, Prentice saw the professional manner

* This observation is one undoubtedly made centuries earlier by Xantippe's husband, Socrates. It is also one with which the present authors hasten to proclaim personal disagreement!

practiced. In addition, he felt the need of more knowledge of ocular pathology. This was given him by Dr. William F. Mittendorf. At this time Prentice coined the word "opticist," * which he used to describe his occupation in lieu of optician or refracting optician until the optometry laws were enacted. At first, he could not see the need for the doctor title for optometrists. He adopted the designation "physical eye specialist"; he used this designation in his correspondence and on his stationery.

Prentice became more and more interested in the development of an independent profession. He especially felt the need of teaching aids and literature. This resulted in a model eye that was presented before the American Ophthalmological Society, and later demonstrated before the University Medical College of New York. During this time he spent two winter semesters at the New York Eye and Ear Infirmary. Meanwhile, his writing continued. He published *The Dioptric Formula for Combined Cylindrical Lenses*. It had taken him five months after office hours to complete the text, illustrations, and a set of five gilded models. This was followed by the publication of *Metric System of Numbering and Measuring Prisms* in the *Archives of Ophthalmology* in 1890.

Prentice was an idealist. Although he attempted to deny this fact in his writings, he deplored anyone who compromised at any stage of his existence. Throughout his memoirs, he criticized his optometric colleagues, his political friends, and his friends in ophthalmology for their compromising attitudes.

The foregoing observations of Prentice's early childhood, education, unfortunate marriage, and intense desire to excel serve as background.

A challenge in the form of a letter written in December, 1892, served to launch Prentice on the crusade which was to occupy much of his time throughout the next several years. He received a letter from Henry Noyes, a physician in New York City, thanking Prentice for referring a patient to Noyes. The patient had an inflammation of an eye causing defective sight. This, of course, Prentice knew; it was the reason for the original referral. In the last part of this historic letter Noyes wrote:

> I know of an instance in which you are said to have charged a fee for the examination as a separate item, in addition to the charge for the glasses. . . . You thereby place yourself in direct competition with them [the oculists], not only, but you assume

---

* The choice of the word *optometrist* instead of *opticist* was an unfortunate one. Prentice's term was far the better one for the profession which was to develop, since it did not imply a restriction to *metrics* or measurement.

their functions without having their training and general education. I think you must see the impropriety of such practice.

I consider the matter to be serious, not because a competition is set up, but because an injustice is done the public by the fact that in charging a fee you assume that you have the qualifications which entitle you to a fee for advice. To this I strenuously object and I beg to call your attention to the subject most seriously and yet kindly.

Very sincerely yours,
Henry D. Noyes

Prentice's answering letter to Noyes clearly sets out a philosophy of practice and establishes a viewpoint which optometry as a profession was to follow. Interestingly, several of the premises on which Prentice based his conclusions are still the sources of interprofessional squabbles today, some 75 years later. Prentice states in the first part of his answer to Noyes that, in spite of his (Prentice's) training in optics and his publication of a treatise on ophthalmic lenses, the oculists of New York City were not sending him sufficient prescriptions for him to operate successfully as an optician. He said:

> You must admit that, with my scientific training and sense of justice, I could hardly be expected to starve, merely in deference to the opinions of these scientific men, oculists, who remained wholly indifferent to my welfare, while lending their undivided support to my less worthy competitors. Only one course suggested itself to me, and that is the one I have pursued for the past five years; namely, to fit glasses myself, and to charge a fee of $3.00 for my services, comprising the time and skill necessary in ascertaining the proper optical correction for persons not afflicted with disease of the eyes.
>
> All my patrons are distinctly given to understand that I am not a physician, that I do not prescribe medicine, or give advice in a medical sense; but that the fee is intended to cover my scientifically conducted mechanical services, precisely in the same manner that a designer charges for his services in preparing his plans and specifications. In this sense every artisan is privileged to put his own price upon his time and skill. . . . Besides, if I did not charge a fee for services rendered, I should be obliged to exact an extortionate price for the glasses, which is the method generally practiced by the charlatan.

Prentice's thinking was indeed far ahead of his time, since this observation was made in 1892. In the same letter, Prentice expresses his attitude toward referral of ocular pathology:

> . . . in many instances when I have taken an examination for glasses I have discovered a condition of disease which promptly led me to advise consultation with an oculist. This is the limit of my advice for which I have never yet charged a fee. It has been my pleasure to refer many of these persons to you.

There followed a series of letters between Prentice and Noyes. Dr. D. B. St. John Roosa was brought into the correspondence, and he accused Prentice of violating a law by charging a fee relative to the practice of medicine—that is, in prescribing glasses. While there were undoubtedly personality conflicts in this correspondence, the issues were basic and the practice of many of the early opticians came under the scrutiny of the medical societies.

In 1895, one of Prentice's physician friends informed him that Dr. Roosa had appealed to the New York County Medical Society. Roosa asked the Society to reject members who sent patients to opticians to have glasses fitted. Moreover, Roosa declared he would have the medical practice act so amended as to prevent men of Prentice's "cult" from meddling with ophthalmology.

Prentice was greatly concerned with the trend of affairs. He consulted Frederick Boger, editor of the *Optical Journal*, concerning Roosa's threat. The need for a national organization was becoming apparent. In the March issue of his journal, Boger wrote:

> There has been no combined effort thus far to effect such an organization but we propose now to do whatever we can to bring about such a thing. The New England Association, the pioneer in its line, is meeting with success, and we intend to aid it all we can but an American Association covering the whole country is what is needed and the men to run it should step forward and organize.

This editorial brought a large response from prominent opticians throughout the country, and at this point Prentice became somewhat concerned about the ability of the opticians to organize into full professional status. He felt more education should be obtained before a full-fledged national organization was formed. He stated:

> . . . in my opinion it is premature to think of organizing a national association of opticians. I am in favor of associations being formed in each state, but purely for the purpose of advancing the scientific qualifications of opticians. I am watching the New England Association with interest and hope soon to see a similar movement on the part of New York and other states.

Prentice was practical enough, however, to recognize that the opticians were in serious danger. The rights which opticians had obtained by established practice over the years—working with lenses, adapting lenses to defects of the eye, ruling out diseased conditions before proceeding with lenses, and charging a separate fee for these services—all would go for naught if the oculists could have their way. Therefore, he decided, immediate legislation would be necessary in the state of New York to protect these rights; there was no legislation regulating vision care in effect any place in America.

Thus began a long series of legal battles to establish optometry as a profession. Here was a group of men who, in their chosen vocation, were rendering a service to mankind. Years of tradition had gone into the work they were doing with lenses. The adaptation of these lenses to the human eye had made tremendous strides during the 1800's. The medical profession had been slow to recognize the correction of eye defects by lenses. Many physicians even at this late date still preferred to prescribe medicines for the eye strains created by the increasing visual demands of society. At the same time, hundreds of optometrists throughout the United States had felt the need for something beyond a purely mechanical approach to adapting lenses to the eye. The need for an approach in which the whole patient was considered was beginning to make itself felt. This was brought out in the events which followed.

Prentice knew that the first step in any legislative activity would have to be the formation of a group of representative opticians. An organizational meeting was called consisting of Prentice, Cross, MacKeown, and others who met at Boger's office. At this meeting there were present only nine opticians, six of whom were interested exclusively in dispensing. At this organizational meeting, Prentice presented the need for a major optometric organization and listed the functions of an optometric organization as follows:

1. The motive for organizing should be to elevate the optician to the highest proficiency of his calling.

2. Bringing reputable opticians together should help eliminate many petty jealousies now existing.

3. There are a few incompetent opticians. The group should do its own pruning. The organization is in a better position to know who is competent than anyone else.

4. Generally, trade organizations have less lofty motives, but optometry requires something more than commercial ability. Business sagacity is necessary; more importantly, scientific knowledge is required. More and more time is needed to acquire the technical knowledge and to practice the skill necessary for this growing profession.

5. Organization affords opportunities for the discussion of scientific subjects not to be obtained in any other way.

In this short talk, Prentice outlined the basis of present-day professional organizations. Most state legislators now realize that *professions should have the responsibility of governing themselves under the framework of the laws of that state.* Prentice recognized that the men within a profession know better than anyone else who is competent and who is not. A professional organization must exist for the advancement of the scientific knowledge of its members—and thereby for the public's good—or it would soon cease to fill its place in society.

Shortly after this meeting, an attorney, Mr. T. Channon Press, thought it feasible to incorporate a society, similar to the dental society, with powers to regulate the practice of opticians. This would insure opticians against molestation from the medical profession. The Optical Society of the State of New York was then organized in February, 1896.

The attorney, Mr. Press, had informed several ophthalmologists that the organization was being formed. Dr. Roosa, hearing of it, angrily declared, "I know who is at the bottom of this—that man, Prentice; he is foxy and I am only waiting for the opportunity to put him behind prison bars; and if any optician undertakes to join this movement I shall see that he is punished; besides I shall fight you in Albany to the last ditch." Although a large number of opticians from all parts of the state attended the first meeting, the quoting of this statement and other events that had taken place resulted in all of the dispensing opticians leaving the meeting. Only the men who were to form the basis of optometry's first battle for legal recognition remained. The officers elected were: President—Charles F. Prentice, New York; Vice-President—George R. Bausch, Rochester; Treasurer —A. Jay Cross, New York; Secretary—Frederick Boger, New York. In view of Roosa's threats and the organized opposition of the medical society, this move took a great deal of courage. The first step was to organize the material for presentation before the state legislature. This task was performed mainly by Prentice.

Among opticians, there were those who wished to establish a new independent profession whose members would test vision in addition to supplying the device for correcting vision. Other opticians, however, were content with supplying the spectacles only. The clear disagreement between these two groups was the basis for many early fights, and characterizes the period of transition. Prentice was well aware of the opposing philosophies of the two groups of opticians in New York in 1896. This difference of opinion did not end with the establishment of legalized optometry in New York, and became the basis for a bitter fight in Pennsylvania in 1914. Fitch (1955) described the division of opinion among the new optometrists in that state, many of whom preferred to accept licensure under the Medical Board as members of a "minor branch of medical technology" rather than to become part of an independent profession. Fitch had led the fight for an independent profession in Pennsylvania.

Backman (1965), commenting on the possible emergence of an optometric profession in France, noted: "The most disappointing impression of optometry in present day France is that opticians are satisfied with their dispensing role and are not at all interested in developing their refractive techniques out of fear of losing the prescriptions sent to them by ophthalmologists." Thus, not only did Prentice and other American optometric leaders encounter unwillingness on the part of some opticians to establish an independent profession, but in most countries where optometry evolves from opticianry, the same phenomenon will be encountered.

Prentice's defense of opticians before the Committee on Public Health in 1896 was a masterpiece of logic. He made many vital points which established the position of the profession soon to be known as optometry, as a unique, independent profession dedicated to visual welfare. He mentioned that, although spectacles were invented before 1300, it was not until Donders published his treatise in 1864 that medical men began to give the subject of spectacles their attention. He called attention to the fact that the optician McAllister of Philadelphia first corrected astigmatism in America and that the optician Chamblant of Paris had made a cylindrical correction in 1849. He then said, "He [the optometrist] was then the only eye refractionist known to the world and always has been since the invention of spectacles, a period of more than five hundred years." It was Prentice's feeling that 1865 was the year that marked the beginning of a profession truly devoted to eye care. In America, men such as John McAllister and J. W. Queen of Philadelphia, Widdefield of Boston, and Charles Lembke and James Prentice of New York led the way in adapting cylindrical lenses for the correction of astigmatism. The fact that a few oculists also saw this possibility in no way detracted from optometry's pioneering in this era nor from its establishing a completely new profession.*

---

* In the early days of optometry's becoming an independent profession, a great deal of emphasis was placed on the precedence in the field of the group of "sight testing opticians." Optometry's defense today would be much less on the basis of precedence and more on being the best way in which to supply vision service to the American public. In Chapter 12 this concept will be explored in some depth.

Perhaps the most famous defense of optometry's position on the basis of precedence was the testimony offered by James Cook McAllister before the Pennsylvania Court of Common Pleas in 1913. A portion cited by Fitch (1955) follows:

Question: What is your profession?
Answer: Optician.
Q. How long have you been engaged in that profession?
A. Forty-three years.
Q. You are of the house of McAllister that has been an optician house since some time in 1700?
A. Yes.
Q. Do you happen to know who was the first man that measured the first pair of eyes in Pennsylvania for glasses and fitted them?
A. My grandfather, John McAllister, Jr.
Q. Do you happen to know the first man who taught the oculists in Philadelphia how to measure eyes?

Prentice in his memorable statement to the Committee on Public Health asserted that oculists should confine their work to the recognition and treatment of eye disease. Such pursuit would leave them little time to become proficient in optics. He criticized at great length the use of atropine in refraction and mentioned that a difference of opinion existed even among members of the medical profession on such a procedure. Again, Prentice was demonstrating that his thinking was far in advance of his time.

Prentice made an extremely strong point, still valid today, near the closing parts of his statement.

> The oculist who would deny the optician the right to make use of the ophthalmoscope clearly has not the public welfare at heart.* By his objections he is guilty of criminal complicity, because he advocates that the patient's eyes should be endangered by the optician's failure to use precaution in adapting glasses to diseased eyes. The optician who has been instructed in the use of the ophthalmoscope will be far more competent to discriminate between those whom he would serve than the general medical practitioner who fails to use the instrument yet who has the oculist's consent to prescribe glasses at all hazards.

In his concluding statements Prentice made a strong case of the optician's use of prisms in correcting muscular anomalies and mentioned specifically that several oculists had denied the value of these corrections. He further stated that it is only an independent profession working in this direction that can produce the necessary research and experience to correct this type of eye defect.

This first attempt of the New York State Optical Society to in-

A. My father, William Young McAllister, and James W. Queen.
Q. That is to your personal knowledge, you were in the store at that time?
A. Yes.
Q. Who were the first oculists to your knowledge in Philadelphia?
A. Peter Keyser, George Strawbridge, Richard Levis.
Q. After they had acquired their degree of Doctor of Medicine, to whom did they go to learn refracting?
A. They got their knowledge of lenses and the use of the test case from my father principally, and other members went to James W. Queen. Those three men came to my father.
Q. Then the profession of oculist came in as a separate profession, or as a specialty in medical work, about when to your personal knowledge?
A. In the 70's, early 70's.
Q. And the work of what is called the optometrists was done up to that time entirely by whom?
A. By the opticians.

* In some European countries, optometrists today are not allowed to use the ophthalmoscope. Perhaps the greatest vindication of Prentice's premises is a comparison of the level of eye care available to the public in such areas with that in the United States. (See Chapter 8.)

troduce a bill establishing a profession of optometry met with failure. It was the first of a long series of legislative battles in the state of New York. It is not surprising that the opposition from oculists, dispensing opticians, and misinformed laymen would be at its highest in the most heavily populated area in the country. When New York actually enacted an optometry law in 1908, it was the thirteenth state to do so.

During the long legislative battle, Prentice became disenchanted with many of his friends in opticianry and began to wonder if an independent optical profession was the ideal solution. He was accused by some of deserting optometry and suggesting a new medical specialty that would combine the qualifications of both the eye physician and the optician. He wrote letters to medical societies in 1897 hoping to find a way to stop incompetent persons from entering the field. He proposed a board of examiners to regulate both opticians (optometrists) and oculists. This was not what many of the other leading refracting opticians of this time had in mind at all. At this point, other leaders, well versed in political procedures, began to take over. Prentice's leadership and drive had resulted in well-conceived arguments which were to form the basis of future legislative action; now others would carry on in the establishment of an independent profession.

The long series of legislative battles begun in New York spread throughout the United States. There were over 2,000 opticians in the state of New York alone. Some type of legislation would have to be forthcoming in every state. Protection for the public was sorely needed. Many of the schools of that time were little better than crude trade schools, but professional development was under way. The era of legislation to regulate vision care for the public welfare had begun.

ANDREW J. CROSS

Andrew J. Cross was the next to assume optometric leadership in the United States. Cross was an unusual man. It is doubtful that without his vision optometry would have made the legislative hurdle as early as it did.

Cross was born in 1855 in Antwerp, New York. As a young man, he felt the call of the West and moved to California, starting optical practice in 1876. He also practiced for a few years in the state of Washington before returning to New York City.

Before the break between the dispensing opticians and the refracting opticians, who were shortly to be known as optometrists, Cross recognized that more education was needed for these men who were soon to be legislated as professional people. Legislation was proceeding faster than education, and Cross did everything he could to help in the educational area. His discovery of dynamic skiametry established a way of thinking which affects the practice of optometry to this day. Optometry's premise, that the eye is part of a living organism subject to rules of physiology and influenced by all physical changes, was beginning to emerge. Cross also took the lead in establishing training courses for the practicing optometrists of that time. He helped establish the New York Institute of Optometry in association with E. LeRoy Ryer and Robert M. Lockwood.

Cross's contribution, however, consisted of more than his scientific ability and teaching interests. His strength was in the ability to make men work together as a group. He also recognized potential abilities and leadership of other men in this early professional organization. In E. E. Arrington of Rochester, New York, he saw a man of the driving energy and force needed to obtain legislative actions in New York. Together they formed an excellent team not only locally, but also on the national scale.

The American Optometric Association was founded in 1898 first as the American Association of Opticians. Cross was elected as leader of the optometrists; in 1900, when the group became entirely optometric, Cross served as its first president. Arrington also became nationally important and eventually became secretary of the American Optometric Association. As a gifted speaker, he was of considerable help in other states in their legislative battles.

THE LEGISLATIVE ERA

Minnesota in 1901 was the first state to obtain an optometry law (Appendix A). Legislative activity followed in every state, as optometrists recognized their responsibility to society and to the individual patients whom they served.

Twenty-three years were to pass before all states succeeded in passing legislation regulating the practice of optometry. The District of Columbia in 1924 was the last legal entity to regulate optometric care. These years were filled with many interesting and unusual legislative battles. This progress to control the practice of optometry by legislation must have seemed very slow to the men involved in it. Actually, however, to encompass the idea that a new profession was needed and to bring it into being in so short a period was indeed one of the modern social miracles.*

---

* Hutchins and Adler (1963) discussed the speed with which scientific and sociological changes take place. They note that Professor Lewis S. Morgan wrote in 1877, "Human progress from first to last, has been in a ratio not rigorously but essentially geometrical." Fifty years ago historian James Harvey Robinson said,

Social change comes about much more slowly than technical or scientific change. Man has a tendency to resist social change because of the intensity of his prejudices as well as the comfort of the status quo. Even after its cause has been eliminated, a prejudice may persist. Optometry had to overcome many prejudices in its early legislative days. Some of these prejudices still exist, particularly on the part of a few medical politicians, even though most of the reasons for their existence have been removed.

Each state presented its own unique problem in professional regulation. The early twentieth century in the United States was still an era of strong individual states' rights. The federal government did not engage in the regulation of professions and businesses to the extent that it does at present. As a result, some states were much more successful in certain types of legislation than others, and the need for different kinds of legislation for each state was obvious. The first laws did little more than define the profession of optometry and limit its scope. The actual details of regulations on what constitutes day-by-day professional practice were not to come into existence until near the middle of the twentieth century.

Professions on the state level usually have two distinctly independent official organizational groups. One group is the state association and the other is the state board. In most states, this system developed in optometry as in other professions.

The state association is a group of men gathered together for educational, social, and general professional improvement programs. The state board, on the other hand, is a group of men appointed by the state to regulate the conduct and licensing of men practicing the profession within the jurisdiction of the state. At times, there can be

"Man's progress was well-nigh imperceptible for tens of thousands of years—but it tends to increase in rapidity with an ever-increasing tempo."

They also quoted the anthropologist Lewis H. Lowie, who, in 1917, expressed the phenomenon in this vivid fashion:

We may liken the progress of mankind to that of a man one hundred years old who dawdles through kindergarten for eighty-five years, then takes ten years to go through the primary grades, then rushes with lightning rapidity through grammar school, high school and college. Considering the nature of developments the past few years one might add, "and graduate research."

The term progress may be moot. What is not moot is the fact of social change. And what staggers the imagination is not change itself, or the spectacular character of individual change but the "ever-accelerating tempo." It is as if human history were a machine moving along in low gear with occasional bumps, blow-outs, and breakdowns—and then having always before resumed its journey in the same gear, suddenly shifting into high gear and then after a short interval into a still higher and then after a shorter interval into a still higher. To the spectator (more awesomely), the sight is marvelous and also terrifying: will it go on accelerating? Is it out of control, roaring forward faster and faster unto some sort of grand smash-up? Will it burn itself out like a rocket? Will it ever slow down again?

a wide split between these two groups. This, of course, should not be, but it is revealed in the past history of optometry as well as other professions.

As a general rule, the governor of the state makes appointments to the state board. The recommendations for these appointments usually come from the state association. In most states, however, the governor has the prerogative of appointing whomever he wishes. Quite often if there is any disagreement within the state association as to the best candidate for state board member, the governor ignores all recommendations and makes his own appointment. Often appointments to state boards are made on political grounds as much as on grounds of technical competency.

The importance of the state board regulating the practice of optometry cannot be overlooked. The practice of the individual members of the medical profession can be controlled to a great extent by various voluntary associations within medicine. One way of accomplishing this is by withdrawal of hospital privileges from members who do not conform to the accepted standards of practice. Optometry does not have this type of leverage over its individual members. Therefore, it has found it necessary to legislate rules of practice and to control its members within the legal framework of the constitutions of the various states and of the federal government. Legislation and control of professions are quite difficult at times; the citizens of the United States are known for their differences of opinion as to who and what shall be regulated and by what methods.

During the early legislative battles, each state had different problems of regulation. In some areas, the greatest opposition came from members of the medical profession (oculists). Sometimes a fear of economic competition prompted such action; sometimes sincere men believed they were battling for the public good in not allowing anyone without a medical background to practice in any area of health care. Wilensky (1964) in his studies of professionalization makes the observation that all professions have only a "tenuous claim to exclusive competence in their fields. Late in the stages of professionalization other occupations begin to compete with the established profession." He feels that the causes of this competition are the newness of the service, uncertain standards, the embryonic state of the social and psychological sciences on which they draw, and the fact that the problems with which they deal are part of everyday living. He cites as evidence the competition between clinical psychology, psychiatry, and other brands of psychotherapy, and states that "even more clearly technical occupations, like medicine, find themselves doing battle with marginal practitioners—with peaceful absorption as one outcome (osteopathy) and all-out war as another (chiropractic)."

Medical eye practitioners probably had a reason in this early stage of optometric development to fear the beginning of a new vision care profession in the health care field. They were aware of optometry's background and development as an independent entity, and admitted their dependence on the early opticians who did the exploratory work in developing lenses, prisms, and other optical means of correcting visual defects. But what medicine disliked was the appearance on the social scene of a *new profession*. Members of this young upstart group even wanted to be called doctors; some of them (like Prentice) wanted to charge fees in the same manner as members of the established profession of medicine. This new profession was also developing a code of ethics based on many of the tenets which medicine had used for years. Moreover, this young profession was trying to establish overnight what it had taken medicine nearly 2,000 years to do. No wonder so much opposition came from medicine in this era.

According to Fitch (1959), the argument with ophthalmology began as a result of five or six medical men persuading the optometrists of the early 1870's to teach them how to refract. It was obvious to these early oculists that refraction would be a nice side-line to the medical treatment of the eye. The interest of ophthalmology in refraction continued to expand.

The first legal attempt by ophthalmology to control optometry began in 1914. A law had been passed in 1913 in Pennsylvania which gave the medical examining board the right to take over control of all professions which it considered to be minor branches of medicine. Optometrists attacked the constitutionality of this law.* Fitch (1959) quoted the opinion in the Lower Court:

> It might be said with a great deal of force that the evil which the legislature intended to provide against was the incompetent physicians and surgeons. Those who hold themselves out to the public as physicians and surgeons, either generally or in a limited sphere, should be subjected to examination by the medical board to the necessity of obtaining a license to practice medicine and surgery . . .
>
> We cannot regard the fact that the work done by the eye specialist physician and that done by the optometrist, to a certain limited extent, lap over each other, constitutes the optometrist a practitioner in medicine. Such work on the part of the optometrist was done by him perhaps and probably long before the eye specialist among physicians had either the knowledge or the skill to do the work which is now done by both physician and optometrist.

Albert Fitch, founder and president for a number of years of the Pennsylvania State College of Optometry, led the fight against medi-

---

* The testimony of the optician McAllister in this famous court case has been cited earlier in this chapter.

cal control of optometry in Pennsylvania. In evaluating medicine's opposition to optometry, Fitch observed that most of the general medical practitioners were tolerant and fair-minded toward optometry. He was, however, highly critical of certain oculists. Some of these men "have shown themselves to be more economy-minded than fair-minded." Fitch accused them of acting more like members of a union or trust and says that few leaders of trade unions would attempt to carry out some of the actions of these men.

Fitch credited the American public and especially the American judiciary for seeing through such efforts to obtain a monopoly. He was critical of medicine's attempt to pass "one board" bills, which would have eliminated independent professions. He paid tribute to the state legislatures which refused to pass such legislation. He felt that in "their efforts to eliminate optometry the oculists ignored the history of both medicine and optometry. They failed to recognize that the knowledge and practice of optometry are based on the science of optics, especially on physiological optics, and that training in physio logical optics requires a preliminary knowledge of mathematics, geometrical optics, chemistry, anatomy, physiology, neural anatomy, myology and pathology." He says that optics emanated from ancient times. He correctly stated that "learned men in every period in history have added to our store of knowledge about optics."

This first attempt at medical control was defeated by the Pennsylvania optometrists but was to form a background for much further legal wrangling and distrust among the medical eye specialty and the profession of optometry. A decision in 1938 by the Pennsylvania Supreme Court helped establish optometry's place as a profession. This decision was an outgrowth of this legal fight for the control of which profession should care for human vision and by what method.

Pennsylvania was not the only state in which there were attempts to bring optometry under the medical laws. In Ohio, a similar basic law was passed in 1916, giving the medical board the authority to decide which professions were to practice minor branches of medicine; in 1919, the medical board in Ohio actually began to issue licenses to optometrists for a fee. However, as a result of legal action by optometrists, the medical board, without waiting for court action, admitted its error in classifying optometry as a branch of medicine.

These early court and medical board decisions were extremely important to optometry. Most states eventually passed basic science laws or laws similar to the Pennsylvania and Ohio laws. Optometry was exempted in these laws as a result of decisions in Pennsylvania and Ohio that optometry is *not* a branch of medicine.

It is interesting to conjecture the extent of the effect on vision care that these court decisions brought about. Had optometry lost these decisions, it is doubtful that an independent profession would have developed. Optometry might have been a separate organization, ancillary to medicine, such as nursing or medical technology. It would not have been an *independent profession* directly responsible to the American people. Medicine would have assumed this responsibility.

Outright opposition from organized medicine did not occur in all states. In states where economic pressures and competition were not so great (as in the western United States), the general medical practitioners actually assisted and encouraged optometry in its early efforts. In recent years, one of the present authors (REW) had the privilege of working with a general physician who assisted greatly in amending one state's public health law. This legislation was introduced by optometry to regulate optometrists, opticians, and ophthalmologists who might be tempted to publicize themselves in a nonprofessional manner.

Great opposition to early optometric legislation also came from within the profession. This, of course, follows the historical progression of any profession. Wilensky (1964), though not particularly concerned with optometry, makes the point that:

> Activists in the association engage in much soul-searching—on whether the occupation is a profession, what the professional tasks are, how to raise the quality of recruits, and so on. At this point they may change the name of the occupation. In this way hospital superintendents have become hospital administrators; relief investigators, caseworkers; newspaper reporters, journalists. The change in label may function to reduce identification with the previous, less-professional occupation. Many, of course, are unsuccessful in this effort. Thus funeral directors or morticians have not escaped the public image of undertaker, and salvage consultants are, alas, still confused with junk dealers.
>
> All this is accompanied by a campaign to separate the competent from the incompetent. This involves further definition of essential professional tasks, the development of internal conflict among practitioners of varying background,* and some competition with outsiders who do similar work.

Because the optometrist evolved from the optician, the question of jurisdiction naturally caused many conflicts. The majority of optometrists initially considered themselves opticians as well as optometrists.† A few of the leaders of the various associations, state and

---

* This internal conflict to which Wilensky refers has been mentioned previously in this volume. Those who have limited competence or a vested interest in limited practice are invariably opposed to increased scope.

† Within the personal memory of both of the present authors, the phrase "optometrist and optician" was used on shingles and stationery to describe the scope of practitioners. Even today, a few recalcitrant optometrists still hold themselves out to be opticians as well.

national, had the foresight to recognize that these two groups must be separated. Naturally, each of the men who made this early decision faced inner personal economic conflicts. The lost income from the sale of optical merchandise would have to be replaced with professional fees for vision care; this was to be a long struggle. Many of the problems that beset optometry today are still deeply involved with ophthalmic materials. Several years passed before optometrists gave up their dependence on the sale of glasses, binoculars, telescopes, microscopes, barometers, and many other items displayed for sale by the early optometrist-optician in his optical shop. Many of these men bitterly opposed the first optometry laws that attempted to separate the optician from the optometrist. With sophistication of legislation and with improvement in the education of the optometrist in vision care, this opposition became less. It was a vital factor, however, in the opposition to optometric legislation in the early 1900's.

The first optometry laws barely defined the scope of the profession of optometry; very little regulation was done. As time passed, certain general patterns began to appear in the state optometry laws. The early leaders realized that if optometry was to obtain full professional recognition, then standards of honesty, competency, and behavior had to be in keeping with those of other professions.

Professional honesty is a virtue that cannot be legislated. Legislation can be passed, however, which makes it *easier* for one to be honest. There is no place in a profession for *caveat emptor* (let the purchaser beware; that is, let him examine the article he is buying and act on his own judgment at his own risk) . Even in most well-run business enterprises, this type of policy is not followed in a literal sense. The implications in a profession, however, are deeper than in an ethical business. Because of the more serious and technical nature of any health profession, the patient is completely at the mercy of the doctor. In no instance is any recommendation ever made for the profit that will accrue to the professional man. In optometric practice, for example, the patient either needs a lens correction and/or vision training or he does not. The patient might be given a choice of two or three methods of treatment, but the benefits which would in each instance occur are carefully explained. In no instance is any treatment ever recommended except that which will benefit the patient.

Corporations are a typical American institution. They are designed for making money for the officers and stockholders. This is as it should be, and they have made a great contribution to the American standard of living. They do not, however, fit in with a profession the chosen aim of which should be to render a service to its patients. In the era when corporations practiced optometry or employed optometrists in department stores, the professional man's behavior was dictated by the corporation. For example, it was not unusual for the optometrist working in these surroundings to be told that his chief function was the selling of glasses. The selling of more than one pair of spectacles was not based on the needs of the patient as much as on the "professional man's" ability to "sell" extra pairs of glasses. In some instances, employed optometrists were told that no "customer" should leave the store without spectacles. Although some corporations acted in this manner, others did not. False promises or statements, after all, do not result in repeat business. Recognizing this situation, American courts and legislatures for the most part have become aware that professions cannot be practiced in corporate surroundings and have so ruled. In most states, it is illegal for a corporation to engage in the practice of optometry and/or optometrists are not allowed to work for corporations.

Professional competency is another area difficult to control by legislation. Again, however, the need for trying to improve professional competency was felt by early optometric leaders. Legislation has now been passed, and is still under consideration in a number of states, requiring that optometrists take postgraduate courses yearly to retain their licenses. Should true professional men require action by a state regulatory body to make them keep up with professional advancement? The need for such laws was much more apparent a few years ago in optometry because of the lack of professional training. Extensive education seems to promote the desire for still more education; with the present six-year university course, the trend toward legal requirements of compulsory education will probably lessen as it has in the older established professions. Such regulations are no problem to the professional man who does keep up with professional advancement; he takes many more hours than the legal minimum anyway. Such legislation probably serves as a stimulus to a few men who otherwise would never go to the trouble were such requirements not mandatory.

SUMMARY

One facet of the process of professionalization is the legal aspect. In optometry, this phase began with the adoption of the first state law in 1901. By 1924 all states had a basic optometry law. These early laws mainly established the area of practice and the scope of optometry. They had some regulations, particularly those which forbade practice of the profession by itinerant peddlers or others with improper training. Some requirements for the education of the optometrist were also included.

In the early years, several cases were battled through the courts to establish the independence of optometry as a profession. Not only was the scope delineated in the laws, but the jurisdiction of the profession was vested by law in an independent entity—and not within the framework of any then-existing profession.

Since 1925 or so, most state laws have been revised and have become more inclusive. Attempts were made to regulate professional behavior. Educational requirements were increased by statute. Corporate practice was abolished. Throughout this period, each of the states has had laws somewhat different from those of the others. Although all such laws have the same aim, to protect the vision of the public, the various states have enacted greater or lesser amounts of restriction. Perhaps the most comprehensive law in modern days is that of New Jersey. (See Appendix B.) Comparison of the New Jersey law with the first law, that of Minnesota (Appendix A), will give the reader some idea of the degree of complexity that has been added through the legislative process.

CHAPTER 7

EMERGENCE OF A PROFESSION— ORGANIZATIONAL, EDUCATIONAL, AND ETHICAL ASPECTS

In his analysis of the route followed by professions which have achieved professional status in the United States, Wilensky (1964) listed three major areas in addition to those described in the previous chapter. These are education, organizational activity, and a formalized code of ethics or mode of behavior. The present chapter is a discussion of the role of each of these factors in the emergence of optometry as a profession.

Wilensky has pointed out the sequence of events generally followed. All of the different professionalizing activities, however, are ongoing. Thus, there is the establishment of not only the first college, but also the second and the third; not only does the first state adopt legislation, but other states follow suit. Marked overlap occurs; for a period, events are occurring in all steps of the professionalization process more or less simultaneously.

ORGANIZATIONS

In the Wilensky timetable, a local professional association is formed first, then a national association, and then the first state license law is passed. In optometry, this was the sequence; the first state association was that formed in New York in 1896, the national association was formed in 1897–8, and the first state law was passed by Minnesota in 1901.

AMERICAN OPTOMETRIC ASSOCIATION

A strong organization was necessary to accomplish the aims of the men who had chosen the correction of visual defects by optical means as their vocation. In several states, the opticians began to form associations. New York State, because of the large number of opticians there who were measuring vision, had a strong state association. It was organized while Prentice was waging his early battles. The idea of organizing a national association came from Frederick Boger, founder of the magazine now known as *The Optical Journal and Review of Optometry*. Such an organization came into being in 1898 under the name of the American Association of Opticians. Initially, anyone engaged in the manufacture or sale of optical goods was eligible for membership. The first president, Charles Lembke of New York City, was, in fact, a dispensing optician. When the group became entirely optometric and membership was limited to refracting opticians in 1900, Andrew J. Cross was elected president and served a two-year term. In 1910, with 42 states as members, the name of the group was changed to the American Optical Association. Although in 1903 the association had endorsed the title "optometrist" to designate its members, the national body was not so named until 1918.

The American Optometric Association served a valuable purpose in the early legislative struggles of optometry. To understand the impact of the national association in those days, one must understand the construction of the organization. Membership in the American Optometric Association is not on a personal basis. The individual becomes a member of the American Optometric Association by joining his state association. The American Optometric Association consists of state *associations*. The representatives of the various state organizations gain training in politics and committee work through activity in their own state associations. In 1907, 22 state associations were members of the national association; by that time, the value of state licensing laws was making itself felt. According to Gregg (1965), 11 states passed optometry laws in the year 1909, making a total of 24 state boards giving examinations to applicants. The national association took the lead in that same year by helping to create the National Board of State Examiners in Optometry. The assembling of various state officers with like interests and desires resulted in more uniform legislation and a valuable interchange of ideas.

The value of the national organization began to make itself felt in other fields. In 1915, a resolution was passed recommending the minimum length of optometry courses. Five years later, the American Optometric Association approved the newly organized International Federation of Optometry Schools. Eventually, a counselor on optometric education was appointed, and an examiner was hired to work with the boards of optometry to upgrade optometric schools.

Although optometric legislation was proceeding rapidly, many shortcomings were noticed by these early legislative pioneers. Lack of knowledge on the part of the public as to what an optometrist is remained one of the chief stumbling blocks whenever optometric legislation was proposed. The national organization established a Department of Publicity, which eventually developed into the Department of Public Information with a full-time public relations counsel.*

---

* Educating the public on the intricacies of a profession is a long, difficult task. Today, for example, the majority of laymen do not know that optometry is an inde-

Over the next 25 years, the American Optometric Association met the challenge provided by a rapidly growing profession. Optometry has always been fortunate in having many dedicated men contributing to its progress. One of these, Dr. Ernest Kiekenapp, was secretary during this period, and his office did much to hold the young, growing organization together. With changes in leadership taking place every year or two, it was very important that a central office continue to run the many detailed projects that had to be maintained from year to year.

Most of the pioneering legislative work and advancement of optometry was done on the state level. With gradual centralization of government in Washington, D.C., however, the American Optometric Association increased its activities on the national level to perform the necessary work that no state organization could undertake. Such organization was needed if optometry was to fit into the national health care picture. In 1952, a professional administrative director was employed. A Washington office was established, and work really began on a national level.

The several facets of the professionalization process might appear to be quite separate (legislation, organization, education, and ethical or behavioral standards). Not so. There is a great deal of overlap. The state optometric associations and the American Optometric Association became the prime professional organizations. These organizations worked toward obtaining legislation; they sought to improve educational standards; and they sought to upgrade the mode of practice of the individual optometrists. During some periods of the past three quarters of a century, greater emphasis has been placed on one or the other of these aspects of professional evolution. But almost always, the lead came from the professional organizations.

Three other organizations had a marked impact on the professionalization of optometry. All three were mainly educational in nature, stressing postgraduate education. They are the Optometric Extension Program, the American Academy of Optometry, and the American Optometric Foundation. All three played an important role in the development of optometry in the United States; all three are still very much alive and still contribute to the expansion of knowledge.

pendent profession whose graduates receive a doctorate after 6 years' study at some of the nation's major universities. Worse yet, many laymen still do not know the difference between an optometrist, an optician, and an ophthalmologist. The vast majority of people, however, now can identify an optometrist as one who works with vision and the eye (Chapter 9).

THE OPTOMETRIC EXTENSION PROGRAM

The first optometrists to receive licenses from the various states had little formal optometric training. They had learned through apprenticeship or, at best, through short, formal courses. In the transitional period, when optical shops were being converted into professional offices, the need for education of the practicing optometrists was great. Travel was neither as rapid nor as simple as it is today, so that education had to be brought to the men in or near their home localities. Most social problems of this era were solved by individuals, private organizations, and if necessary, by state governments; federal projects were scarce. It is understandable, therefore, that a private organization was formed and was highly successful in bringing postgraduate education to the optometrists. This was the Oklahoma Extension Program, started by E. B. Alexander, a young Oklahoma optometrist, who was secretary of the state association. Because of the need and desire of the early optometrists for education, this program was expanded and became known as the Optometric Extension Program. Traveling lecturers visited study groups in all of the various states where the Optometric Extension Program existed. Synonymous with the early development of this program was A. M. Skeffington, a Nebraska optometrist, who had the ability to assimilate knowledge from the various disciplines related to optometry and to present it in an interesting and challenging manner. This group supplied the main source of postgraduate optometric education, particularly in the western states, for many years. It was organized in 1928 with 51 members as a state association program and gradually grew to a membership of nearly 4,000 members. This growth attests to the need it filled in the development of the profession.

It is interesting to compare the problems of self-education on a postgraduate level of today's optometrist with those of the early optometrists. Today's optometrist is highly trained by years of college as compared to the early optometrist, who had little formal optometric training. In the early days, there was almost no optometric literature; today, in addition to a growing number of optometric textbooks, there are several optometric journals. Today's optometric colleges all offer postgraduate courses during the school year and during the summer, and several organizations offer series of courses during the year. The needs met by many organizations and institutions today were all met by the Optometric Extension Program in its early days.

To make up for the absence of texts and periodicals, the Optometric Extension Program mailed its members a series of papers each month. The optometrists in various localities around the country formed small study groups that met periodically—some as often as weekly, others, monthly. Optometrists studied together and helped each other improve their skills. To fulfill the need for formal post-graduate lectures, the Optometric Extension Program sponsored speakers who visited the various areas; Skeffington was for years the major traveling lecturer to work with the various groups. Even today, with optometrists as well trained as they are and with courses and literature abounding, many optometrists still prefer this method of group study to any other. The role of the Optometric Extension Program has changed over the years as conditions have changed, but the idea of small groups which meet periodically for study together still holds great attraction for many optometrists.

The American Academy of Optometry

Another primarily educational organization is the American Academy of Optometry; like the Optometric Extension Program, it has had a change in emphasis over the years, although from its very first official meeting in 1922, under the chairmanship of Dr. M. Steinfeld, the Academy has stressed the scientific aspects of vision care as well as the highest type of professional conduct of its members.

Impatience with the progress of organized optometry toward the status of a true profession had much to do with the formation of the Academy. This impatience was natural; it must have been disheartening indeed to see many of the early state associations, and even the national association, dominated by men who were interested more in the business aspects of optometry than in the scientific and professional facets. Some definite professional goals were badly needed in the early 1920's. Dr. Eugene G. Wiseman, in his address before the Academy in 1925, put it this way:

> Since progress proved so slow and valuable opportunities were lost and the time and effort spent at most meetings largely wasted, it became evident that if a reasonably ideal association with others was to be consummated there must be formed a group of selected practitioners whose ideals were harmonious and whose sincere devotion to optometric science was beyond ordinary doubt. On the theory that he travels fastest who travels alone, a small choice group with a specific idea and program can progress much faster and further than a large conglomerate mass, especially if the latter has no concrete plans but possesses antagonistic interests pulling in different directions and thus arriving at nowhere in particular.

It is true that in this era optometry was sometimes practiced as a profession; more often it was conducted as a business. An association of men with like ideals was needed. As Wiseman said:

But, until the formation of the Academy, these men did not have available a group in which they could feel entirely at home and free to express themselves with the confidence that they were in harmony with those around them. There was no group with whom they could associate with the assurance that they could learn from each as well as perhaps instruct each.

They could not very well discuss fees with men who charged no fees. They could not speak of the requirements of publicity with men who blazened out in crass display advertisements. They could not interchange ideas concerning the psychology of surroundings with men who conducted stores. They could not safely advance ideas and conclusions relative to their scientific work for fear "store" men would seize them and prostitute them so as to bring discredit upon Optometry. They could not converse about technical subjects with even some of the best known and most prosperous optometrists in the country because they could not be sure that these men were either interested in or had the slightest idea of what they were speaking. And often, when their consultants went to distant cities, they could not refer them to a particular individual because they could not be sure of the particular type of practice and service of that individual.

The organization of the American Academy of Optometry helps to solve all of these problems.

Initially, the three basic requirements for membership in the Academy were: (1) The candidate must practice in an office; (2) he must charge an examination fee of $3.00 or more; * and (3) he must not engage in advertising—window display, blotters, billboards, handbills, or even newspaper advertising. While these requirements seem quite elementary by present-day standards, they were considerably ahead of the average practice of optometry as conducted in the early 1920's.

At the second formation meeting of the Academy, in 1922, it was decided to invite a small group of optometric educators to accept fellowship in the Academy. From its inception, the Academy has attempted to maintain a balance between optometric educators or scientists on the one hand and practicing clinicians on the other. This it has done very well.

Again, the Academy was most fortunate in selecting, early in its existence, as secretary Dr. Carel C. Koch, † who dedicated a large

---

* This was more than 30 years after Prentice had begun the fight for legislation which was set off by the accusation that in doing exactly this, charging a fee of $3.00 for his examination, he was practicing medicine. By this date, every state in the union had laws recognizing optometry—yet most of the optometrists still had not adopted the behavior of Prentice, the founder.

† Dr. Koch, whose professional life has spanned much of the total lifespan of the optometric profession in the United States, has done more perhaps than any other to further the dissemination of knowledge in the field of visual science. A charter member of the Academy, he has acted as its secretary for 25 years; he founded

share of his professional career to the formation and growth of the Academy. It is quite a tribute to the wisdom of these early pioneers of professionalism that such an organization as the Academy should come into existence. It is also a tribute to optometry that enough of its early membership supported this organization so that it could continue to exist and become one of the leading scientific organizations devoted to vision care in the world.

In addition to supplying the sounding board for research reports at its annual meeting, the Academy conducts postgraduate courses * for members and non-members, publishes home study manuals, encourages the formation of local chapters throughout the world, encourages the application of scientific methods to daily practice, provides discussion facilities for various optometric specialties in its sections at the annual meeting, engages in a scientific information program for the public, assists in research projects, and provides a scientific journal of the highest caliber.

The Academy's greatest contribution to the profession, however, still remains the gathering together of men of like interests. Whereas it is an honor to be invited and accepted to Academy fellowship, the benefit of membership, as in any organization, comes only through participation. The annual meetings have grown so that every interest within the profession is now represented. Although the Academy consists largely of optometrists, members of other related professions also attend the annual meetings; membership in the Academy includes educators, illuminating engineers, ophthalmologists, psychologists, physicists, physiologists, reading teachers, librarians, and others interested in visual science. Membership in the Academy is really a way of thinking; it continues to be that as much today as when the organization was originally formed. The yearly contact of research scientists and faculty people with clinicians keeps an avenue of communication open in a way not possible by any other means. The professional advancement accomplished by this means, although difficult to measure, has been very great.

The shifting of emphasis in organizations which was described

the *American Journal of Optometry*, the profession's major scientific publication, over 40 years ago and still serves as its publisher. He merged his Journal with the Academy's *Transactions*, the new publication being known as *The American Journal of Optometry and Archives of the American Academy of Optometry*. Up to the present date, this journal is read by all who would keep abreast of vision science.

* The 1966 series of courses offered by the American Academy of Optometry, for example, included 96 different courses offered by 58 leading optometric educators and representing 173 hours of instruction. During the three days alloted for this activity, the optometrist was able to choose any one of five courses given during each of the 35 hours. The courses in 1966 were dedicated to Vincent J. Ellerbrock who served for ten years as director prior to his untimely death.

earlier is well illustrated in the Academy. Fellows in the Academy, from the beginning, were required to practice in the most professional manner. Over the 40 or so years of its existence, the Academy has made few changes in its rules of behavior, indicating clearly that there is little change on a day-to-day basis of professional standards. However, more and more optometrists have adopted the professional mode of practice; whereas only a handful of optometrists could qualify for membership in the 1920's, today most optometrists follow the Academy mode of practice. Over the years, the shift has been toward the scientific and educational aspects of the Academy. Today, the Academy takes the professional behavior of its members for granted; although rigid rules apply, little enforcement is needed. The 1500 optometrists who are Fellows observe the Academy Code scrupulously. The punishment for failing to do so is no more than loss of membership. The members' esteem for the organization and the profession which it represents is great; for a member to lose membership for misconduct is extremely rare.

THE AMERICAN OPTOMETRIC FOUNDATION

Organized optometry has recognized its responsibility to encourage research and develop trained educators. Graduate facilities were available, but it was necessary to finance the education of these future leaders.

After ten years of planning by officers of the American Optometric Association and educational leaders, the American Optometric Foundation was formed in 1947. The chairman of the founding committee, William C. Ezell, devoted many years to developing this organization into a true foundation. Optometrists supported this Foundation in its beginning so that it could make a substantial contribution to optometry.

A report of the Foundation's activities in the *Journal of the American Optometric Association* in December of 1958, 11 years after the Foundation's inception, showed its progress. Thirteen men had been given grants; ten had been assisted in completing their Ph.D. requirements. Eight of the men were teaching in various optometry schools. This had been accomplished with limited financial resources.

The directors realized that the Foundation must gain wide support throughout the profession. Early in the history of the American Optometric Foundation, it adopted a policy of "encouraging research in physiological and psychological optics and their application in the practice of optometry and related fields such as vision in schools, industry, and transportation in which the practicing optometrist is called upon to participate."

Harold Kohn, legal counsel of the American Optometric Association for many years, was active in forming this new Foundation. His statement concerning its purpose and need was well expressed.

> The need for a Foundation for research, education and the professional advancement of optometry is self-evident. A profession which fails to recognize and provide for this need must die. Optometry is too progressive and virile not to embrace and achieve the aspirations of creating a Foundation second to none which will provide students, optometrists, and more importantly, the public, with the latest and greatest in the care of vision.

The Foundation's main support over the years has been from within the profession. Optometry is now assuming its place as one of the major health care professions. The general public and governmental agencies are turning more and more to optometry for guidance in vision research and care. Support of the Foundation should be assumed in greater proportion by the public which it serves. Steps are being taken to assure a broader support of the Foundation's present activities and to enlarge the scope of its work.

The Foundation's activities helped establish first-class optometric education. A large number of men with advanced degrees were needed for the formation of new optometry schools within major universities.* This was made possible by the continued support of career teachers and research personnel as a major project of the American Optometric Foundation.

In addition to the four major organizations which have been described, there are many local groups. The American Optometric Association is made up of state societies. The members of the state societies are also members of county, city, or zone societies. The American Optometric Association and its affiliated societies form the official organization of professional optometry today. The other three organizations all concern themselves with education: the Academy through dissemination, by a variety of means, of all new techniques and fruits of research in vision; the Optometric Extension Program through individual study and study groups; the American Optometric Foundation through underwriting part of the costs of educating teachers, of conducting research, and even of writing textbooks.†

* See, also, Chapter 12 for a discussion of optometry's need for teachers.

† Part of the expenses for preparation of the manuscript for this text was supplied by a grant from the American Optometric Foundation. The authors acknowledge this help with gratitude.

EDUCATION

The education of its members is one of the prime characteristics of a profession. Two of Wilensky's milestones along the professionalization pathway deal with the establishment of educational institutions. Most optometrists have looked to education as the panacea for all of the growing profession's ills. They argue, for example, that education will even eliminate personal behavioral and ethical problems. They assume that anyone who spends the number of years required to complete professional training in optometry would be willing to discipline himself enough to establish a professional practice.

The view of the educational scene from the pinnacle of the present six-year university program leading to the doctorate degree is quite encouraging. Five of the ten optometric schools are now university affiliated; three of these are in state-supported universities; at least one independent school receives grants from the state to assist in its educational plans. The students entering optometry today are more carefully selected than at any time in the past. The physical plants, for the most part, are in excellent shape. Optometry is now training teachers and research personnel in its own colleges. Plans are underway in every optometric college for enlargement of facilities to accommodate the increasing number of students expressing an interest in optometry as a profession. Most important, plans are being made for the development of new schools of optometry in areas somewhat isolated from optometric education at present. A present goal of optometric leaders is to increase materially the number of optometric colleges. This pleasant scene makes the view of the past all the more remarkable, since formal education has only been with us for three quarters of a century. The first optometry college was formed in 1892; the first university-affiliated school, in 1910. There was, however, instruction in optics for the many hundred years that the optometric service was offered by spectaclemakers and opticians.

The skilled craft of optics that developed in Holland, Germany, France, Italy, and England in the early 1400's followed the course of most trades of that era (Chapter 4). A major function of the guilds was to improve the training of workmen, which was by apprenticeship. The completion of apprenticeships in these guilds was not a simple matter. The training was tedious, and high standards of workmanship were required. Official recognition of spectaclemaking by the courts of Europe and England in this era is the first recorded governmental acknowledgment of the importance of training workmen in applied optics.

The peddlers and general merchants who distributed spectacles in Europe contributed little to the skill of optics and did little to pass on knowledge in the field of optics. However, the opticians who distributed spectacles themselves did contribute both research and the spread of learning. The first optical shop was established as early as 1600 in Germany, at which time the term *opticus* (optician) came into use. Such optical shops became established in most of the large cities throughout Europe, and the proprietors, themselves members of the optical guilds, passed on knowledge of optics through the apprenticeship system. Although in the early training in optics there were no formal courses, it would be improper to assume that there was no education. Apprenticeship training was often rigorous. The method of individual instruction was probably the most efficient at that time for teaching the practical applications of optics.

In America, too, individual instruction was the method of education in optics. Education as we now know it was not even dreamed of at that time. Formal education was reserved for the wealthy few. There was little or no optical literature available in America.* This was the period of Yankee ingenuity, epitomized by Benjamin Franklin, of whom Haight (1941) wrote:

> He had also a remarkable endowment of Yankee ingenuity, which he applied to the improvement of everything about him. He invented the Franklin stove to warm houses and the lightning rod to protect them, a combined chair and ladder to reach books and bifocal glasses for reading them . . .

Franklin was a friend and client of John McAllister, who founded the first optical shop in the United States, in 1783. Cox (1947) credits Franklin with having encouraged John McAllister to begin the business that thrived as a family venture for a hundred years. McAllisters, members of America's first optical family, also supplied vision care to Thomas Jefferson and Andrew Jackson. They are credited by most authorities with making the first successful correction of astigmatism in America in 1828. (See Chapter 5.) Cox (1947), in his excellent review of this era, observes that this correction was made 40 years before the first prescription for an astigmatic lens was written by an oculist in America.

American business ingenuity made itself felt in optics as well as in most other fields of endeavor in the early 1800's. James W. Queen,

---

* *The Handbook for Opticians* by William Bohne in 1888 was one of the first American optical textbooks. Bohne, an optician of the German school, was thoroughly trained in Europe in the guild tradition. His book appeared at an appropriate time and was used in the first formal courses in optometry.

a partner of the McAllisters for many years, decided to start his own business of importing and distributing optical instruments. Within a short time, he began manufacturing his own materials. He imported skilled workmen from Germany and also trained his own personnel. Queen evidently combined business ability with an ability to select and train good workmen. His business prospered and continued to grow until it became one of the largest equipment and instrument distributors in America.

Cox (1947) credits Queen with the training of the first generation of several families that contributed greatly to the development of professional optometry in America. Some of the examples he cites are Drs. John W. Jarvis, Harry Pine, Sr., William W. Russell, Henry Kaiser, and William G. Walton. All these families, even the second and third generation, made substantial contributions of an organizational nature, as well as establishing and continuing successful practices.

This era of American optometry is unique from another viewpoint. The guild tradition was never established in American optics as it had been in Europe. Nevertheless, training was on an individual, on-the-job basis. The absence of the rigidity of the apprenticeship system, the free enterprise system prevalent in America, and the existence of an open frontier made it possible for anyone to start his own business as soon as he felt he had obtained sufficient training. Men were free to go where they wished—to fail or prosper according to their ability. Under this freedom, new businesses and professions developed in America on a grand scale. The stronger traditions of Europe, the lack of stable and dependable governments in many countries, the absence of an open frontier, and the firmly entrenched class system of most European countries combined to inhibit the development of optometry as an independent profession there. In the United States, on the other hand, the proper climate existed for a new profession to develop.

Education during the nineteenth century was on a private, individual basis. Research, too, was informal and on an individual basis. Charles A. Spencer brought the principles of scientific design to the making of microscopes in America. His business, like so many others of this period, was passed along in the family and later became the Scientific Instrument Division of the American Optical Company. In addition to its effect on clinical optometry, the scientific lens designing started by Spencer and expanded by his student, Robert B. Tolles, made great contributions to medical and related research.

The combination of scientific instruments such as telescopes and microscopes with ophthalmic lenses in these early days of the profession's development was fortunate. These men had to know optics from both a theoretical design viewpoint and a practical application viewpoint. It gave optometry a scientific background which was to be of immense help as the young profession began to mature educationally.

The close association between making or selling scientific instruments, such as microscopes, and the ophthalmic aspects of the practice of the early opticians is exemplified in the history of two interesting optical families in America. The Bausch and the Lomb families contributed to both facets of optical endeavor. Because of the lack of optical establishments, John Jacob Bausch, a German emigrant, could not find work in Buffalo, New York, in 1850, then a city of 42,000. He went to Rochester, New York, where, in 1853, he established an optical shop. In addition to spectacles, he sold microscopes, telescopes, magnifiers, and other optical products purchased in Germany. Along with his retailing activities, Bausch conducted a workshop and a laboratory and began manufacturing his own optical products. Henry Lomb joined him in the business, which had difficult times in its early days. When Lomb entered the Union army in the Civil War, his pay was contributed to keep the struggling business going. The Civil War had a fortunate effect, also, in that it reduced the supply of European optical goods. By 1886, the partners had rented a factory and were manufacturing optical goods to distribute to other opticians. Today, Bausch & Lomb is one of the major American manufacturers of optical materials.

During most of the nineteenth century in America, knowledge in optics was passed on by individual instruction. There was also an importation of European workers, primarily German, who had been trained under the guild apprenticeship system. Toward the end of the century, however, several German institutions were offering formal instruction in optics, and some Americans, like Prentice, went to Europe to be educated. Finally, a sufficiently widespread interest in optics made on-the-job individual training no longer a satisfactory solution to the need for education. Various "courses" began to appear on the American scene in the 1890's. This was the start of formal optometric education in America and the first step away from the European tradition of guild and family training in optics.

Before discussing formal optometric education, we should examine the general professional training that existed at the end of the nineteenth century. The established professions of medicine and dentistry were just beginning to institute education as we know it today. The idea of studying people and of using laboratories in scientific study was just coming into existence.

Deitrick and Berson (1953) state:

It was not until the last two decades of the 19th century that a significant number of medical schools began to introduce their students to the study of patients. This method of teaching proved so effective that hospital facilities were seen to be a great advantage to a medical school.

Scientific knowledge in Europe was developing rapidly. Medical training as well as optical training was more advanced in Europe at this time than it was in America. The laboratory sciences were just coming into scientific acceptance. Bacteriology, chemistry, pathology, and physiology—so essential to the study of medicine—became established in recognized universities in Europe.

The United States soon followed the pattern of European education. Medical schools began to develop their own laboratories. The advantage of hospital affiliation could be seen, and the leading medical schools soon adopted this method of training students.

The number of proprietary schools with widely differing standards of admission and curriculum was apparent to medical leaders. In 1876, the Association of American Medical Colleges consisted of only 22 medical schools out of nearly 150 schools then in existence. This association had its problems and, after a period of inactivity, was reorganized in 1891. It set minimum requirements for admission to membership and soon had 55 schools which qualified.

At that time, medicine did not have the organizational control over its members that it was to exert a few years later. It was necessary to pass legislation controlling licensure requirements; by 1895, nearly every state had its state board of examiners. This was the same procedure optometry followed 25 years later.

In 1904, the American Medical Association established its own Council on Medical Education and Hospitals. There were approximately 160 medical schools of all kinds in existence at this time, and the problem of setting standards of medical education was a serious one. Optometry later faced the same problems when it attempted to make reason out of the large number of its own proprietary schools which had come into existence.

It took the jolt of the Flexner report to bring any semblance of organization to the medical curriculum. The Carnegie Foundation for the Advancement of Teaching surveyed the field of medical education in the United States and Canada. The Foundation's report was prepared by Abraham Flexner and published in 1910. Organized medicine realized its weakness in education and adopted the Flexner report to the extent that many of the weaker schools were unable to continue. It can truly be said that the Flexner report helped change the whole face of health education in the United States.

Much of the same service was rendered the dental profession by the Carnegie Foundation in its report by William J. Gies (1926).

The first optometric colleges were merely an extension of the individual instruction process. These schools often took on the names of their founders. Education was very elementary by present-day standards. Among the first of these courses was one by Spencer Optical Manufacturing Company, which offered a two-week course for $25.00. Most of the actual training in "refraction" was done by the use of the Audemaire Trial Case of Test Lenses. Another prominent course of this time was given by the Julius King Optical Company at its offices in Cleveland, Ohio, and New York City; the Elite Test Case and Optician's Outfit was supplied with this course. The course required a week and, in all probability, existed for the main purpose of teaching the use of optical equipment sold by the company.

One interesting development took place at this time in the training process for eye refraction. Medicine was using the same type of training in optics for its members as was optometry. It was only natural that the two should merge. In 1872, Drs. George W. and J. B. McFatrich organized the Northern Illinois College of Ophthalmology and Otology in Chicago. Classes were given on Sunday mornings and for a while were limited to physicians; for a number of years after 1898, however, refracting opticians took the same courses with physicians. This was to be the start of what was later known as Northern Illinois College of Optometry and finally, the present Illinois College of Optometry.

This same phenomenon, the simultaneous education of both opticians and physicians by an individual, characterized the school, founded by Dr. M. B. Ketchum, that preceded the Los Angeles College of Optometry (Bergin, 1965). Dr. Ketchum, a Canadian by birth, was trained in pharmacy and in medicine. He had practiced and taught general medicine. He also practiced in the field of eye, ear, nose, and throat. At the turn of the century, Ketchum established the Los Angeles School of Ophthalmology and Optometry, of which he was the sole faculty member. His students were physicians and nonmedical men. They studied with Ketchum in his office in Los Angeles. Instruction was informal and individual. The school was incorporated in 1911 and was distinctly a profit-making venture. Ketchum and two other physicians were the stockholders. A number of similar "schools," also individually owned, was operated throughout the United States. In Los Angeles alone, there were three schools, of which one was Ketchum's. The other two had the impressive names of California Eye College, and Southern California College of Optometry and Ophthalmology. These two, operated by physicians M. M. Ring and T. J. Ruddy, and popularly known as the "Ring and

Ruddy" schools, were sold lock, stock, and charters to Ketchum in 1914 for the sum of $200!

This was the commencement of an era which brought the development of many private schools in optometry; at the end of the 1890's and into the early 1900's, over 60 flourished at one time or another. Most of these were proprietary schools and existed mainly as businesses engaged in educating future refractionists, both medical men and optometrists.

The year 1910 was a milestone in optometric education. The first university optometric course was opened at Columbia University as a two-year course. The first-year subjects were trigonometry, physics, theoretic and physiologic optics, and anatomy and physiology of the eye. The second year was devoted to physics, theoretic and practical optics, and physiologic optics and theoretic optometry. Andrew J. Cross and Charles Prentice were among those instrumental in setting up the first curriculum.*

The next 15 years of optometric education saw the development of educational standards throughout the profession. Optometric leaders could see that they must establish their own schools. Optometry was following the lead of the older, established professions in installing its courses of instruction in universities. This process was taking place across the United States. In 1915, a four-year course in applied optics was started at The Ohio State University. This was the first four-year university optometric course granting a degree, which was then Bachelor of Science in Optometry. The school was under the direction of Charles Sheard, Ph.D. Schools were also established at the University of Rochester and the University of California, and, for a brief period, at the University of Illinois.

The establishment of the School of Optometry at the University of California in 1923 was another high mark in optometric education. Members of the California Optometric Association gave $9,000 to finance the first year of the program. In addition to this, the association sponsored a law requiring that part of the annual license fee paid by each registered optometrist would be used to support the optometry course at the state university. This voluntary action of a professional group with a state university was to set a model to be followed by the other universities across the United States as optometry grew.

---

* One gains a greater respect for the phenomenal foresight of such leaders as Prentice and Cross when he recognizes that their establishment of a university curriculum was met with resistance from many proprietors of schools. Bergin (1965) cites the blunt statement of Ketchum in 1914, "There is not enough to optometry to call for two years of nine months each."

During this period of university affiliation, the private schools made their own educational advances. All of them departed eventually from their proprietary organizational setup and developed into non-profit institutions. Klein's school eventually became the Massachusetts College of Optometry; Ketchum's school became the Los Angeles School of Optometry and still later, the Los Angeles College of Optometry. The Pennsylvania College of Optometrists was replaced by the Pennsylvania State College of Optometry under the direction of Albert Fitch. Today it is known as the Pennsylvania College of Optometry. Southern College, started by J. J. Horton as a proprietary school, was purchased by Wilbur Cramer and managed by him and his wife until it was eventually converted to a non-profit institution several years later.

Dr. Albert Fitch was among the first optometric educational leaders to realize that proprietary schools of optometry could not continue to exist. The Pennsylvania State College of Optometry was chartered as a non-profit private college of optometry, the first of its kind.

The state of Pennsylvania has been unique in its support of all professional health schools. In 1899, this state passed a law that resulted in grants to all medical schools of the state to help meet yearly deficits. Since that time, many medical schools in Pennsylvania have functioned as privately controlled schools that develop their own endowments but whose income is supplemented by the state. The Pennsylvania College of Optometry has obtained funds from the state to support the school. This is unique among schools that have no state university affiliation.

The Pennsylvania State College of Optometry pioneered in another area. It was the first college of optometry to grant a degree of Doctor of Optometry. Fitch fought for this achievement for a number of years. His graduation address in June of 1927 expresses his opinion of the need for the doctorate degree in optometry. He said:

> In speaking of degrees, I find a great many who hold erroneous ideas on the subject of college degrees. I am speaking, of course, of the earned degrees and not of the honorary degree.
>
> Today, however, all degrees have an economic value because of the great demand in almost all vocations for highly trained men, and the various degrees are evidence of the completion of so much fundamental training, either special or general.
>
> The physician, perhaps, was the first to realize the true economic value of a degree and adopted the doctorate degree even when he read and studied medicine in another physician's office, much as the lawyer formerly studied law in the office of another lawyer.

Fitch goes on to say that, while all degrees have an economic value, it is only those in the healing arts who use them in this way. He says that this way of belief has become so fixed in the public mind that patients expect this title to be used by their health practitioner.

He concludes this discussion of the doctorate degree with the statement that optometry had both the moral and scholastic right to use this degree. His school had been in existence four years before it received the power to give this degree; a special action of the state legislature was necessary to grant it.

The 15-year period between 1910 and 1925 had indeed been a productive one in optometric education. Many of the proprietary schools were on the way out. The profession had to take control of its education. There were still 30 of these schools in existence and the time for a weeding out process had come.

In January of 1922, the American Optometric Association financed a conference on optometric education. As a result of this conference, many of the optometric schools were eliminated or rated in such a way as to eventually bring about their elimination. Representatives from the International Association of Board of Examiners and the Federation of Optometry Schools met with a member of the Council on Optometric Education of the American Optometric Association. A schedule for grading optometry schools was adopted; the points stressed were the qualifications of the faculty, the administration, supervision, buildings, equipment, and the product of the schools, that is, the records of its students. Preliminary educational requirements of four years of high school education or the equivalent were established. Frederic A. Woll of Columbia prepared syllabuses that served as guide lines for the conference and for the subsequent grading of schools. Action was taken at this conference by concluding: (1) that efforts be made to have the laws of the various states changed to make possible the standardization of optometric education; (2) that all apprenticeship clauses be removed; and (3) that all correspondence courses in optometry be discontinued and that the syllabuses of optometric education as prepared by Dr. Woll serve as guides.

With its guide lines established, optometry made progress. A committee was appointed to survey and inspect the schools for the purpose of accrediting and rating them. Of 30 schools in existence, only 16 met preliminary inspection requirements. The International Association of Boards of Examiners gave six schools an "A" rating, two a "B" rating, and one a "C" rating. The rest of the schools were listed as "unclassified." The requirements for an "A" rating were:

1. The school must be a non-profit institution.

2. It must have adequate teaching staff and administration facilities.

3. Only students with high school training would be admitted.

4. A minimum curriculum of two years was in effect.

5. Subjects as outlined in Dr. Woll's syllabuses must be properly taught.

The "B" rating was reserved for schools that showed intentions of meeting the "A" requirements within a reasonable time. The "C" rated institution needed extensive alteration to qualify. This was a probationary measure to allow the "C" rated school time to qualify by a series of necessary improvements.

Perhaps the most unusual aspect of this meeting was that it was voluntarily instituted by the profession of optometry and carried on without any outside help or subsidy. What the Flexner report accomplished for medicine twenty years previously, and what the Gies report accomplished for dentistry was now achieved for optometry.

The next decade, 1925 to 1935, showed a steady advancement in optometric education. The American Optometric Association appointed a Council on Education to make a three-year study. This council was to take over the work of the International Association of Boards in accrediting and rating the schools. The optometric syllabuses were revised as the length of optometric courses increased. Educational requirements increased to three years and eventually to four years in all accredited schools by 1936.

Another milestone in optometric education was reached in 1936, when the program of graduate work leading to a Ph.D. degree in physiological optics started at The Ohio State University under the direction of Glenn A. Fry. Optometric educators up to then, although truly dedicated teachers, had been recruited from related sciences and disciplines, such as physics, physiology, optics, medicine, and psychology. The optometric profession needed its own heritage if it was to continue to grow as an independent health profession. This meant that career teachers, optometrically oriented research personnel, and trained authors capable of producing optometric literature had to be produced by optometry. The training would have to be at a recognized university where graduate students could be produced; yet the identity of optometry must be maintained if the profession was to benefit. A graduate training program had been a dream of Glenn A. Fry at The Ohio State University for many years. The result of the program he started can now be seen in every school of optometry in the United States.

In the next two decades, 1935 to 1955, optometric education made a steady and mature growth. This era saw the beginning of a curriculum which was truly professional in nature. Several new schools came into existence, and some of the older, weaker ones fell by the wayside.

The College of Optometry at Pacific University was established in 1945. The assets and charter of a former proprietary college, the North Pacific College of Optometry, were transferred to Pacific University. These assets, coupled with the help of the Oregon Optometric Association, brought an optometric educational institution to the Northwest.

Optometric schools were established in Indiana and Texas in 1952. The Indiana Optometric Association followed the pattern of the California organization by donating funds to start the school and by encouraging the state legislature to pass a law requiring each optometrist to pay an additional fee with his annual license renewal fee. These funds go directly to Indiana University marked for support of the department of optometry.

The College of Optometry at the University of Houston was started by a pledge of $100,000 from the optometrists of Texas. Although richly endowed originally, the University of Houston became a state-supported school in 1963. Optometry thus obtained the security of another state-supported institution for its educational program.

The addition of these three university-affiliated schools brought the number of schools to the present-day total of ten.* (See Appendix C.)

With the establishment of optometry schools in independent optometric colleges, in small private universities, and as part of major universities, optometry colleges developed their own character. Over the years, optometry has been taught in independent schools, physics departments, engineering departments, and separate schools within a university. Independent schools, free to develop as they wished, sometimes put more emphasis on physiology and anatomy as contrasted with the emphasis on mathematics and physics in the early university-affiliated schools. The independent colleges often developed their clinical instruction to a high degree. Although clinical training was not lacking in the university-affiliated schools, the emphasis was more on academic than on clinical material. This is no longer true, nor has it been for many years. All of the ten accredited schools have very strong clinical programs, and students receive a great deal of training with patients.

---

* As this book is receiving its final editing, the announcement has been made of the passage by the Alabama legislature of a bill stating the intention of establishing an optometry school at the University of Alabama. This state university-affiliated school will be unique in that it will be located on the campus of the medical center in Birmingham. The School of Optometry will be one of the professional schools on that campus.

The clinics in some schools have been largely non-profit clinics. In other schools, they have been used as a means to help support the academic program of the school.

In spite of minor variations in the curriculum, most optometric colleges have now become quite well standardized. It is hoped, however, that individual differences in schools will always exist to some degree in the electives that are supplied. Interchange of professors has helped to bring on healthy changes in various departments of the optometric institutions.

In the last ten years, optometric education has matured to the present six-year professional course. It has now been standardized in all optometric institutions as a two-year pre-professional course and a four-year optometry curriculum. This type of education—the traditional liberal arts education plus specialized professional education —is now in keeping with the standard education of the older, established professions in the United States. The basic arts and sciences of the first two years of pre-optometry not only prepare the student for the optometric curriculum, but contain enough of the humanities to produce a well-rounded professional man.

Pre-optometry requirements vary somewhat from state to state, depending on the particular requirements of that state. A typical four-year specialized optometric course of the present six-year optometric program is contained in Appendix D.

Standardizing the optometric curriculum as a six-year professional doctorate degree course establishes this minimum requirement at least for the next few years. The optometric trained educator, the high caliber research program of the optometric schools, and more carefully selected students point toward a continuation and improvement of optometry's growth.

One characteristic of the established health professions in the United States is the ultimate disappearance of all independent colleges. In medicine, only a few of the over 150 medical schools are not affiliated with a general university. In dentistry, during the 1960's, the last of the independent colleges, Physicians and Surgeons of San Francisco, became affiliated with the University of the Pacific at Stockton, California; every one of the over 50 dental colleges is now university affiliated. Veterinary medicine is now taught at 20 colleges—all university affiliated. Since optometry to date has followed the process of these other professions, one would expect a decline in the ratio of independent colleges to university-affiliated schools to ensue. However, there are problems peculiar to optometry to be considered.

At this time, there are five university-affiliated colleges and five independent colleges. The classes in the independent colleges are markedly larger than those in the university schools; the latter have traditionally insisted on smaller classes. In the optometry schools which are part of a university, the classes are between 40 and 60 students; classes in independent colleges are often twice this size. Thus, the simple affiliation of the present independent colleges with universities will not solve the optometric manpower problem. Two affiliated schools will be needed for every present independent college.

A second problem is the attitude of political medicine * toward optometry. Once dentistry was established as a profession, cooperation between it and medicine followed. Optometry has not yet been completely accepted as a profession by medicine, despite the fact that it has attained almost complete professionalization by all the criteria of those (like Wilensky) who study the sociology of professionalization. There is, therefore, a fear among optometrists that, if they do not retain some independent colleges owned and controlled within the profession, optometry could be seriously hurt by a concerted drive to have optometry no longer taught at universities.

This fear is not without some foundation. After 40 years of operation, the School of Optometry at Columbia University was discontinued, leaving the New York area devoid of optometric educational institutions. After a few years of affiliation with the University of Southern California, the Los Angeles College of Optometry was reestablished as an independent college in the 1930's; had the charter not been retained, the Southern California area, too, would have been without an optometry school.

The leaders in optometry today are aware that the ultimate step in educational professionalization will be the existence of between 20 and 30 strong optometric colleges, all university affiliated. They have set as an immediate goal the creation of ten new university-affiliated optometric colleges. However, in the interim, the independent schools are being strengthened and are continuing to train optometrists.

An interesting solution to the problem of making the transition without increasing the vulnerability of optometric education has been suggested by the turn of events in New York State. Optometric colleges, in addition to training undergraduates for professional practice, have several other important functions. The clinics of an optometry

---

* The term "political medicine" is used here to differentiate medical organizations and leaders from physicians in general. In most communities, practicing optometrists and practicing physicians enjoy splendid relationships characterized by complete cooperation in the patient's behalf and by mutual respect. Some medical organizations and/or some medical leaders have not exhibited this same degree of cooperation. It must also be noted that some optometric organizations and/or leaders have also reacted at times in a destructive fashion. Although organizations should reflect the thinking of the members, it is nevertheless a fact that group actions have often been hostile while individual actions have been cooperative.

college often serve patients who cannot afford private practitioners; research is carried on at colleges; postgraduate education is usually a major function of optometric colleges. When the optometry college at Columbia University was closed, several of those who had been active in the optometry school founded the Optometric Center of New York. For ten years, this institution has carried on all of the functions of a college of optometry *except* undergraduate education. It has clinics, conducts postgraduate classes, and conducts an ambitious research program. Because the Center plays an important role in making vision care available to those of limited means, it will be discussed in greater detail in Chapter 11, dealing with the problem of making care available to all.

The present independent colleges of optometry may possibly in the future become optometric centers, retaining their charters to teach undergraduates but voluntarily relinquishing this function when it is filled by university-affiliated colleges. These centers would fill important roles in making service available to clinic patients, in research, and in postgraduate education. Most important, however, during the transition period, they would assure the profession of its own teaching institutions if it ever became necessary for the profession again to assume the responsibility for undergraduate education. The role of the independent colleges in supplying manpower for the future is discussed again in Chapter 12.

A review of the past three quarters of a century in optometric education reveals tremendous changes. Starting with on-the-job training, education progressed to a one-week course, then to short courses in proprietary schools usually centering around a single instructor, then to larger proprietary schools, then to independent colleges of high caliber, and finally to the existence of five university-affiliated colleges and five independent colleges. At this time, optometric leaders are cognizant of the final step which must be taken and are proceeding in that direction. That so much has been accomplished in so short a period is truly awesome and bodes well for the future of the optometric profession.

ETHICS AND PROFESSIONAL BEHAVIOR

In ten of the 13 established professions which Wilensky (1964) studied, the adoption of a formal code of ethics came at the end of the process. Such codes, Wilensky describes as "rules to eliminate the unqualified and unscrupulous, rules to reduce internal competition, rules to protect clients and emphasize the service ideal . . ." In optometry, the adoption of a formal code of ethics followed the pattern typical of other professions, occurring "ca. 1935" according to Wilensky.* The well-established professions of law and medicine adopted formal codes of ethics in 1908 and 1912, respectively, about a quarter of a century before optometry.

The control of behavior and ethics, the most recent step in professionalization, is the least nearly complete. Legislation, education, and organization have attained relative stability and completion; personal behavior and ethical standards alone remain in a stage of incomplete development.

Tawney (1920) described the moral basis of professions:

> . . . [a profession] is not simply a collection of individuals who get a living for themselves by the same kind of work. Nor is it merely a group which is organized exclusively for the economic protection of its members, though that is normally among its purposes . . . Its essence is that it assumes certain responsibilities for the competence of it members and the quality of its wares, and that it deliberately prohibits certain kinds of conduct on the ground that, though they may be profitable to the individual, they are calculated to bring into disrepute the organization to which he belongs.

The terms morality, ethics, and professional behavior, although sometimes used interchangeably, imply different concepts. Morality of a professional person or a businessman would include such attributes as trustworthiness, honesty, and integrity. Morality is not the sole property of the professions. Professional people should be moral—but so should business people.

In general usage, ethical and moral behavior are almost synonymous. In the professions, ethics has come to mean the broad guide lines for professional activity. The Code of Ethics of the American Optometric Association, finally adopted by that organization's House of Delegates in 1944, is similar to the codes of other professions. Although this Code has nine separate statements, there are only two major themes: (1) to keep the patient's welfare uppermost at all times, and (2) to see that no person shall lack care regardless of his financial status (See Appendix E). The other seven points may be considered as means of attaining these two goals. Thus, the patient is advised of the need for consultation because it is in his best interest; the patient's records are kept confidential because it is in his best interest; the optometrist obtains education and improves his proficiency to benefit the patient.

The same two broad statements appear in the codes of most pro-

---

* Although Wilensky lists *ca.* 1935 as the date, the official Code of Ethics of the American Optometric Association was not adopted by its House of Delegates until 1944; the Rules of Practice were not adopted by that body until 1950.

fessions, and are a major difference between professions and business or trade. The businessman, one for example who sells clothing, should be as moral as a professional man. He should be honest, should not misrepresent his merchandise, should not cheat his clients. However, he does not accept the responsibility of considering his client's overall welfare. If the client wants a particular suit of clothing, the merchant will sell it to him whether or not he needs it. The difference between *caveat emptor* and professional ethics has been discussed previously, in Chapter 6. The tradesman also does not assume the responsibility for seeing that all persons are clothed; he is concerned only with those who can pay for their clothing.

The professional behavior or rules of professional practice deal with the day-to-day behavior of the professional man. They are the ways in which he will conduct his practice so as to attain his ethical standards. The American Optometric Association Rules of Practice adopted in 1950 contain 14 separate rules; again, however, there are only two major themes which cover all of the rules. (See Appendix F.) These are: (1) the professional man obtains his clients by means other than advertising, and (2) the professional man emphasizes service rather than merchandise.

Regulation of corporate practice and professional competency is primarily for the good of the public. The reason for the regulation of certain aspects of professional behavior, however, is not always so apparent to the layman. Why, for example, should a professional man not run advertisements in the newspaper stating his competency? Why should an optometrist not display spectacles—or a dentist teeth—so that they can be seen by the public? Why should the professional man be so careful in his statements to newspaper reporters regarding his methods of treatment?

Methods of advertising do illustrate some fundamental differences between a business and a profession. The professional man must depend on his competency and ability to work with his patients rather than on his ability to advertise. The time spent in building up advertising campaigns of any kind could much better be spent in developing professional competency. Attracting patients to a doctor's office, by tradition, has been done by word-of-mouth recommendation. Somehow, even to the general public, it seems a bit out of place for a professional man to brag about how good he is, either in paid advertisements or personal interviews. The same philosophy can be applied to the displaying of merchandise by a professional man. The patient should be attracted to the doctor's office by the professional services available and not by the display of fancy spectacle frames, teeth, drugs, or whatever the professional man might be dispensing. This tradition, common to all professions, has been handed down through the years and has influenced much of optometry's legislative activities to control advertising.

The strongest statement of justification for rules of practice in professions and for insisting on adherence to them was made by Chief Justice Hughes in a Supreme Court case involving dentistry.* Justice Hughes noted that "it could not be doubted that practitioners who were not willing to abide by the ethics of their profession often resorted to such advertising methods 'to lure the credulous and ignorant members of the public for the purpose of fleecing them.'"

The Hughes decision further notes that the community is concerned with guarding against "practices which would tend to demoralize the profession by forcing its members into an unseemly rivalry which would enlarge the opportunities of the least scrupulous." He finally notes that the ethics of a profession are "but the consensus of expert opinion as to the necessity of such standards."

In this opinion, three very important aspects of professional behavior are enunciated. First is the fact that rules of practice are "the consensus of expert opinion." It therefore follows that they may change from time to time as the consensus changes. The display of merchandise, for example, so much frowned on today in the health professions, was the accepted pattern of the *ocularii* in ancient Rome (Chapter 3). Proclaiming one's own excellence was accepted behavior at another time in history; it is not now.

The second major point in this Supreme Court decision is the observation that those who do not abide by the rules of their profession invariably break the rules "to fleece the public." There is a constantly recurring argument within the professions whether it is possible for a professional man to display merchandise or to advertise and still treat the individual patient with the greatest degree of honesty and morality. The answer is that it is obviously possible, but it rarely happens. One goes against the consensus of his profession for personal gain; one *might* do so through altruism; but experience throughout the ages has shown that *in fact,* one does not.

The third major point is found in Justice Hughes' phrase, "tend to demoralize the profession" to describe behavior not in accord with accepted rules. This is similar to Tawney's phrase, "bring into disrepute the organization to which he belongs." Implicit in this concept is the fact that the deviant from accepted professional behavior acts in such a fashion as to bring discredit to the majority of the members of his profession. The total effect of his acts is contrary to the public's welfare. This is apparent to today's professionally practicing optometrists who represent the majority of the profession. The deviant be-

* This decision is cited in full in Chapter 8.

havior of the few is often sufficiently blatant to influence the public in a manner not in the public's own interest. The public is best served in the health professions when it seeks advice and service rather than teeth, spectacles, or penicillin shots. The advertising dentist or optometrist counteracts efforts to make the public service-conscious rather than merchandise-conscious.

What constitutes ethical practice is a topic very much alive today—one which has been but incompletely resolved. Yet, even in this area, optometry has made tremendous strides during its history.

From the date of the first optometry laws up to the present, there has been an attempt to control professional behavior through legislation. A good deal has been accomplished. One of the first modes of practice to be legislated out of existence was that of the itinerant optometrist, whose methods were similar to those of the earlier spectacle peddler. Many optometrists in the early days traveled from town to town on regularly scheduled trips. The promotion necessary to sustain this type of practice brought disfavor upon many of these early itinerant practitioners. Many means were used to publicize the arrival in town of an optometrist in this period. Handbills, banners outside of the hotel where the practice was conducted, and even calliopes to herald the visit of the "doctor" were not uncommon. This practice continued in many areas for years longer than necessary. When automobile transportation became more common, the need for itinerant practice of optometry lessened. It was carried on in some areas, however, until legislation was enacted to abolish it. The image created in the public eye by this type of practice was intolerable to organized optometry.

Optometry was still a young profession; with its youth came many growing-pains. The self-consciousness of its members during this time prompted much of the legislation. If optometry was to be accepted as an "established profession," it had to give the appearance of being one to the general public. It did no good for the early optometric professional leader to say, "We are professional men," if throughout his city and state most of the optometrists still appeared to be practicing as merchants or storekeepers. Therefore, it became necessary to legislate the behavior of the optometrist already in practice so that he more closely approached in appearance other professional men. This legislation, of course, was a source of bitterness within the profession; it meant a great change in the accepted way of doing things for many optometrists.

Legislation was necessary to control the itinerant practitioner of this early era. Different problems existed in the larger cities and more densely populated areas. The transition from jewelry stores and optical shops proved to be a much more serious problem. In time, education would eliminate this practice. The rapidly developing profession, however, could not wait until everyone was educated to professional status. Details of professional conduct had to be legislated for a large number of men who had not had a professional background in college.

The first optometry laws were quite simple. First one state, then another, added sections to control professional behavior. A number of states enacted laws limiting the type and amount of advertising; corporate practice was eliminated in many states; branch offices were forbidden in some states in order to end the chain-store type of practice; price advertising was forbidden. These additions were designed to regulate the mode of practice of the less professionally oriented or more commercially minded practitioners.

In some instances, legislation worked quite well. Itinerant optometrists were essentially legislated out of practice, and the more flagrant examples of "bait" advertising were curtailed in most states. At the time laws were being enacted, improved education was having some effect. Optometrists trained in a longer college curriculum were less interested in "off-brand" practice; they had too much of an investment in their education. Also, simultaneously, official organizations of optometrists worked to educate members. A formal code of ethics and rules of practice were adopted.

Ultimately, the state legislatures tired of the representatives of various professions, including optometry, coming to them at each session to demand new rules and regulations. Many of these rules seemed petty to the average layman because their importance to the public was difficult to see. The trend in recent years has been to pass "enabling legislation." It is so termed because it enables the various state boards to regulate the professional conduct of men in practice. State boards having such power can pass any necessary regulations, provided such regulations do not interfere with constitutional rights of individuals.

Although the level of optometric practice has advanced markedly in the period of professionalization, the profession is still plagued by its renegades. In the broad overview, however, the progress has been encouraging. When the American Academy of Optometry was formed in the 1920's, only a handful of optometrists could qualify for membership based on the Academy's rigid standards of practice; today, although the membership is only 1500, about 70 percent of optometrists could qualify insofar as mode of practice is concerned. Optometry has passed through periods of earnest debate on the need for professional behavior. Today there is no longer such debate. The only question is when and how to obtain total conformity to professional rules. Most recently, the American Optometric Association set a target date in the 1970's for the total disappearance of commercial practice.

Optometry followed much the same pattern as the established health professions of medicine and dentistry. The era in which this was accomplished for optometry, however, resulted in a greatly speeded up process. When any process as complex as professionalization takes place rapidly, there are certain to be omissions and regressions. The commercialism which still plagues optometry today is one of these regressions.

All professions have their unscrupulous practitioners. Those violations of the present code of ethics committed by a dentist or a physician are now, for the most part, not so obvious to the public. Wilensky (1964) quotes a definition from Everett Hughes: "The quack is the man who continues through time to please his customers but not his colleagues." Wilensky then continues:

> In any work context where the professional lacks strong colleague constraints, the customer's complaints, real or imaginary, are likely to receive prompt and costly attention; his real problems, if they require professional skill, may be overlooked. In the extreme case, the client-oriented practitioner makes a point of maligning the techniques and motives of his professional competitors and, like the proverbial ambulance chaser, solicits work where no work needs doing.

Optometrists today are beginning to recognize the behavior of the commercialists as regressive. Behavior which might have been acceptable in another time and place is regressive today. The display of merchandise in the window was acceptable in fifth century Rome, but is not in twentieth century United States; advertising was not contrary to guilds or opticianry, but it constitutes abnormal behavior among present-day professional people. With greater recognition of its regressive aspect, commercial practice will continue to diminish. Concomitantly, the level of service that the public receives will continue to improve.

Optometry has arrived at the last steps in the total process of professionalization. Legislation has gone as far as it has in the other professions. Education has reached the point where both the length and content of the curriculum necessary for the terminal doctorate degree have been attained. No further increase in these aspects need be contemplated for a time—only an increase in the number of schools. Organizationally, optometry has the same structure as other professions. Even in the field of personal behavior, 70 percent of the present practitioners meet all requirements. They stress service, rather than merchandise, and abide by rules of practice essentially the same as those for other professions. One differentiation between optometry

and any other of the established professions is the more apparent regressive behavior of some of its practitioners. These, however, amount
to less than a third of the optometrists. The proportion of deviants,
moreover, has continually decreased through the years. The total
emergence of optometry as a profession in the United States awaits
only the disappearance or marked decrease in the number of its own
"failures." Everything in history points to achievement of the final
step within the next decade. Unless there is a reversal in established
trends, it will occur. The emergence of a new profession, a remarkable sociological phenomenon in so short a period, is now all but
complete.

CHAPTER 8

DEVELOPMENT OF HEALTH PROFESSIONS IN THE UNITED STATES AND OF OPTOMETRY IN OTHER COUNTRIES

No profession exists within a vacuum. Therefore, a complete understanding of the professional emergence of optometry requires comparison to the emergence of other health professions in the United States. The professionalization of optometry has been primarily an American phenomenon. Insight into the overall professionalization process may be gained, however, from considering optometric service in other countries of the world, even though in many countries a true profession has not emerged and the service remains a skilled trade.

OTHER PROFESSIONS IN THE UNITED STATES

MEDICINE

Of all the professions, the oldest ones, medicine and law, are the most firmly established. In the health field, medicine is unquestionably the broadest-based profession.

Although only three or four physicians resided in the American colonies before 1700 and practiced a primitive form of service, medicine as a profession emerged during the eighteenth century (Wilensky, 1964). By 1735, there was a local professional association in the colonies; and by 1765, the first training school was established. The first university school which taught medical science was established in 1779. The first state license laws had been enacted at a still earlier date. By 1847, there was a national professional association.

For many years medicine was the only health profession. It is therefore understandable that all other health professions had to establish their field of competency and scope over the protestations of the medical profession. Dentistry, optometry, pharmacy, osteopathy, chiropractic, and clinical psychology each had to defend its claims to professional status in the face of opposition from the already established profession. These several health services have established their claims with varying degrees of success. However, any group which has worked in the field of health has been invariably resisted by the medical profession as a whole because traditional medical thinking has held that medicine embraces the entire field of health. Often, the medical profession recognized the need for a new special aspect of health practice but held that those who practiced it should be technologists acting under medical supervision. Medicine's opposition has been to independence of the other health professions.

Today there are many technologists who practice within the health field and who do so under medical supervision. Laboratory technicians, physiotherapists, and other medical assistants pursue their occupations in this fashion. Other occupational groups, however, have striven for the establishment of independent professional status.

Many books have been written on the history of medicine and it would be of little value to summarize them in the present text. Since historically the pattern for professionalization in the health field has been set by the medical profession, many of the convictions held by the allied health professions, such as optometry, had first been enunciated by medicine. The importance of the doctor-patient relationship and the importance of patients having a free choice of doctors are concepts first established by the medical profession and later adopted by all other health professions.

The problems faced by the medical profession, such as prepayment plans and preventive practices, are also challenges to the other health professions. Society's challenges to optometry and to all other health professions will be discussed in Chapters 11 and 12.

DENTISTRY

The profession of dentistry offers a classical example of a group's development to full independent professional status. It is the profession whose pattern of emergence and development is closest to that of optometry. Dental service, like optometric service, goes back to antiquity. Skulls from the new stone age show evidence that teeth had been extracted, possibly by placing a spear head against the offending tooth and shoving it inward. For a long period in history, and in fact until the second quarter of the nineteenth century, dentistry was practiced in a primitive fashion. There was no dental profession and no formal schooling, but a form of dentistry was practiced. The need for the service—the first requisite of a profession—was clearly present.

Atkinson (1956) has summarized the emergence of the dental profession:

> Until this time (1839), the medical colleges of the United
> States, as of all countries, failed to see the importance of caring for

diseased conditions of the mouth and teeth. Attempts had been made to have chairs established in the various medical colleges of the country for the purpose of providing a foundation not only for the study of teeth but also the mechanical means of improving conditions of the mouth. These all ended in failure because the colleges could not see the importance of such a step. In Baltimore, Dr. Horace Hayden, after much opposition, during the years of 1837–38 succeeded in giving a course of dental instruction to the students of the University of Maryland, and in 1839, finding so little cooperation among the medical profession, Hayden established the Baltimore College of Dental Surgery. This was the first dental school to be founded in the world, and it proved to be such a popular venture that in 1845 the Ohio College of Dentistry was founded in Cincinnati, this being followed in Philadelphia by the establishment of the Pennsylvania College of Dental Surgery and, in 1863, the Philadelphia Dental College. Harvard College, seeing the success of these first schools of dentistry, soon after this time established in Boston its own school, the Harvard Dental College.

Several of the states in 1868 passed laws regarding registration in dentistry as a requisite to taking up practice of the dental profession, but not until 1900 did all the states require a license of those who wished to practice dentistry. It will be seen by this that the United States gave origin to the profession of dentistry as we now know it, and this lead of American dentists has not lost any ground since it was first acquired, as nearly all countries in the world now have dentists of American training who are leaders in this profession. At this time there are few dentists in the United States who have not had at least one year in preliminary college work and three years devoted to practical study and to training on the various steps of mechanical dentistry. The dental courses have now been extended to four years in most of the better schools.

Thus, dentistry, like optometry, followed the sequence outlined by Wilensky (1964) very closely; dentistry and optometry had another similarity. Each group supplied a service which could have been met by the medical profession but which was not. Yet, as each profession emerged, it was actively opposed by medicine. An important difference is that once dentistry emerged, medicine gave up all claim to the dental service; it has not, however, relinquished the practice of the optometric service.

Since dentistry and optometry have followed such similar courses of development, a comparison of the time sequences of each profession is interesting. In the establishment of the first school and in the establishment of the first professional association, optometry was 52 years behind dentistry (Wilensky's data). However, the first university-affiliated school of optometry was established only 43 years after the similar event in dentistry's history, and the first optometry law was enacted only 33 years after the first dental law. Thus, in education and legislation, optometry moved ahead of schedule.

This rapid legislation that furthered the development of optometry as a profession was brought about by many factors. The large number of exempt optometrists admitted to practice necessitated immediate development of state laws to control the activities of these men. The early fathers of optometric legislation had the advantage of being able to study and profit by dentistry's mistakes in many areas of professionalization. The first optometry law passed in New York State, for example, was patterned to quite a large degree on the legislation first introduced by dentistry.

Although optometry was ahead of schedule in legislation and education, it was well behind dentistry's schedule in another area. The first optometric code of ethics came 78 years after dentistry had adopted such a code. Clearly, then, in the area of personal professional behavior, optometry was behind schedule.

Both dentistry and optometry had had much the same problem in trying to control their practitioners. Unlike medicine, optometry and dentistry involved no hospital privileges to be withdrawn as a disciplinary measure for unprofessional behavior. All of the rules on conduct had to be spelled out in dental laws. Dentistry's early battle with its commercial elements provided many guide lines for subsequent optometric legislation. The Semler case, which was fought through local courts and on into the United States Supreme Court, was a keystone in establishing the right of a profession to control its members in all aspects of professional behavior, including advertising.

The Semler case has been important to the professions in their attempts to regulate behavior. Subsequent attitudes have depended on it. Semler, a dentist in Oregon, brought action against the Oregon State Board of Dental Examiners because of the attempts of the board to control his professional activities. The case went through the lower courts before finally being heard by the United States Supreme Court. The following description of the basis for the action is quoted directly from the early court records:

> It appears from the complaint that while plaintiff was engaged in the practice of dentistry he (1) employed the services of advertising solicitors; (2) used as advertising mediums large display signs and glaring light signs showing illustrations of a tooth, teeth and bridge work; and (3) advertised in the daily newspapers as follows: (a) That he had acquired superior skill and ability and knowledge in the practice of dentistry and his ability to perform the professional services of dentistry in a superior manner; (b) the prices that he would charge for various services to be rendered; (c) that he makes examinations for prospective patients without making any charge therefor; (d) that he guarantees all dental work performed by him; and (e) that dental operations are performed painlessly.

Plaintiff alleges in substance that by reason of the methods of advertising above mentioned he has acquired a large and lucrative practice; that he and his employed assistants—who are licensed practitioners and working under his supervision—have treated daily at his offices approximately 150 patients; and that on account of such volume of business he has been enabled to render service to his patients at a much lower price than charged by most practitioners. Plaintiff also alleges that all of his advertisements were made in good faith and honestly express his "intention of carrying out each and every of the representations contained therein." It is also averred that if the above statutory provisions are enforced the plaintiff will sustain irreparable loss and injury.

Plaintiff alleges as conclusions of law that the above portion of chapter 166, Laws of Oregon for 1933, is unconstitutional and void because it (1) deprives him of property without due process of law; (2) impairs the obligation of contracts; (3) constitutes class legislation; (4) is so indefinite and uncertain as to be incapable of enforcement; and (5) denies to him equal protection of the law.

The history of legislation in the various states regulating the conduct of practitioners in the learned professions—law, medicine, and dentistry—discloses a marked tendency in recent years to enact more stringent regulations, that the standards of these professions be raised and the ignorant, gullible members of the public be protected from quacks and charlatans who spurn the ethics of their profession and thrive by flamboyant methods of advertising and "high powered salesmanship."

Semler lost this case in the State of Oregon and appealed to the United States Supreme Court. Chief Justice Hughes delivered the opinion of the court. This case established beyond any doubt the legal right of a profession through its state board to control its members. Justice Hughes grasped the importance of regulating professional behavior, especially advertising. In his opinions, he stated:

This case presents the question of the validity of a statute of the state of Oregon, enacted in 1933, relating to the conduct of dentists. Oregon Laws 1933, c. 166, p. 208. Previous legislation had provided for the revocation of licenses for unprofessional conduct, which, as then defined, included advertising of an untruthful and misleading nature. The Act of 1933 amended the definition so as to provide the following additional grounds for revocation: "advertising professional superiority or the performance of professional services in a superior manner; advertising prices for professional service; advertising by means of large display, glaring light signs, or containing as a part thereof the representation of a tooth, teeth, bridge work or any portion of the human head; employing or making use of advertising solicitors or free publicity press agents; or advertising any free dental work, or free examination; or advertising to guarantee any dental service, or to perform any dental operation painlessly." Laws 1933, p. 210, §2 . . .

(3) The question is whether the challenged restrictions amount to an arbitrary interference with liberty and property and thus violate the requirement of due process of law. That the state may regulate the practice of dentistry, prescribing the qualifications that are reasonably necessary, and to that end may require licenses and establish supervision by an administrative board, is not open to dispute . . .

(4) Recognizing state power as to such matters, appellant insists that the statute in question goes too far because it prohibits advertising of the described character, although it may be truthful. He contends that the superiority he advertises exists in fact, that by his methods he is able to offer low prices and to render a beneficial public service contributing to the comfort and happiness of a large number of persons.

We do not doubt the authority of the state to estimate the baleful effects of such methods and to put a stop to them. The legislature was not dealing with traders in commodities, but with the vital interest of public health, and with a profession treating bodily ills and demanding different standards of conduct from those which are traditional in the competition of the market place. The community is concerned with the maintenance of professional standards which will insure not only competency in individual practitioners, but protection against those who would prey upon a public peculiarly susceptible to imposition through alluring promises of physical relief. And the community is concerned in providing safeguards not only against deception, but against practice which would tend to demoralize the profession by forcing its members into an unseemly rivalry which would enlarge the opportunities of the least scrupulous. What is generally called the "ethics" of the profession is but the consensus of expert opinion as to the necessity of such standards.

It is no answer to say, as regards appellant's claim of right to advertise his "professional superiority" or his "performance of professional services in a superior manner," that he is telling the truth. In framing its policy the legislature was not bound to provide for determinations of the relative proficiency of particular practitioners. The legislature was entitled to consider the general effects of the practices which it described, and if these effects were injurious in facilitating unwarranted and misleading claims, to counteract them by a general rule even though in particular instances there might be no actual deception or misstatement.

The state court defined the policy of the statute. The court said that while, in itself, there was nothing harmful in merely advertising prices for dental work or in displaying glaring signs illustrating teeth and bridge work, it could not be doubted that practitioners who were not willing to abide by the ethics of their profession often resorted to such advertising methods "to lure the credulous and ignorant members of the public to their offices for the purpose of fleecing them." The legislature was aiming at "bait advertising." "Inducing patronage," said the court, "by representations of 'painless dentistry,' 'professional superiority,' 'free examinations,' and 'guaranteed' dental work" was, as a general rule, "the practice of the charlatan and the quack to entice the public."

This decision of the United States Supreme Court in 1935 had far-reaching effects on all professional behavior. Added impetus was given to state professional organizations in all professions to pass legislation to standardize the conduct of their members. Optometry was to find this approach particularly effective in speeding up the progress of professionalization.

State boards could regulate such behavior as newspaper, radio, and television advertising, office cleanliness and appearance, office location, the keeping of patients' records, equipment required for minimum optometric examinations, the minimum examination procedures, the type of education professional men should pursue after graduation, and virtually every aspect of professional life. Legislation of this sort was not passed without many battles.

Not all behavior, however, could be controlled by legislation. The most flagrant offenses in both dentistry and optometry were controlled by legislation. But when behavioral problems were more equivocal, some recalcitrant member of the group would find a way to circumvent a law as soon as it was passed. Today, more and more emphasis is being placed on the societal relationships of the members of the group. The few dentists who to this day practice in a manner not calculated to bring credit upon the group as a whole are shunned and disregarded by the organized profession. In optometry, the group of deviants is larger but is rapidly diminishing in size.

PHARMACY

Establishment of any independent profession in the health care field was opposed at the time of its emergence by medicine and to some extent still is. Organized medicine believes that most of the health professions should be composed of technicians under the control of medicine rather than independent professional groups. Even as ancient an occupation as pharmacy, in its recent struggle toward professionalism, has been opposed by some physicians. This is difficult to understand, inasmuch as professional pharmacy recognizes the physician as the source of all prescriptions; until a prescription is written, most potent drugs cannot be released. The professional pharmacist regards himself as the legal custodian of *all* drugs. Professionalization of this custodial power could only result in improved health care for all people. Many minor physical ills could be better handled by a professional pharmacist's recommendations than by those of a "store manager" druggist.

Pharmacy's drive toward professionalization offers an interesting view of a group of dedicated men trying to solve what dentistry and optometry did many years ago. Plans to professionalize the appearance of the pharmacy have been offered (American Pharmaceutical

Association, 1966) . The trend is toward pharmaceutical centers. Other recommendations include the family record system, health education centers, the absence of displayed products, and the recommended use of a professional fee method to determine charges.

One of professional pharmacy's goals is to separate the practice of pharmacy from the commercial surroundings of the drug store that stocks all items from hair pins to lawn furniture. This is to be replaced by a pharmaceutical center, which would be similar to the professional offices of the dentist, optometrist, or physician. The optometrist need only look at the present appearance of pharmacy dispensaries in most localities to realize how far optometry has professionalized.

White (1965) in the *Journal of the American Pharmaceutical Association* graphically portrays the problem of converting from a store atmosphere and commercial surroundings to a professional office or center. It took him four years by a series of planned stages to eliminate the commercialism of a store. He emphasized professional services and developed personal relationships with his clients. He eliminated all evidence of commercialism by removing displays and merchandise from public view.

Pharmacy in the past, both in the United States and in many foreign countries, has been much more professional in appearance than it is at present. The recent drive toward professionalism, however, is a somewhat different approach. Present-day pioneers in this struggle wish to enlarge the scope of pharmacy to include *regulation* of all professional behavior as well as *expansion* of the professional responsibility in the release of many non-potent medications to patients. According to this concept, well-trained professional pharmacists can assume responsibility for certain treatments much better than the drug store managers of the past; a professional atmosphere is almost a necessity in this respect.

White, one of the present leaders in the process of professionalization of pharmacy, goes on to say, "Our guiding rule in all of our planning has been to ask if a physician or an attorney would do this in his practice. If the answers were negative we dropped the idea." * He changed his sign to a small dignified colonial sign, discarded the awning on his store, and hung an attractive drape inside. No newspaper, radio, or television advertising was engaged in, since it "would

---

* This method of resolving questions of professional behavior by emulating other well established professions is quite common. The American Academy of Optometry, faced with the problem of judging behavior which was professional in one sector of the country but considered unprofessional in other areas used the same yardstick that White used in pharmacy. Optometric professional behavior is considered to be professional by the Academy if physicians and dentists in the same locale engage in the same behavior.

destroy our professional image." The externals are important but they are still secondary. The primary element is the "personal professional relationship between the pharmacist and his patient based on the sincere interest of the pharmacist in the health and welfare of his patient and his family."

The concept of the pharmaceutical center is surely a step in the direction of professionalization. The development of a fee system rather than a mark-up on drugs, a code of ethics, and more professional training in pharmacy colleges are the next steps. Obviously, pharmacy has a long way to go for complete professional recognition.

Pharmacy will find, as optometry did before it, that legislation will be necessary to accomplish many of its aims. The struggle will be a hard one until many more professional centers are voluntarily established. Great opposition will come from the large employers of pharmacists. They will not want to lose the obvious financial gain effected by the management of the present-day drug-and-variety-store combination. Pharmacy will probably exist as part business and part profession for many years to come. The legislatures will help the professional adherents when legislators are convinced that the more stringent regulations are primarily for the good of the public; but legislatures need many more examples of successful professional pharmacists before they will feel justified in regulating any group with the strictness used by a profession to attempt to regulate its members.

CHIROPRACTIC

Unlike optometry and dentistry, each of which deals with only one part of the human organism, chiropractic deals with the entire organism, as does medicine. The difference between established medical practice and chiropractic lies in the approach to disease rather than in specialization in specific organ systems or areas of the body.

Chiropractic is primarily an American phenomenon. It has attained all the milestones of professionalization but one. Failure to attain this one criterion, however, has seriously militated against the acceptance of this vocation as a true profession. No university has had an affiliated school of chiropractic. This vocation has been taught at independent colleges only.

Chiropractic has two basic tenets which differ from accepted medical thinking. One of these is the emphasis on physiotherapy in the treatment of patients. The second is a difference in concept of the nature of disease. Chiropractors tend to attribute many diseases to abnormalities of the spine. The latter view has been found unacceptable at an academic level. This rejection accounts, in part at least, for the fact that chiropractic never has been integrated into traditional higher education. Thus, chiropractic has failed to attain professionalization in the United States because it has failed to gain university recognition; it has failed to gain this recognition because the body of knowledge on which the science is based is not acceptable to the academic community.

OSTEOPATHY

The vocation of osteopathy has in common with chiropractic its sphere of interest in the entire human organism and an interest in physiotherapy. The similarity ends here, however, for the basic body of knowledge on which osteopathy has been based is the same as that on which medical practice rests. Osteopathy has attained all of the steps of professionalization except the integration of its education with traditional higher education in universities.

Osteopathic education, although not incorporated into any university, has been recognized for its excellence. Nonetheless, the lack of educational acceptance has hampered the osteopathic profession. In 1964 in one large state, California, a pattern was established which may well mark the end of osteopathy as an independent health profession. By law, the osteopathic state board was terminated, thereby preventing the licensing of new osteopaths. Simultaneously, all osteopaths who chose to do so were taken in under the medical board and permitted to use the M.D. degree rather than the D.O. As a result, in California osteopathy has been assimilated by medicine; its schools, hospitals, and practitioners are being incorporated into medical organizations.

If nothing else, the problems encountered by the two paramedical vocations of chiropractic and osteopathy serve as an object lesson to other groups. The two basic weaknesses of these vocations are: (1) the total overlap in scope with established medicine, and (2) the lack of integration with the university system of education. These two phenomena have been sufficient to keep one vocation (chiropractic) from full emergence and acceptance as a profession and to lead to assimilation of the other vocation (osteopathy) by medicine. These two weaknesses have hampered these vocations, despite the fact that osteopaths in every respect have been as capable and as dedicated as any group of paramedical practitioners. It is clear that in order for a vocation to emerge as a totally accepted profession in the United States, it must meet every one of the criteria of professionalization—regardless of how much its existence may be justified.

CLINICAL PSYCHOLOGY

Clinical psychology is an occupation which is emerging rapidly as a health profession. The subject matter of this field has recognized validity, and psychology has long been a subject taught in universities throughout the United States and Europe. Unlike the other health professions, clinical psychology never had to depend on independent colleges to teach the occupation; it grew out of the university curriculum. For many clinical psychologists, the terminal degree is the Ph.D., recognized academically as the highest earned degree.

A competing medical specialty does exist in the form of psychiatry. Yet clinical psychologists seem to be attaining complete professionalization in a very brief period of time. Magraw (1966) discusses the overlap between clinical psychology and psychiatry and offers an explanation for the rapid rise of the former:

> Clinical psychologists have made particularly rapid progress toward professional acceptance in comparison to other groups. The length of their training, the fact that they had doctors' degrees (Ph.D.'s), the fact that their direct competition with physicians was restricted to psychiatrists (at that time a low status specialty), and that they were predominantly males may explain their relatively rapid acceptance in comparison to other health professions.

Another factor which undoubtedly has contributed to the rapid progress of clinical psychology is the absence within the group of commercial deviants.

Summary of Other Professions in the United States

In a study of the status of the various independent health groups in the United States, two aspects stand out as having the greatest importance in determining the degree of acceptance as professions. First is the acceptance by the academic community. Complete emergence as a profession seems to depend on integration into the nation's universities.

The second important aspect in determining the successful establishment of a health occupation as an independent health profession is the degree of overlap with medical practice. Chiropractic and osteopathy, essentially in competition with all of medicine, have had the greatest obstacles to overcome. When the lack of university affiliation is added, the chances for success of these two groups become very small. Dentistry, faced with no competing medical specialty, has attained independent professional status. Clinical psychology, as noted by Magraw (1966), was fortunate in that it competed with a "low status" medical group. The future relationship of optometry to established medical practice will be discussed in Chapter 12.

The effect which social trends in health care will exert on the health professions will be of considerable importance and may change existing patterns leading to professional success. Up to the present, however, the acceptance of independent health professions has been clearly most affected by education and by the degree of overlap with existing medical practice.

THE OPTOMETRIC SERVICE IN OTHER COUNTRIES

During the present century, optometry in the United States developed from a trade into an independent health profession (Chapters 6 and 7). In few other countries, however, has optometry reached this same status; in most other countries, optometry is still practiced as a skilled trade, and in many areas there is no optometry at all. Optometry has not evolved to quite so high a form in any other part of the world as it has in the United States.

No useful purpose would be served by listing each country and the form in which its optometrists practice. But for illustrative purposes, the broad categories of type of service will be described as they apply in several countries. It is not the purpose of the present chapter to regard with chauvinism the lesser development of optometry in foreign countries; rather it is our purpose to understand optometry in the United States better by noting how it is practiced in other areas.

In various countries of the world, some evolution toward an optometric profession can be seen. The range extends from nations where there is little optometric service or evidence of professionalization to the United States, where a profession has clearly emerged and become established. Four broad categories within this range will be considered: (1) underdeveloped nations: (2) nations with no optometric profession; (3) nations with optometrists but no profession yet established; and (4) the English-speaking nations in which an optometric profession has definitely emerged.

Underdeveloped Nations

A large majority of the world's population lives in underdeveloped countries. Two major characteristics of such countries (aside from the obvious poverty of the people) are illiteracy * and lack of industrialization. Since the development of optometry goes hand-in-hand with literacy and industrialization, optometry in such countries might be expected to be very primitive. In countries where literacy is low and where agriculture is primitive, there is little need for sophisticated ophthalmic care. Just as there was less need for the optometric service in earlier times in Europe and the United States (Chapter 1), so today there is still little need for optometry in many countries.

---

* In 1966, 40 percent of the people of the world were illiterate (*Britannica Book of the Year*, 1966). The figure is as high as 93 percent in Egypt, 77 percent in India, and 82 percent in Burma (*Encyclopaedia Britannica*, 1958).

The effects of minor refractive errors are of no great concern to those who eke out a bare subsistence through primitive agriculture.

In many formerly underdeveloped countries, industrialization is advancing rapidly. In such countries, changes in optometry are occurring simultaneously. When farming with a pointed stick or an ox-drawn plow gives way to farming with tractors and complex machinery, better vision is needed. Adjusting the carburetor or reading the book of instructions on how to operate the tractor is more demanding of visual accuracy. As underdeveloped nations emerge, so optometry as a profession begins to emerge in these areas.

In many large underdeveloped countries, the only visual service is found in larger cities. Unlike the United States, where optometrists practice even in small communities, these nations offer no service in moderately sized towns and cities. Even in the larger cities of the underdeveloped nations, there is little legal control of ophthalmic practice; anyone who wishes to do so may set up shop and sell spectacles, make spectacles, or test vision. In parts of the Middle East where much of the retail business is conducted in outdoor market places, a native optician with a primitive grinding stone and a stock of lenses and frames (sometimes of American manufacture) may be found conducting his business in the open air much as did a peddler in eighteenth century Europe or the United States. These same cities, however, may have several well trained optometrists practicing professionally. This lack of uniformity of service within metropolitan areas and between metropolitan areas and rural areas is one major difference between optometry in the United States and optometry in many of the emerging nations. In the United States, the quality of the service is far more homogeneous; the optometrist in a small town is as well trained and offers the same high quality of service as the optometrist in the city.

India is a typical example of an underdeveloped nation. One fifth of the total population of the world lives there. In the cities of India, one finds optometrists who have been trained abroad and who practice in a highly professional manner side by side with those who practice in a very primitive fashion. Braff (1965) has stated:

> Requirements for calling oneself an optician or optometrist in India are hardly any. There are qualified and unqualified opticians and there is no license required to open an optician shop. [There are] qualified opticians and optometrists in India but . . . their number is not very many.
>
> Some of the . . . offices were rather nice, being clean and containing relatively modern equipment. . . . Many other "offices" were rather dirty places with antiquated equipment. . . . I remember seeing a place in Old Delhi with an optician and an aide, both

in pajamas (the Indian dress of those without much money) doing a "refraction" in a hovel which looked as though it had been bombed many years ago and had never been cleaned up.

The wide divergence of types of practice in India has also been described by Dastoor (1966). Some areas of the country are served by free eye camps serviced by mobile units. In these units, surgeons perform eye surgery; some refractive services may also be performed. Dastoor also mentions eyeglass banks in various parts of the country. Spectacles donated locally or by people from other countries are sorted by technicians and stored for later distribution.

A person in India who requires optometric service may obtain it in any one of several ways. He may obtain it from a well trained optometrist who practices much like his colleagues in the United States. He may obtain the service from a poorly trained ophthalmic optician who tests vision with test types and trial lenses. He may obtain the service from a traveling mobile unit with operators who may be quite well trained. He may obtain a pair of spectacles of approximately the required strength from an eyeglass bank. Most likely, he does not obtain any service and lives with his visual anomaly, as most people have done for thousands of years.

In Colombia, South America, the level of optometric practice in large cities like Bogotá is not greatly different from that in the United States; in the smaller towns and back country, however, there is little or no optometric service. The optometric service received by a resident of Bogotá, Colombia, and a resident of New York City is not greatly different, but there is a vast difference in the service available to a Colombian who lives a hundred miles from Bogotá and the service available to the upstate New Yorker. In the former locale, there is little or no optometric service; in the latter, the service is like that in the city.

A major difference between optometric service in an underdeveloped country and that in the United States is the degree of control of standards and the uniformity of the service. Another very significant difference is the availability of the service to the population. In Colombia, for example, there is one optometrist for about every 100,000 persons. This is about one eighth the ratio in the United States. Even correcting for the fact that literate persons are more apt to need or demand the service than illiterates, the number of optometrists in Colombia per potential users of the service is one fourth that in the United States.

In countries like India or Colombia, two things stand out insofar as the optometric service is concerned:

1. A high quality of service, not unlike that in the United States,

is available, but only in large cities and only to a small percentage of the population.

2. There are few laws governing practice; therefore, an inferior type of service is supplied in many areas by peddlers, ill-trained opticians, and others.

NATIONS WITH NO OPTOMETRIC PROFESSION

In some countries of the world, the optometric service is performed only by physicians. The largest country with such a system is the Soviet Union.* There are no optometrists in the Soviet Union. In the United States, optometry is an *independent* health profession. In the Soviet Union, no profession is independent, and the absence of optometry is not as surprising as it might at first appear. Training health personnel and administering health services are government functions.

The Soviet student who wishes to enter the health service professions attends medical college for six years. During four of these years, all students take the same basic course. The last two years are devoted to specialization. The eye practitioner learns about his field during the last two years; the dentist learns his specialty during this period. Thus, all health practitioners, including dentists and eye practitioners, take the same four-year basic biological-medical course and two years of specialization. Upon graduation, the new doctor usually works in a polyclinic, the basic public health facility which serves partly in a screening capacity.

After he has served for five years in the polyclinic, the Soviet eye doctor can pursue further studies and advance to a hospital post, where he will practice eye medicine and eye surgery. Thus, apprenticeship, training, and limited practice are combined. The same system is used in other branches of health practice, and the system of training doctors is integrated into the system of supplying health care. The doctor during his career passes through different steps; the patient seeking care goes through the same steps. A patient with an eye problem visits the polyclinic first. If he requires minor medical care or refraction, he is given this care at the polyclinic; if the problem is more complex, he is referred to the hospital. At the hospital, the more complex care is given by a doctor who has completed his years at the polyclinic and has, by further study, advanced to a hospital post.

Many people receive optometric service in the Soviet Union,

---

* The description of the optometric service in the Soviet Union is from Eglin (1966–1967) . The present authors have discussed the Soviet optometric service with Eglin, whose visit to the Soviet Union was under a professional information exchange program, The Citizen Exchange Corps, through which American volunteers in the program meet individual Russians who are their counterparts in occupation.

since all persons can attend the polyclinic as a matter of governmental procedure; the service is free. Spectacles are obtained from an optical shop at a reasonable price. Eglin (1966–1967) describes a visit to such a shop. There were two signs in the waiting room. One announced which lenses were available on that date; the other announced which lenses already in frames were available. These were all spherical corrections; cylindrical lenses must be ordered from the factory and cost about three times as much as spherical lenses. The previously framed lenses were of equal power for each eye. These ready-made spectacles, therefore, are similar to those sold across the counter in a seventeenth century English haberdashery shop, in a twentieth century general merchandise store in the United States, or by a sixteenth century European peddler. The difference is that the Russian receives a test of his vision at the polyclinic and knows specifically which lens power he is to seek. However, such refinements as small degrees of difference between the power required by the two eyes, small degrees of cylinder, centering of the lenses, correct facial fitting of the frame, and small degrees of prism are all as absent for the Soviet patient as for the seventeenth century English patient.*

A comparison between health care in the Soviet Union and in the United States is interesting. Although in the Soviet Union there is no optometric profession *per se,* there is also no independent dental profession. The eye doctor who completes the six-year course and practices in the polyclinic is the counterpart of the American optometrist. His six-year training program is probably not greatly different from the six-year training program of the American optometrist. The scope of his practice is not greatly different. He treats some minor eye pathology which the American optometrist does not; but unlike his American counterpart, he does not refract children. † Optometry does not exist as an independent profession more because of the nature of Soviet governmental structure than because of a difference in the need for the service.

The Soviet doctor who has completed his five years in the polyclinic and has pursued further studies advances to the hospital. There he learns and practices eye medicine and eye surgery. This interesting

* In the final two chapters of this book, we shall deal with the challenge of the present period: how to make optometric service available to all people *and* not impair its quality. Clearly, the Russians have met half of the challenge: the service is available to all Soviet citizens. Equally clearly, they have not met the second half of the challenge; optometric service is not equal in quality to that offered in the United States.

† In several European countries, including France, optometrists are forbidden to examine children's vision. That function is reserved for eye physicians. The Soviet eye physician who works in the polyclinic is similarly restricted; only the specialist in the hospital may examine children.

system is on rare occasions followed in the United States. Sometimes an optometrist, after practicing a few years, obtains further schooling and becomes an ophthalmologist. In the Soviet Union, however, this is the rule rather than the exception. After practicing optometry for five years in Russia and then by further schooling and study, one may become an ophthalmologist. Such a system is calculated to avoid duplication or unnecessary training. The American optometrist who decides to become an eye physician must take many years of additional basic science and general medical courses; the Russian takes only those additional courses that pertain directly to his field.

The major conceptual fallacy, however, of the Soviet system is the basic assumption that the skills required for optometry and for eye medicine are similar. This is far from the truth. The practice of ophthalmology is *not* a higher form of optometric practice; it is a different profession, requiring different interests, skills, and approaches. Lack of recognition of this fact more than anything else accounts for the relatively unsophisticated type of optometric service offered in the Soviet Union.

The Soviet Union is the only *large* country in the world with no independent optometric profession. There is probably no one reason for this phenomenon other than the fact that optometry was within the sphere of medicine at the time the Soviet government took control of all education. In lacking independence, optometry is no different from the other health specialties within the Soviet Union.

Several smaller countries also have no optometric profession. These are usually poor countries in which optometric service is supplied by medical eye practitioners. In Greece (Magoulas, 1966), where 30 percent of the 8.5 million people are illiterate and most are engaged in agriculture, there is not a great need for optometric service. Despite the fact that there are no vision-testing opticians in Greece, contact lenses are, nonetheless, fitted by opticians.* In Greece, as in other poorer nations, what service is offered is concentrated in the larger cities. The ten opticians who fit contact lenses are all located in Athens, the capital city (Magoulas, 1966).

Israel, a small country with a population of about two million, is of interest optometrically because it is an exception to several rules. There are very few optometrists (about 25), and yet Israel is *not* a

---

* The view held in countries like Greece is somewhat difficult for an American optometrist to understand. In these countries, optometrists (opticians) are not permitted to examine the eyes, since this is deemed to be a part of medical practice. Yet opticians *do* fit contact lenses. The American optometrist would argue that there is far more potential danger to the patient from contact lenses which rest directly on the eye for long periods of time than there is in a pair of conventional spectacles. Spain (Tato, 1966) is another country in which opticians do no sight-testing but do fit contact lenses.

country of high illiteracy. It is one of the few countries in the world in which the number of medical men performing optometric service far exceeds the number of optometrists. There are six ophthalmologists in Israel for every optometrist. The ratio of physicians per capita is the highest in the world (one to 430), according to Raphael (1966). Public medical services in Israel also run contrary to common patterns. In Europe and America, public medicine has evolved to fill the gaps left by private medical services; in Israel, the state from its beginnings planned for medical services (Raphael, 1966).

There are no laws governing the practice of optometry in Israel, and the 25 optometrists who do practice have been trained in Europe or the United States. Raphael (1966) attributes the lack of controlling legislation to the small number of optometrists. He points out that ". . . no government is likely to legislate for such a small number of optometrists in the midst of strong medical opposition." The majority of the optometrists practice in hospitals or clinics, and only a few have any private practice at all.

Although the status of optometry in Israel seems to run counter to several general observations, it does demonstrate a phenomenon of which American optometrists are aware. The profession, as well as the public it serves, is very much dependent on the supply of optometric manpower. Since American optometrists are highly cognizant of this fact, they have worked diligently for many years to increase the ranks of optometrists. The situation in Israel tends to confirm the belief that development of an optometric profession can be hindered by insufficient manpower.*

Countries like the Soviet Union or Israel, in which there is no optometric profession but in which the optometric service is offered to a literate populace by medical practitioners, are countries in which the health needs are met by government. Furthermore, this was true *before* an optometric profession as such developed. In England, there is a national health plan, but there is also a strong optometric profession that had developed *before* the government entered into the health field. But in the Soviet Union and Israel, the governments had planned to supply health services before an optometric profession had developed in their countries. It seems quite obvious that the optometric profession developed as strongly as it did in the United States because of the climate of "free enterprise."

As has been noted in earlier chapters, optometry developed because an unfulfilled need existed—that is, medicine was not supplying the needed service. The need alone would not have been sufficient, however, had the climate for the development of a competing

* For a discussion of optometry's future manpower needs and plans, see Chapter 12.

independent profession not also existed. A new independent profession can develop to compete with an existing independent profession, but there is far less likelihood that a new independent profession will develop if it must compete with an existing profession which has the support of the state.*

NATIONS WITH OPTOMETRISTS BUT WITHOUT AN OPTOMETRIC PROFESSION

Spectacles and the science of optics as it applies to the optometric service were developed in Europe. For many years, the optometric service was supplied in Europe by guild spectaclemakers—the direct antecedents of the modern optometrist (Chapters 4 and 5). Today, continental Europe (exclusive of the Soviet Union) has an area and population less than those of the United States, but it has over 25 different countries, each differing with respect to the status of the optometric profession. A range of degrees of professionalization of optometry exists not only throughout the world, but also within continental Europe. In Greece, as noted earlier, there is no optometric profession; in Switzerland or Denmark, many optometrists practice on almost the same high level as optometrists in the United States. Between these two degrees, there are as many subtle differences in development of the profession as there are countries.

Spectacles were manufactured in many of the countries of Europe by the fifteenth century. The guild opticians who made spectacles (Chapter 4) in these countries became dispensing opticians. Many countries of Europe arrived at the same situation as prevailed in the United States or Great Britain at the turn of the century. In these two countries, a profession of sight-testing opticians evolved; in many continental countries, it did not. In France today, opticians both dispense spectacles prescribed by physicians *and* do some sight testing. The optometrist, if he can be called that, is an optician *and* optometrist.

Giles (1966) offered the opinion that the stronger the influence of the guilds, the less chance there was for an optometric profession to evolve. He attributed the failure of a profession to evolve in many continental European countries to strong guild influences; the emergence of a profession in the United States and in the other English-speaking countries, on the other hand, is attributed by him to the weakness of the guild system in these countries. A second factor, ac-

---

* The reader cannot help but have observed the anomalous position taken by some American medical politicians whose two pet "hates" are the independent paramedical professions and state control. They desire the total control of all health fields which medicine has in state-controlled plans, but they do not want state interference. The "free enterprise" whose virtues they extoll is the one thing that has made independent paramedical professions possible.

cording to Giles, is that "the dispensing optician . . . is able purely by supplying spectacles to prescriptions to make as much or even more money than the optician who carries on the combined functions of refraction and dispensing." Backman (1965) arrived at a similar conclusion. He stated:

> The most disappointing impression of optometry in France is that opticians are satisfied with their dispensing role and are not at all interested in developing their refractive techniques out of fear of losing the prescriptions sent to them by ophthalmologists.

In many European countries, the opticians do no testing of vision. In addition to the Soviet Union and Greece, this is true in Czechoslovakia, Portugal, Spain, and Austria (Backman, 1965). In several countries, opticians test vision *and* fill ophthalmic prescriptions (making more money on the latter practice), but are restricted in the type of examination they can perform. In France, Finland, Sweden, Poland, Holland, and Belgium (Backman, 1965), the optician may test vision by subjective means (Chapter 2) but may not use a retinoscope or ophthalmoscope. The use of these instruments is considered to be part of the practice of medicine.

In France, the optician may not supply spectacles for anyone under the age of 16 without a physician's prescription; a similar restriction is placed on the eye physician in the polyclinic in the Soviet Union. In Italy, the optician may test vision and prescribe lenses for presbyopia and for myopia of less than 4.00 D., but may not prescribe for hypermetropia, astigmatism, or aphakia. Backman (1965) questions how the Italian optician is expected to know what is wrong with a patient *before* he examines him. Nonetheless, the Italian optician may examine a patient only if the patient has certain anomalies.

Clearly, there is some optometric occupation, but no profession in these countries. The status of the optician in these countries today is not unlike that of the American or British optician at the turn of the century. The optometric profession simply has not evolved beyond this point. The lack of development is attributed to: (1) strong medical opposition; (2) the strong guild system and tradition; and (3) the optician's dependence on income from dispensing spectacles for physicians.

In a few European countries such as West Germany, Switzerland, Yugoslavia, and Denmark, an optometric profession is evolving but has not reached the stage of professionalism found in the United States or Great Britain.

The impetus in most European countries to develop an optometric profession by teaching opticians to do vision testing usually depends on German or English influences. Schools for refraction are available in these two European countries only. In Germany, Denmark, Switzerland, and Yugoslavia, the optometric examination is conducted by opticians. In Germany (Gunkel, 1966), Switzerland (Lienberger, 1966), and Denmark (Nielsen, 1965), the state health plan will not pay for an eye examination when it is performed by an optometrist. State health plans cover a large number of patients. The optometric profession, therefore, has not attained any degree of security in these countries.

Nielsen (1965) describes an interesting situation in Denmark. Outside Copenhagen there are only 40 ophthalmologists to care for over three million people. Since this is clearly impossible, the "Health Scheme" does pay optometrists for the spectacles which they prescribe and supply, even though the law states that it will do so only if the prescription is written by a physician. In Copenhagen itself, however, where there are enough physicians, the plan does not pay the optometrist for spectacles which he prescribes.

In Yugoslavia there is also a severe shortage of practitioners who can write an ophthalmic prescription. Although there are no regulations giving the optician the right to refract, he may do so if he is qualified (Grims, 1966). Clearly, the optometrists in Yugoslavia and Denmark are beginning to achieve professional status, and for one of the same basic reasons that optometry evolved into a profession in the United States and England: need exists, and optometrists are filling this need.

On continental Europe, it is clear that an optometric profession has not emerged. In a few countries, there are signs that a profession may evolve. In Denmark, Germany, Switzerland, and Yugoslavia, there are now some optometrists, usually trained in England, Germany, or the United States, who are pioneering. They are testing vision in offices with modern equipment, using modern techniques, and they are charging a fee for their services. But this handful of optometrists performs only a fraction of the vision tests performed in Europe. Generally, these men are not included in the state health plans.

Another populous country in which optometry has evolved as an occupation, if not as a profession, is Japan. Greenspoon (1966) describes optometric service in Japan:

> There is no such thing as an optometrist. There are opticians and refracting opticians. There is no law controlling the vision care professions. Out of 12,000 opticians, approximately 10% refract. They learn refraction through an apprenticeship program and courses given at various times under the auspices of the Optical Consultants Association.

Greenspoon notes that the refracting opticians often have well equipped offices and use both objective and subjective techniques. Iwasaki (1966) points out that a vision examination is paid for by the various health schemes if it is performed by a physician but not if it is performed by an "optometrist." Thus, in Japan there is a sizeable number of optometric practitioners (refracting opticians). The occupation of optometrist may be said to exist, and its members do well financially. However, governmental recognition is lacking; there is no controlling legislation. Willingness to pay through governmental health plans for examinations performed by optometrists has not been demonstrated.

In many countries having an optometric occupation (but not profession), government health care plans cover a large number of the citizens. Almost invariably, the government does not recognize the service performed by an optometrist (refracting optician). Such is the case even in Norway, where the majority of the population is covered for a multitude of services. Although the insurance system in Norway covers physiotherapy and the services of a midwife, it does not cover a vision examination by an ophthalmic (refracting) optician (Muller, 1966). The same service in Norway, as in so many other countries, is covered only if it is performed by a physician.

Optometric Professionalization in the English-speaking Nations

Certain practical criteria for determining the degree of evolution of the optometric profession are apparent. Simple yardsticks may be applied to estimate the stability and degree of professionalization that has been attained in any country. These are:

1. The occupation is practiced by individuals as their sole occupation. In many countries, this is not true; refraction is practiced as an adjunct to the business of selling spectacles prescribed by someone else.

2. Laws control how optometry shall be practiced.

3. Schools or training institutions exist within the country.

4. The government is willing to pay for the service and to recognize it in governmental health programs where such programs exist.

The first three criteria are used by Wilensky (1964) for any profession. The last criterion is met in very few countries of the world. In the United States, however, most of the state, county, and federal plans for health coverage do include the services of the optometrist. This criterion of professional acceptance by government is also characteristic of many other English-speaking nations. In England and Canada, optometrists are recognized, and the optometric service is paid for by government. In some countries, such as Australia, all criteria but this one are met (Attiwill, 1966). Australia has two fine optometric colleges, and optometry has attained professional recognition in all spheres except inclusion in the national health plan.*

In Canada, New Zealand, Australia and, to a lesser extent, Great Britain, more and more optometrists are practicing in office premises or in premises without any display of spectacles (Giles, 1966). This trend toward professional behavior in these countries, Giles felt, is part of an evolutionary process; he predicted that professional behavior will become universal in these countries. Giles also described the optometric educational institutions in the various other English-speaking countries. Canada has two optometry schools, both of which are university affiliated. There are two university-affiliated colleges in Australia; one of these is the recently-established optometry department at the University of New South Wales. In England, Giles (1966) notes that "the colleges of Technology, in which the courses of optometry are housed, are now upgraded as Colleges of Advanced Technology and [are] able to grant Diplomas equivalent to Honours Degrees." †

The evolution of the optometric profession in the various English-speaking countries has been similar to the evolution of the profession in the United States. Each country has had a slightly different history, but the various criteria for the professionalization of any occupation have been met. Several other countries, particularly those markedly influenced by the United States or by Great Britain, have also seen the development to some degree of an optometric profession. In many Latin American countries, a clearly delineated optometric occupation controlled by legislation exists. Giles (1966)

* The evolution of the optometric profession and of optometric educational institutions in Australia parallels that in the United States very closely. Because the country was less populated, Australia did not have a phase of proprietary schools, but had independent (paid) tutors serving the same purpose. De Lacey (1967) has summarized the situation very nicely:

> For a century after the founding of the colony of New South Wales . . . , spectacles were sold by vendors who were usually untrained. The first optometric teaching was provided by wholesale supply houses, and then by a few tutors, the quality of whose instruction was not always outstanding. Subsequently the professional bodies, which were formed from the turn of the century, began to provide courses of instruction and, later, examinations. As registration Acts were passed by the State parliaments, the courses and examinations became more formal and standardized. In New South Wales and Victoria, they eventually became part of a university department or a university faculty, a pattern of precedent which New Zealand is at present following.

† There are at present six optometry schools following the pattern of university affiliation and achieving a high degree of excellence. They are: (1) University of Manchester Institute of Science and Technology, (2) The City University (London), (3) University of Aston in Birmingham, (4) Stow College, (5) Welsh College of Advanced Technology, (6) Bradford Institute of Technology.

notes that this is true in Brazil. In Colombia and Venezuela, there is an optometric profession with legal controls placed upon it. In much of Latin America, however, the number of optometrists is sufficient only to supply the needs of a small segment of the population.

Giles also notes that countries like Cuba and the Philippines, which were highly influenced by the United States during the period when optometry was developing in the United States, have laws similar to those of the various states.

Optometry as an independent profession exists only in a part of the world, mainly the English-speaking countries and those nations that have been markedly influenced by the United States and Great Britain.* In these countries, representing less than a quarter of the world's population, the optometric service that the patient receives is excellent. There is a close relationship between the degree of professionalization of optometry and the quality of the service. This same relationship holds not only in optometry but in dentistry as well; the quality of dental service received by patients in the United States is the best in the world.

The same factors that worked against the development of optometry as an independent profession in the United States or England have succeeded in preventing the emergence of the profession in many parts of the world. Tradition, medical opposition, absence of governmental recognition of the service, and absence of control of those practicing it have acted to prevent the emergence of a true profession. On the other hand, in much of the world, literacy is increasing and society is becoming more complex. The need for optometric service may be expected to increase markedly throughout the world. With this increase, optometry may be expected to emerge as a profession in many countries. The responsibility for leadership and help in developing the profession will fall upon English-speaking optometrists and, possibly, some German optometrists. In a worldwide view of the optometric picture, there are tremendous horizons. At the same time, there is an overwhelming amount of work yet to be done if all people are to benefit by the body of knowledge encompassed in optometry.

There is a close relationship between extent of professionalization of optometry and the quality of the service received. A quarter of a century ago, Justice Holmes noted of professions in general (Chap-

---

* De Lacey (1967), for example, cites two instances in which Australian optometry was influenced by the United States optometric profession. In 1906, the Code of Ethics adopted in Australia was that of the Rochester (New York) Optical Society. Later, precedents in the United States were quoted in preparation of the case for optometric instruction in Australian universities. It is clear that the strong optometric profession in the United States has helped the development of the profession in many other countries.

ter 7) the relationship between quality of service and professional conduct. Admitting that theoretically it was possible to have high quality service in commercial surroundings, Justice Holmes went on to note that in actuality this was never the case. It is one of the facts of life that the quality of the health care the patient receives is in direct relationship to the degree of professionalization that has occurred. This phenomenon obtains not only *within* a country, as Justice Holmes noted, but also for the various countries of the world. For all of the countries of the world, two variables can be determined: (1) the degree of professionalization of optometry (using criteria such as those of Wilensky), and (2) the quality of the service which the populace receives. If this is done, significant positive correlation will be found. That is, there will be a very close relationship between the two variables. As in the opinion of Justice Holmes, it may be argued that this need not be the case, but in actuality it *is*.

This relationship between professionalization and quality of service is a very important one for professional optometrists to understand. It is the real justification for professionalization. Professions require education, governmental control and recognition, codes of conduct, and professional associations for only one reason: *it is in this way that the public may receive the highest quality of service.* Individual rules may seem arbitrary; the importance of any step in the total concept of professionalism may be questioned. Nevertheless, the fact remains that total professionalization yields the highest quality of service to the public. A comparison of professionalization and of quality of service in all countries of the world bears out this observation.

CHAPTER 9

THE PRACTICE
OF OPTOMETRY TODAY—
OFFICE AND STAFF

The optometric service (described in Chapter 2) is rendered to patients in the United States today on a professional basis by the majority of practicing optometrists. To the sociologist, professionalism implies high educational standards and continuing postgraduate education; it implies emphasis on service rather than on incidental materials; it implies placing the patient's well-being ahead of the professional man's personal gain; it implies the existence of a professional association that works to upgrade the quality of the service. The criteria which sociologists use to determine the degree of professionalization that an occupation has attained have been studied by Wilensky (1964); modern optometry meets these criteria. (See Chapters 6 and 7.)

The layman often uses the same criteria as the sociologist for judging professionalism. He is aware that services rather than materials are associated with professions and that *caveat emptor* is a basis of business and trade but not of professional behavior. However, he depends more on other criteria, such as the physical surroundings. The layman is cognizant of the differences between a professional assistant (nurse, receptionist, secretary) and a sales clerk in a shop. The environment in which an occupation is conducted greatly influences the layman's judgment of whether that occupation is a profession or a trade.

Most optometrists in the United States practice in a physical environment that present-day society considers typical of a profession. Physical surroundings and optometric assistants in most practices convey to the patient the professional nature of optometry. But not all optometrists have evolved to this point.

A range of modes of practice exists that in a sense recapitulates all of the stages through which optometry has passed. The majority of optometrists practice in an advanced manner, representing the upper end of this range. Others, comprising a minority, practice in surroundings typical of various periods of the past. In Roman times, some 1500 years ago, vision service was offered by the *ocularii,* who kept shops with eye-catching window displays to attract clients (Chapter 3); some optometrists still use similar methods. In seventeenth century England, spectacles could be purchased from a haberdasher; a few optometrists in the United States still practice in stores of general merchandise, attempting vainly to reconcile modern society's concept of professional service with the mode of practicing the optometric profession in Shakespeare's time.

Over the past 75 years in the United States, the trend has been steadily in the direction of the professional practice of optometry. At the time of Prentice, almost all optometrists were shopkeepers. Today, approximately three quarters of the optometrists practice in surroundings similar to those of the established professions of dentistry or medicine. Year by year over the past 75 years, the ratio of professional offices to shops has steadily increased.

Optometric leaders have recognized the evolutionary process that has been operating. Now that optometry is well advanced, they have called for the complete disappearance of those vestigial environments representing the early stages through which optometry has passed. The American Optometric Association has set target dates a few years hence for the complete disappearance of practices that are completely outmoded in present-day society.

The physical environment of the professional 70 percent of optometrists is a factor in their professionalism. The remaining 30 percent of the optometrists, a group which annually declines in number, still practices in many different unacceptable environments. All of these environments have (in addition to unacceptability) one thing in common—all are vestiges of former periods in the development of the optometric profession in the United States and Europe. In some countries, all optometrists still practice in the commercial manner (Chapter 8). Optometry in those countries has not evolved past the point of being a trade.*

Since the various forms of commercial practice are remnants of the past, the best method of describing them would be to review briefly the development of optometric environments embodying all of the unacceptable types of practice of the present day.

---

* In a sense, there is something basically dishonest about the commercial optometrist in countries like the United States. He practices in an outmoded manner—yet shares the prestige of a profession which his colleagues have earned. He is "cashing in" on the prestige he does nothing to earn.

DEVELOPMENT OF OPTOMETRIC OFFICES

The optical shops of Europe and the United States prior to the present century sold binoculars, cameras, telescopes and microscopes, hand magnifiers, and other optical devices. The itinerant peddler of spectacles distributed his wares in the less populated areas. Little was known of scientific refraction and case analysis; the emphasis was largely on the sale of spectacles and not on the services performed in connection with them. There was no need for specially designed offices as we know them today. The office was primarily an area for selling merchandise similar to other retail stores. A tiny dark room was added, in which a few tests were hurriedly performed before getting down to the business at hand—that of selling a pair of spectacles.

The change in office design in the last 30 years reflects both changes in optometry and changes in general professional practice as well. Some professional optometric offices at the beginning of this era were located in upstairs suites usually in the business district. Physicians and dentists practiced in similar locations. Such offices were maintained by young optometric graduates and a few of the older graduates who had caught the spirit of professionalism. In the same community, optometry might be found as a department in a jewelry store (because of the silver and gold used in the frames and the jeweler's facility in making repairs), in a photography store (because of optometry's connection with lenses and other optical supplies), in the back of a drug store or department store (a throwback to the English haberdasher as spectacle purveyor), and in a hotel room or an extra room of another professional man because these locations were convenient for the itinerant optometrist (peddler) traveling from town to town.

Some hold-overs from this era are still seen today. Among the 30 percent of optometrists who have not yet fully evolved professionally, a few have offices in department stores, a very few are still in jewelry stores, and many occupy individually owned shops (which nevertheless have all of the physical characteristics of general merchandise shops).

In the early part of this century in the United States, there was a phenomenon in general merchandising that had its effect on optometry. Merchants found that advertising was a valuable stimulus to retail trade. However, the cost of advertising was prohibitive for a small shop. If, however, several small shops had similar ownership, merchandise, and physical characteristics, one unit of advertising could be used for all of the shops. This phenomenon was particularly prevalent in the large cities, where a chain of several shops could be advertised in the large city daily newspapers. Enterprising opticians in the early twentieth century availed themselves of this method of selling spectacles. In most populous areas, chains of optical shops under single ownership and with single advertising offices were opened. In some states, one owner might own as many as a hundred optical shops, each run by an employed optometrist or optician. In a few areas today, this chain store type of optometric practice still exists. Legislative efforts have been made to eliminate this unhealthy mode of practice. In California, for example, an optometrist may not be employed by a layman or a corporation, nor may one optometrist operate more than two offices at one time. In some states, however, the chain store type of practice still exists. A few individuals have tremendous financial holdings in optical chains and usually will not give them up willingly or graciously. The chain store optometry shop, however, is disappearing today mostly because young optometrists are refusing to be employed by chains or to practice in this regressive fashion.

The change in all professional offices in the last 30 years has also been marked. Almost all professional offices 30 years ago were in downtown office buildings. They were generally located on the upper floors to avoid the high rent involved in ground-floor locations.

Advertising in medicine and dentistry was already out of favor at the turn of the century. There were in these professions a few notable exceptions in the larger cities, but, for the most part, few professional men advertised in any way. In keeping with this practice, it was no longer necessary to have a location noticeable to the public. Patients were referred by recommendations of their friends and by other physicians or dentists. Optometry soon followed the patterns established by these other professions.

With improved transportation and more people owning cars, a new trend followed in professional offices. Parking became a problem in the downtown area. Older people had trouble climbing the stairs or were reluctant to use self-operated elevators. It was often necessary to walk long distances from the parking lot to the offices. Professional office buildings began to be built on the edge of the business areas in the smaller towns. In larger cities, shopping centers were built in outlying areas, and many professional offices moved near these centers. The clinic building occupied by several doctors forming a group practice became a popular type of office for medical practice. Some optometrists joined these professional groups, finding advantages as well as disadvantages. Perhaps the biggest advantage was that, with a source of referral from other professionals, the young optometrist was able to make a living at an earlier stage of life.

Upstairs offices in modern office buildings continued in the larger business areas. Elevators were made available, and many buildings were provided with their own parking areas. With improved city planning, professional offices were obliged to provide their own off-street parking.

In outward appearance, the modern optometric office is similar to the office of the dentist or the physician. The interior design, however, differs because of the type of professional services performed.

At the end of the nineteenth century in the United States, optometry was practiced in the environment of the retail merchant. Over the past 75 years, the optometric environment has increasingly become similar to that of the dentist and physician. But during this period, the environment of the physician and dentist was also changing. Professional offices moved from private residences and from downtown office buildings to offices designed specifically for the professional practice of healing arts and sciences.

Optometry today is mostly an individual practice; the environment of the optometrist is his own independent office. There may be possible future expansion as the practice grows and becomes a multi-optometrist practice. There are some principles of present-day office design that distinguish modern optometric offices from those of other professions.

This environment is that of the majority of optometrists in the United States today; it is being adopted by more and more optometrists annually. If present trends continue, this environment will be almost universally accepted by optometrists in the foreseeable future.

THE OPTOMETRIC OFFICES TODAY

The optometric office is planned for the function it performs and the patients it serves. In recent years, there have been noticeable trends toward preventive optometry and toward the study of developing vision in children; modern optometric offices are designed with these trends in mind. The major visual-system defect that develops eventually in everyone who survives long enough is presbyopia. This condition becomes noticeable when the patient is in his forties; it was largely responsible for the early development of the profession and for many of the profession's advancements. Thus offices are also designed for the older patient. With the increase of longevity among the American people and the larger number of children, optometric offices will be geared even more toward these two age groups in the future.

The styling of eyewear has undergone many rapid changes. It is not uncommon today for a child to falsify symptoms in order to obtain spectacles as attractive as those of a classmate. Attractive facial features can be accentuated by proper styling of eyewear; some facial defects can be made less noticeable by properly designed spectacles. Since style is a part of modern optometric practice, the modern office is designed accordingly.

Scientific optometric instruments are being developed in greater numbers each year. Instruments now found in the optometrist's office not in common use ten years ago include: electronic tonometers, biomicroscopes, vision field screening devices, and in the field of contact lens work, such inspection devices as radiuscopes, illuminated binocular microscopes, shadow-spector viewers, and many smaller inspection devices. Special instrument rooms have been designed in modern offices to accommodate this equipment. Refinements of examination procedures, as well as the use of polaroid equipment and other means of binocular refraction, have necessitated changes in the examination room itself.

General Office Design and Location

Location of the optometric office away from the business area is a natural part of professional development. With modern transportation, it is often easier to drive to an outlying location than to a downtown area. Because of the length of time required for an optometric vision examination, parking meters are an inconvenience. Most doctors' offices now have off-street parking so that older people have to walk only a short distance from automobile to office. Modern offices are often built with no steps but with short ramps to accommodate older people.

Offices in the outlying areas often emphasize attractive design. It is easy to direct new patients to an attractive, outstanding type of building. This factor has been found especially helpful when patients call to ask for the location of the office.

Downtown business lots are extremely expensive, so doctors' offices are either in upper stories of office buildings or in outlying locations. In the outlying areas, one still finds space at less cost. Larger rooms are then available for reception areas, examination rooms, and other parts of the optometric office. Buildings can be located on the lot in such a way as to leave room for expansion as the practice grows. The main consideration in this respect has been the location of doors or temporary walls to allow for additional rooms.

Allowing for expansion in an office has been found to be

extremely important. It would have been impossible, for example, in the early 1950's to have foreseen the changes that were to take place in the contact lens field. Few optometrists foresaw the new instruments that were to be designed and used in optometric practice. The space required for frame styling would have been difficult to anticipate a few years ago. Prospective changes in group practice (Chapter 11) and in technology make it essential to plan for the future.

In the optometric office, most of the rooms are used for more than one purpose. The prime example of this is the private office that is used as a consultation room, as an extra room for adjusting or delivering spectacles, and even as an overflow area for patients from the reception room when several members of a family come in at the same time. Few optometrists can afford the luxury of a private office merely for a place to rest between patients or to study, although it may serve these purposes too.

RECEPTION AREA

The waiting *room* of the professional office has now given way to the reception *area*. In the modern optometric office, the reception area is well lighted, has comfortable seating arrangements for several members of the family, includes chairs with arms to accommodate the older patient, and has a children's area to keep the children occupied while waiting for their parents or for their own appointments.

The business office usually overlooks this area. There is a receptionist present to greet patients and to make them feel at home. As soon as the patient is made comfortable, coffee may be served if the patient desires it. This type of treatment is ideal in an optometric office perhaps more so than many other professional offices because of the length of time a patient must be present for the service performed in the office. Many doctors have found it convenient to have the patients fill out a preliminary registration form as soon as they arrive. This form contains such items as: name, address, telephone number, occupation, and by whom referred.

BUSINESS AREA

The business area in the typical one-man optometric office has a receptionist who serves as both business manager and optometric technician. As the practice grows, it is not uncommon to employ both a receptionist and an optometric technician in the business area; it therefore should be large enough to accommodate an extra desk at a later date if needed.

The business area is designed for maximum efficiency of the assistant. Changes in modern business techniques have been as rapid as professional advancements. There are several business procedures and business machines which lend themselves ideally to professional optometric practice. The business office is designed to include these facilities.

The filing system is of great importance in optometric practice. Files are arranged so that expansion is possible both in number of files and in alphabetical dividers within the files.* The filing system should be efficient, since the patient's record must be retrieved from the files each time he visits the office. Even spectacle adjustments are performed with the record present so that the optometrist may know of any unusual facial characteristics, special adjustments, lens specifications, patient's preferences, and the date of the last examination.

Telephones are arranged so that conversations can be conducted without being overheard by others. Speaker systems are awkward in professional offices because of the personal nature of so many of the calls.

The patient arranges in the business area to pay for the services he receives. There should be a desk at which the receptionist can write receipts. Pegboard systems are available and widely used; these units enable the receptionist to prepare a receipt for the patient and at the same time make an entry by carbon on a day ledger. Present-day optometric practices are rarely large enough to require machine bookkeeping systems.

The receipt system, change drawer, and appointment book are all kept in or on a desk available to the patient as well as to the receptionist. A separate large desk or work table is needed for several of the functions that the office assistant performs. Here, the monthly statements are prepared. Here, the letters reminding the patient of the date of his next visit are prepared. Although a professional accountant is usually employed by optometrists, the office assistant does the daily posting and writes checks to pay bills. These various functions are best performed on a desk that is not accessible to patients.

Many business office aids are utilized as the practice grows. These are duplicating machines (widely used now to prepare statements), postage meters, dictating equipment, electric typewriters, specialized machine bookkeeping systems, and other office equipment. The modern optometrist constantly analyzes his practice to determine when the efficiency of his staff can be increased by the use of modern business equipment.

REFRACTION ROOM

The modern refraction room is built to accommodate the newer methods of refracting; polaroid projection equipment operates best

---

* Modern alphabetical files are designed according to the frequency with which names occur in certain geographical locations.

with a full wall aluminized screen; methods of binocular refraction, such as the Turville test, require special room design. There should be enough space around the examining chair for the doctor to move easily and efficiently.

Panel type wiring for equipment is useful. A common mistake in office design is underestimation of the amount of electrical equipment needed in the area of the examining chair. At least eight outlets or a panel type arrangement allowing for this many plug-ins should be in this area; new equipment is certain to be developed in the future.

Most optometrists, once they have acquired confidence in their refracting technique, like to have parents present during the examination of children. It is much easier to explain the child's vision problem if the parents are familiar with the examination that has been performed. Therefore, one or two "spectator" chairs are needed in this room.

A majority of optometrists explain to the patient the tests that are being performed. Patients want to know that their eyes have been examined for cataract, glaucoma, and other eye diseases; unless they are told so by the optometrist, they have no way of knowing whether these examinations were performed. Pictures to demonstrate what is seen by the doctor are often used. Patients should also know that a completely objective method of eye examination is available by the use of the retinoscope. The tests to determine muscular coordination for near work and far work should be explained simply by means of projectors or pictures near the examining chair. Offices should be designed accordingly.

Instrument Room and Visual Training Area

It is obviously impossible to keep all of the specialized examining equipment in the refracting area. The special instrument room may contain such equipment as a biomicroscope, a keratometer, an electronic tonometer, visual skills equipment, visual field instruments, various binocular vision testing and training devices, and other types of specialized equipment not usually used in eye examinations. Patients are taken into this area whenever the eye examination indicates the need for special tests. Many optometrists have an extra ophthalmic chair with an ophthalmoscope and an operating lamp for external examinations. It is then possible to begin an examination in this area if the regular refracting room is occupied. In designing this room, provision for all present equipment must be considered and space for additional instruments as the need may arise must be left.

Although chair-centered operation is efficient, moving the patient to specialized examination areas can prove to be a break from the examination routine and can emphasize to the patient the amount of equipment necessary to perform complete visual examinations when necessary. Wall strip plug-ins should be used to allow for a large number of instruments.

Some optometrists prefer to have a visual training area apart from the instrument room; it depends on the amount of visual training and orthoptics performed in the office. A large visual training practice warrants a special area set aside for this purpose. Since children will be the prime users of these services, consideration is given to their comfort; the room is decorated accordingly.

Most optometrists select visual training patients very carefully and refer difficult cases to other optometrists specializing in this work. With proper arrangement of equipment, most one-man offices can accommodate the visual training equipment in the same room with the other specialized instruments. Proper scheduling of patients also helps to make this room serve several purposes; for example, field charting and tonometry may be scheduled in the morning and visual training after school.

THE PRIVATE OFFICE

The private office is one of the most versatile rooms in the optometric building. Its purpose, as the title implies, is to serve as an area where personal subjects may be discussed with patients, where the results of the examination may be presented to the patient, and where the doctor has a chance to relax or study between appointments. It may also serve as an extra room for adjustments and deliveries of spectacles when the regular room reserved for this purpose is occupied.

The refraction room is not designed for consultation with patients. It is built for efficiency in the performance of vision tests; its lighting and the general form are designed for this function. Moreover, the ophthalmic chair built for the specific purpose of eye examination is not the most relaxing type of chair for the patient. It is possible to have a small desk and chair in the refraction room separate from the ophthalmic chair; some doctors prefer this method. The trend in modern design, however, is toward the private office that serves for consultation before and after the examination.

One of the most important ways in which the optometrist gains information about his patient—more important, perhaps, than any of the tests he performs—is through the case history (Chapter 2). The optometrist listens to the patient; he offers the patient information, reassurance, and advice. The optometrist speaks and explains to his patient. Although the optometrist listens and speaks throughout his relationship with the patient regardless of which room they are in, it is in the private office, designed primarily for these purposes, that most of the listening and speaking is done. Most optometrists meet the patient first in the private office and return to it after the examination has been completed.

The private office is furnished comfortably, much like a den or library in a private home. It is usually carpeted. The optometrist's books are easily available, and the decorations of the room and the diplomas of the doctor are arranged in such a way as to give confidence to the patient and put him at ease. The doctor's desk is the center of attention in the private office. Since this room will be used as an extra room for the adjustment or dispensing of spectacles when the area for these purposes is occupied, an extra set of pliers should be kept in one of the desk drawers.

There should be a comfortable chair for the patient near the doctor's desk. It can be used to measure the patient's usual reading distance and to observe his reading habits. Such habits as tilting of the head to one side, throwing the head back, holding the work to one side, or unusual tilting of the reading matter can be observed only in normal surroundings. It is nearly impossible to make observations of this type when the patient is seated in an ophthalmic chair. The final prescription of bifocal lenses in many instances depends as much on these observations as on the actual tests performed during the examination.

The private office should be large enough to accommodate members of the patient's family.* Many doctors like to have both parents in at the time spectacles or any visual training is prescribed for children. This is particularly true for the first visit of the family to the office. Often an older patient likes to have one of his children along to be sure he understands the doctor's orders.

Since the private office will be used for explaining the patient's vision problem and needs, several teaching aids should be present. Slide viewers, model eyes, drawing materials, and equipment the individual optometrist uses to make his explanations lucid and understandable should be available. The term "case presentation" has been used recently to describe this very important function of the optometrist. The presentation to the patient of an explanation of his vision problems and needs is *not* a "selling" procedure. The optometrist has

---

* Many optometric offices use the family system of record filing. The keeping of individual records in a jacket under the heading of the family name is of considerable help in case discussion and diagnosis. Clinicians of experience have found that many eye defects run in families. Furthermore, they seem to occur at almost the same age in many of the children. This phenomenon is explained to the parents so that examinations can be arranged at the most crucial times. Having the records of the family all in one folder is of considerable help in the discussion of these problems.

the responsibility of telling the patient what is wrong and what is the
ideal solution. If there are alternate solutions to the problem (two
pairs of spectacles versus bifocals, for example), each is described, and
the advantages and disadvantages are discussed. It is not the optometrist's function to sell as much service or as many pairs of spectacles as
he can. For this reason, the term "case presentation," implying as it
does a salesman armed with a "presentation kit" is most unfortunate
and misleading. The discussion following the examination is designed
to lay out a program for the patient and to give him insight into his
problem.

Shana Alexander (1966) expresses what should be accomplished
in the optometrist's private office:

> I would not think of having a doctor I didn't like. The reason
> has nothing to do with professional competence, which I cannot
> judge anyhow. My liking him won't make him a better doctor, but I
> think it will make me a better patient.
>
> I don't require him to have a lollipop up his back, but I do
> want my doctor to listen very carefully to what I have to say; to tell
> me every bit he can about what he is looking for and what he finds;
> and when he doesn't know, say so.

The private office should set the tone for establishing this type of
rapport with the patient. This is one room in the office where the
doctor can be made to seem a bit more human, and not just an optical scientist. The display of certain hobbies, pictures of the family,
and a general home-like atmosphere help to create such an effect.

CONTACT LENS ROOM

Because of the time involved in contact lens fitting, a special area
is used for this purpose. This area can serve as a multi-purpose room
as well. Extra frames may be kept in this room for styling when the
regular style room is occupied. An extra plier set may be used here
for delivering and adjusting spectacles.

The contact lens room is well appointed and comfortable for the
patient. The reaction to the first insertion of a contact lens often determines the ease with which the entire contact lens adaptation is
made. If this area is comfortable and the patient can relax without
the embarrassment of having other patients nearby, much time and
effort can be saved. Thus, a special area is set aside for contact lens
fitting just as soon as it is warranted by the amount of contact lens
work being done.

STYLE ROOM

The style aspect of optometric practice has been much abused
during the evolution of optometry. When optometry was practiced

mainly in stores and shops, the sale of spectacles often was the main goal. As the emphasis came to be placed on the service performed for the patient, the pendulum swung to the opposite extreme. The training in optometric schools was almost solely on the technical aspect of professional practice; little time was spent teaching the styling and designing of frames for the individual patient. Optometrists, however, soon realized that the best professional examination is of no value if the patient does not wear the correction in front of his eyes. Modern eyewear had developed to the point where almost anyone can wear spectacles without detracting from his or her appearance. Many patients have actually found their appearance improved with the proper selection of eyewear.

Opticians and commercial optometrists set up attractive window displays that serve to entice prospective spectacle wearers into their places of business. It is not the purpose of this chapter to discuss the ethics of this type of operation, but it is mentioned to point out that the American public is fully aware of the wide variety of frames available.

The styling of eyewear in the optometrist's office is best accomplished on an individual basis. It is not necessary to display several hundred frames in the style room. The style room is designed so that the doctor or his assistant working under his supervision can assist the patient in the selection of the eyewear that is most flattering cosmetically.

The style area is usually carpeted and well lighted, but not glaring; it often has a full length mirror so that a patient can see how the eyewear looks with the complete ensemble being worn. The style room is usually designed mainly for women patients since they are more style conscious than men. Another area is often set aside for men, for they also appreciate personal attention to the details involved in designing eyewear that is masculine and attractive.

There is a marked individual variation in the methods used in frame selection. Some optometrists prefer to have no frames visible; frames are kept in drawers or shelves and are selected by the optometrist or his assistant and tried on the patient. Other optometrists, recognizing that some patients enjoy seeing many frames and making tentative selections themselves, prefer to have a number of frames simultaneously visible to the patient. Since there are individual differences in patients, some will prefer one method, some another. Some patients prefer to have the trained person help them make a choice; others are unhappy unless they can personally examine many frames. Women purchase dresses with the same individual differences. Some prefer to rummage through hundreds of dresses on racks, while others prefer to have a trained person pick out a few items for them. Op-

tometry differs from all of the other health professions in that this
element of style is present in the choice of the holder for the prosthetic devices, the lenses.

The trend today is to design style rooms that can please either of
the two types of patient just described. No frames are visible, and the
optometrist can help make the selection. However, if a patient wishes
to work alone, the frames can be brought into view and the patient
can be allowed to "browse." Because part of the professionalization
process has been a de-emphasis of materials, a great deal of care and
thought goes into the design of the style room. The optometrist
wishes to have the room convey the concept of a professional office
with emphasis on service. Yet a compromise is reached with the desire
on the part of some patients to see many frames before making a
choice.

The style room is designed for the proper arrangement of frames,
so that they may be located easily by the stylist. Pleasing lighting
conditions, comfortable seating arrangements for the patients, and a relaxed atmosphere for individual eyewear selection are always present.

DISPENSING ROOM

There usually is one room set aside in the office primarily for the
delivery of spectacles and the subsequent adjustments that they require. From the standpoint of office efficiency, this room is as near the
reception area as possible. For minor adjustments encountered frequently during a day's routine, the patient need not be moved
through all of the building. The dispensing and adjusting room is
often small in size, since adjustments are made for only one patient at
a time. On completion of the adjustment, if other consultation is required, the patient may be moved to the private office. The patient's
record is always present when an adjustment is made, so that if an
unusual lens correction is being used this fact can be noted and the
adjustment made accordingly. In high cylinders, for example, if the
spectacles have been bent in any manner, the patient should be taken
to the refraction room for the final adjustment and alignment of the
spectacles.

The dispensing room is also utilized for other purposes—for example, as an extra style room for men's frames or a special display area
of eyewear for teen-agers. Teen-agers appreciate the attention of individual styling, but most of them prefer to try on a large number of
frames by themselves. If they show this inclination, they should be
given the opportunity. For this purpose, a small style room with a
special table and mirror for teen-agers could be provided; it could
also serve as a dispensing area.

This room is well lighted—with more illumination than most

other areas of the office—so that the adjustment can be made with a minimum amount of effort on the part of the optometrist.

The doctor's final instructions to the patient about visual care are given in this room. These instructions include the care of spectacles, how to use new bifocals, the method of putting on and taking off eyewear, and when and how spectacles should be worn. Space is allowed for easily located pliers, instructional material, and reading material for the patient when he tries out his new lenses. When the doctor has an optician or a technical assistant do the dispensing, the final result should be supervised. The doctor himself gives the final instructions.

LABORATORY

In the typical optometric office, the laboratory is small, well lighted, and efficiently designed.

Economically, it does not pay the average optometrist to do his own laboratory work. He has two alternatives. He may send his work out to an optician; or as his practice grows, he may employ his own optician. In the latter instance, the laboratory must be enlarged to accommodate additional equipment.

There is also a question as to how much laboratory work an optician should do in an optometric office. Often the optician's time can be better utilized in frame styling, minor repairs, adjustments, and deliveries. The convenience to the patient is the principal factor involved in employing an optician. The edging and inserting of single vision lenses can be done in the optician's spare time and should not monopolize his day.

The laboratory in a typical one-man optometric practice need not be too large. It is built in such a way that expansion can be made later if desired. It may have to serve as an office and working space for an optician as the practice grows. It is usually located close to the area where most of the adjustments and deliveries are made, although this arrangement is not always possible if the room is added at a later date. The laboratory often serves as a storage space for cases, extra instruments, various repair parts, and the multitude of items that accumulate over a period of time in any practice. Extra storage space can always be used. In this area, storage cabinets are built on all possible walls for utilization in time to come. Additional storage space is arranged in the business area and the private office, but the centrally located laboratory can be especially useful for this purpose.

OFFICE PLANNING

Few optometrists start their practices in new office buildings of their own design. Most optometrists find that it takes a few years in practice to determine what they really desire in the way of individual rooms, arrangement of the various areas, and the size of the rooms. Many optometrists work for a while with an established clinician, and from this association learn what they will require in the way of operating space. Many optometrists starting their own practice find it advisable to rent and remodel a building; later they move to an office of their own design.

Often optometrists planning their own offices require the services of an architect. There are not enough optometric offices in the country, however, to have encouraged architectural firms to specialize in this type of work. Many costly mistakes have been avoided by employing an architect willing to discuss the individual needs of the doctor and the general office requirements.

The major optical manufacturers have departments of office planning. The American Optometric Association also has an active committee which can supply a number of plans, pictures, and suggestions for office design.

Whether optometrists employ an architect or design their own office, they should take into consideration as many ideas as possible.

The optometrist's physical environment, his office, is designed for the patient of today and his many visual needs. The more efficient the office, the better the doctor can serve these needs. The design of the office varies with the scientific knowledge and training of the optometrist and with the manner in which he utilizes his equipment. The best optometric clinician will fall by the wayside, however, if he cannot work properly with his patient as an individual. Proper design and interior decoration of the office make it much easier to establish the rapport and confidence necessary for complete vision service.

OPTOMETRIC ASSISTANTS

With optometry's development as a profession, the need for specialized auxiliary assistants in clinical practice has increased.

There are three capacities in which optometric assistants may be employed: (1) the optometric office assistant (office manager), (2) the technical aide to the optometrist (optometric technician), and (3) the manager and dispenser of ophthalmic materials (optician). There is an overlapping of work in any arbitrary division of responsibility. In the smaller or beginning practice, the optometric office assistant may also at times do technical work and optical work. As the practice grows and the number of aides increases, the staff members become more specialized.

THE OPTOMETRIC OFFICE ASSISTANT

The optometric office assistant is usually the first employee of the optometrist. Elmstrom (1963) found that optometrists tend to employ an assistant when the net income reaches about 6000 dollars a year. However, this is not always the case; many optometrists "go it alone" as long as they can. Elmstrom cites a survey which shows that 40 percent of the practitioners in a large state who had been in practice ten years or more did not have assistants. Thirty percent of a group of optometrists over 19 years in practice did not have an aide. The same survey indicated that, while 50 percent of the optometrists in the lower earning range employed an aide, almost 90 percent of the optometrists in the higher income range found an assistant essential. Apparently, the use of office assistants is associated with practice growth. Some men, however, do not seem to mind interruption of examinations to make appointments, to set up the next patient, to keep books, and to perform the dozens of details necessary in routine office procedures.

What should the optometric office assistant be trained to do in an optometric office? In general, the optometric office assistant has three functions: receptionist, office manager, and housekeeper. In a large clinical practice, two or three individuals could perform these tasks. Just how far the aide is allowed to develop in each area depends on the personalities of the doctor and the assistant. Obviously, all of these functions are extremely important in the management of any successful optometric practice.

THE OPTOMETRIC TECHNICIAN

Many years ago, medicine and dentistry found it necessary to train technicians to assist the professional man in his work. As optometry has grown in scope technically and professionally, more and more activities assignable to trained technicians have become apparent. A few of the activities that are now being delegated are: registering the patient and taking a preliminary history; preparing the patient for the examination; assessing such visual skills as visual acuity or color vision; performing preliminary tests of binocular vision or stereopsis; assisting during the examination by recording the examination findings; aiding in field charting and recording the findings during field measurements; and giving preliminary instructions to the patient in the care, insertion, and removal of contact lenses.

The decision as to which tests may be delegated to the optometric technician is of utmost importance. Before a decision can be made, the nature of the optometric examination must be considered

(Chapter 2). Analogies are often made between the professions of dentistry and optometry. There are many similarities in the development of the two groups as independent professions, yet there is a fundamental difference in clinical practice. *The examination of the patient's vision, the vision analysis performed as a result of that examination, and the writing of a lens formula constitute the major part of the optometric service.* The *productive* time in optometric practice is spent to a great extent in the examination itself. In dentistry, on the other hand, the examination is required only to decide which type of work will be necessary. Most of the productive time in dental practice is spent in doing the actual restorative work.

Because the optometric examination requires professional skill, and because the examination is a unified procedure, parts of it should not be delegated to an assistant. The history, external examination, ophthalmoscopic examination, retinoscopy, subjective examination, muscular coordination tests, and similar tests (Chapter 2) should all be performed by the optometrist.

It is possible that a technician could be trained to perform each of the optometric tests in a routine manner. It is the interpretation of the tests that is a professional skill and not the actual performance of the tests. However, any clinician of experience realizes that it is the *way* in which the patient answers certain questions during these procedures, as much as the results, that determines the final prescription. Responses may be discovered during the administration of one test that may indicate the need to repeat previous tests. A patient's reaction in one test determines whether certain following tests can be eliminated, can be done briefly, or should be amplified. The proper performance of these visual tests, with the intermingling of observation, conversation, test analysis, and lens prescribing, constitutes the practice of optometry. Delegating the performance of these tests can only result in skimpy, improper vision care.

THE OPTICIAN

Some parts of the total optometric service may be performed by a technician such as an optician. The occupation of the optician, however, requires some elucidation, since it includes anyone skilled or trained in the mechanical aspects of lenses. One who makes microscope, telescope, or camera lenses and lens systems is an optician. One who works in the lens manufacturing industry is also an optician. One who processes ophthalmic lenses and places them in a frame is also an optician. And one who takes the lens formula of another person and then produces and fits an appropriate pair of spectacles is also an optician (dispensing optician). Optometrists evolved from the opticians. In many parts of the world, the word optician remains in the language as a remnant of former days to describe the optometrist. In England, for example, the optometrist is called an ophthalmic optician or a refracting optician.

Many opticians, particularly those engaged in the manufacturing aspects of the trade, are still trained by apprenticeship. Schools of optics exist, and some opticians are trained in these institutions. Some colleges offer a two-year vocational or technical course in opticianry, and many well trained people emerge from them. There is little standardization, however, of requirements for licensure of dispensing opticians in the various states (Chapter 12).

Many opticians do not work directly with the public. They make spectacles which an optometrist or ophthalmologist (who assumes the responsibility for accuracy) fits to the patient. The *dispensing* opticians, however, do supply eyewear directly to the public. The role of the dispensing optician is an outgrowth of conditions in the time of Prentice in the United States. At that time, opticians made and sold spectacles directly to the public. As some of the opticians increased their knowledge of the testing procedures, they evolved into the present-day optometric profession. Others preferred to make and sell spectacles only, leaving the testing to others. These men were the forefathers of the present-day dispensing optician.

With the widespread use of contact lenses during the past ten years, an interesting development has occurred within the field of opticianry. Many dispensing opticians have sought to fit contact lenses, to determine the curvature of the surface which would bear on the eye, and to make modifications in the fit of the lens. The opticians maintained that only the determination of the lens power required the professionally trained practitioner. On the surface, this entrance into the field of prescribing might sound like a repetition of optometry's inclusion of certain professional acts into its scope—which occurred at the turn of the century. It might seem that just as optometry adopted sight-testing as part of its scope, so opticianry now is adopting eye measurement. However, there is a major difference. *With optometry's evolution came commensurate education*—not only in the acts to be performed but in the basic sciences upon which the application was justified. The right of opticians to use a keratometer, slit lamp and biomicroscope, and similar instrumentation and techniques is being contested in the courts in many states. In a major decision in one state (New Jersey), opticians have been held by the court as not qualified to engage in contact lens fitting except under direct supervision of one licensed to do such work.

The aspects of opticianry pertinent to the present discussion of optometric aides is the work that can be done by an optician for the patients of an optometrist and under the direct supervision of the optometrist. Eyewear styling, facial measurements, repair and adjustment of spectacles, cutting and insertion of lenses in an ophthalmic frame, and inventory control of ophthalmic materials can become quite time consuming. Good office economics suggests that much of this work should be delegated. Most of the technical aspects of making and fitting spectacles can be handled by a trained optician or an office assistant trained to perform opticianry tasks. A career optician, however, is better qualified by training and experience to perform these tasks than is the average office assistant.

A lens formula is *not* a prescription in the same sense as a physician's order for a drug (Chapter 2). A great deal of judgment must still be exercised after the lens formula has been determined. Traditionally, one of optometry's premises has been that the patient is served best if the same individual who performs the vision examination and analysis also designs and fits the spectacles. How, then, is this concept to be reconciled with the utilization of an optical technician in the optometric office?

The key to the relationship is found in the phrase "under the direct supervision." When an optometrist delegates technical tasks in his office, the entire procedure is still under his direct supervision; the unity of the optometric service is maintained if he assumes the responsibility for the entire service. The relationship analogous to that of optometrist to his optician is not that of the physician to the pharmacist; it is that of the physician to his office nurse, to whom he may delegate, for example, the task of giving hypodermic injections. This practice, common in present-day medicine, in no way implies that physicians sanction independent offices in which nurses "give shots."

Therefore, in the use of opticians in the optometric office, as in the use of any technician, two partly contradictory conditions must be met. The optometrist is to be freed of certain routine tasks, yet the unity of the service, traditionally performed by one person, must be maintained. The conflict is resolved by the concept of the total service being under the optometrist's direct personal supervision. But these words must mean just what they say. Sometimes it is as easy to do the mechanical tasks personally as it is to delegate each step and to supervise it personally. In this area of optometric practice, a great deal of experimentation is being carried on to determine how mechanical aspects of the service may be delegated without adverse effects on the unified service (Chapters 11 and 12).

EDUCATION OF OPTOMETRIC ASSISTANTS

Optometrists encourage the best possible training for their technical assistants. They recommend courses at the college level; the study time required is determined by optometric educators.

At present, the greatest demand is for optometric office assistants who can be of some limited assistance technically to the optometrist and also do some of the work of the optician. There have been many courses given by laboratories, schools, and the Optometric Extension Program in this area. These courses should be enlarged and improved.

Dentistry separated the dental technician from the office secretary many years ago. The income of the average optometrist is increasing. The scope of his professional services continues to expand. The demand for college-trained people in this area is growing. Today, in multi-optometrist practices, where more than one assistant is employed, the trend toward specialization can be seen.

Schools of optometry could provide the best possible education for all technical optometric assistants; opticians especially could receive the best training in these schools. However, in some professional schools at present, such overcrowding already exists that to take in more students would be almost impossible. Were it practicable, the training of opticians in these schools would result in a much better relationship between optometry and the trade from which it originated.

The use of well trained optometric assistants as office managers, optometric technicians, and opticians is being encouraged in optometry. The areas in which they are to work are being carefully defined and supervised. Allowing the professional man to do the work for which he is trained by relieving him of many routine duties can only result in better vision care for everyone; but this must be achieved without destroying the personal nature or the unity of the optometric service.

ASSOCIATE PRACTICES IN OPTOMETRY

The professional practice of optometry has traditionally been a one-man affair. In recent years, however, as optometric practices have flourished, optometrists have found several advantages to practicing in association with one or more other optometrists. This trend is just beginning. The vast majority of optometric professional practices are still solo practices. This trend, however, is another sign of arrival at professional maturity.

The advantages to the public of associate practice include: continuity of service should one optometrist be on vacation or ill; consultation among optometrists in the same practice on difficult problems; and application of advanced techniques through special knowledge, since one optometrist may specialize in contact lenses and another in visual training or another specialty. The advantages to the optometrist are: increased free time; continued earnings in the event of illness; more time for postgraduate education; and, interestingly enough, increased earnings for the same amount of work because of the increased efficiency of a multi-optometrist office.

A major advantage of multi-optometrist offices is the improved quality of care that patients receive. Although optometry is a general practice profession and one optometrist *can* practice all of the special branches, such is usually not the case. Solo practitioners often find themselves too busy with the refractive aspects of the service to offer their patients such special services as visual training, contact lenses, subnormal vision aids, or aniseikonic refraction services. In the multi-optometrist office, each member of the team can practice one of these items in addition to his regular work. In the group situation, peer judgments tend to keep the individuals in the group interested in increased proficiency. The optometrist who practices alone is the sole judge of the quality of the care his patients are receiving; the optometrist in a group has peers who also can judge the quality of care. He therefore tends to seek to improve his skills and knowledge.

Associateships most frequently are the junior-senior type, in which a young optometrist joins an established practice. However, other types are known. Sometimes, two or more optometrists begin practicing in the same office. Sharing the expenses enables them to have more elaborate equipment and better office help from the beginning than either could afford alone. Sometimes, two optometrists with established practices join their practices and build or rent common offices.

There are many aspects to associateship practices which will not be discussed here in detail.* However, the trend away from solo practice, which to date has been almost the exclusive type of professional practice, is worthy of note. Often, especially in the junior-senior type of associateship, one optometrist (the junior) will for a period perform some of the duties of such optometric assistants as the optician or technician.

In recent years, throughout the United States, several excellent associateship practices have been built. These practices have the stability to outlast the life of a single mortal. This continuity of the optometric service will have a marked advantageous effect on the quality of optometric care being received by patients.

Although the present discussion pertains mainly to multi-optometrist offices in private practice, group practice also is a characteristic of the various health care plans (Chapter 11). Such practices

---

* The authors recognize that several aspects of optometric economics require far more detail than can be afforded in this volume. Associateship practice is one such topic. A volume on optometric economics is planned for the future.

have all of the advantages of multi-optometrist offices (peer judgment, specialization) and all the disadvantages (loss of personal contact or fragmentation of the service if the group becomes too large). As the trend toward multi-optometrist offices—both in private and public health practices—continues, the effort will be made to maintain the advantages and to minimize the disadvantages.

CHAPTER 10

THE OPTOMETRIST TODAY— HIS ECONOMIC AND SOCIAL STATUS

In the brief period of three score and ten years, the biblical life span of an individual, the optometric occupation has attained professional status in the United States. What effect has this professionalization had on the men and women who practice optometry? What kind of a living do they make? How are they regarded in their communities? What is their status insofar as the government of our complex society is concerned?

Little is known about the status of the optometrist or optician at the turn of the century. Complete data for that period, such as those that have been obtained for the present-day optometrist, are not available for comparison. We do know that the early optometrist was not recognized as a professional person. He was a merchant, often a financially successful one, and a skilled artisan. His place in the social strata of that early period was not greatly different from that of a successful television repairman of the present day. He had special knowledge not available to most people, and this knowledge was respected. He performed a useful function in society for many people.

Today, the story is quite different. The professionally practicing optometrist is recognized in his community and by governmental agencies as a practitioner of an independent health profession. His income is roughly commensurate with the income of other professional people in the community. If there is still some reluctance toward complete acceptance of the optometrist as a professional in the health care field, it is caused by the actions of the still unprofessionalized minority who practice the same occupation.

ECONOMIC STATUS

Professions traditionally place the welfare of clients above financial gain. However, because of the amount of time necessary to prepare for a professional career, the economic outcome must be considered. Moreover, in the United States, economic status and professional prestige seem to be very closely related.*

The professional optometrist does not practice solely for the income from that endeavor. If there were no personal satisfaction, there would not be so many dedicated men in practice. A certain standard of income must be maintained in a profession, however, not only for the prestige of the individual, but for the advancement of the profession itself. Without adequate income, the optometrist soon finds himself unable to replace equipment, unable to obtain new textbooks, and unable to attend the meetings, seminars, and postgraduate courses so necessary to keep him up to date in his profession. Some thought, then, must be given to the economic status of optometry and its relationship with other professions in the American way of life.

Any study of optometry as a profession must include its relationship to all professional groups, not just the health professions. Although optometry is considered one of the health professions, it is unique in this area. Most health professions treat diseases; optometry is unique in that most of its service is with healthy tissues and healthy people. When pathological conditions are found, the patient is referred to another profession. This fact accounts for the various titles assumed by optometrists over the years vision specialists, eyesight specialists, or vision consultants. These titles connote the process of treating light so that it will focus on the retina rather than the process of treating the eye to make it more nearly normal; they imply the training of visual attributes to enhance the behavior and performance of the total organism.

Recent studies show optometry's economic base relative to other occupations. Table 2 reveals some interesting comparisons. Of most interest to optometrists is the ranking based on income growth. The median income of optometrists in 1949 was $4,343.00; in 1959, $8,772.00. The projected income was extrapolated to show an average income of $17,700.00 by the year 1969. Optometrists rank third of 48 occupational groups on the basis of the most rapid advancement in the median income during the period 1949 to 1959. Only athletes and veterinarians did better. The percentage increase in income from 1949 to 1959 for optometrists was 102 percent, as compared with 92 percent for dentists and 81 percent for physicians and surgeons.

The income projected to 1969 is quite encouraging, and there are indications that this extrapolation is conservative. The 1964 economic survey of members of the American Optometric Association indicated that, at that date, optometrists were ahead of the schedule. It is clear

---

* A common definition of a successful practitioner in the health professions is: "one who has the respect of his colleagues, the gratitude of his patients, *and is a good provider*." Another dimension is added to this definition in Chapter 11.

TABLE 2

INCOMES IN PROFESSIONAL OCCUPATIONS [a]
*Median Income of Men in 48 Professional Occupations, 1949, 1959, and 1969 Projected,[b]
and Percentage Increase 1949 to 1959*

Note: Except for some occupations omitted because of inadequate data or other technical reasons this is the original census list of professional occupations.

Rank (Based on Income Growth)	Occupational Group	Median Income		Projected 1969 [b]	Percent Rise in Income 1949–59
		1949	1959		
1	Athletes	$2,336	$ 5,394	$12,500	131
2	Veterinarians	4,220	9,178 c	19,900 c	117
3	Optometrists	4,343	8,772 c	17,700 c	102
4 °	Airplane pilots & navigators	5,263 c	10,514 c	21,000 c	100
4 °	Librarians	2,294	4,592	9,200	100
6	Photographers	2,941	5,692	11,000	94
7	Dentists	6,448 c	12,392 c	23,800 c	92
8	Aeronautical engineers	4,828 c	9,127 c	17,300 c	89
9 °	Funeral directors & embalmers	3,179	5,967	11,200	88
9 °	Natural scientists (n.e.c.)	4,245	7,965 c, d	15,000 c	88
11	Electrical engineers	4,657 c	8,710 c	16,300 c	87
12 °	Chiropractors	3,471	6,463	12,000	86
12 °	Metallurgical engineers	4,657 c	8,639 c	16,100 c	86
12 °	Therapists & healers (n.e.c.)	3,011	5,591	10,400	86
15	Mechanical engineers	4,594 c	8,497 c	15,700 c	85
16	Physicians & surgeons	8,302 c	15,013 c	27,200 c	81
17 °	Chemical engineers	5,005 c	8,948 c	16,000 c	79
17 °	Lawyers & judges	6,284 c	11,261 c	20,200 c	79
19	Artists & art teachers	3,552	6,333	11,300	78
20 °	Chemists	4,091	7,245	12,800	77
20 °	Pharmacists	4,170	7,385	13,100 c	77
20 °	Social scientists	4,446 c	7,868 c	13,900 c	77
23	Musicians & music teachers	2,700	4,757	8,400	76
24	Actors	3,260	5,640	9,800	73
25 °	Clergymen	2,410	4,151	7,100	72
25 °	College faculty, deans & presidents	4,366	7,510	12,900	72
25 °	Industrial engineers	4,519 c	7,790 c	13,400 c	72
25 °	Miscellaneous engineers (except mining)	4,965 c	8,522 c	14,700	72
29	Social & welfare workers (except group)	3,196	5,481	9,400	71
30	Accountants & auditors	3,977	6,758	11,500	70
31	Civil engineers	4,590 c	7,773 c	13,100 c	69
32 °	Authors	4,033	6,745	11,300	67
32 °	Draftsmen	3,470	5,794	9,700	67
34 °	Entertainers	2,217	3,674	6,100	66
34 °	Nurses, professional	2,645	4,400	7,300	66
34 °	Sports instructors & officials	3,330	5,519	9,200	66
37	Teachers (elem. & second.)	3,465	5,709 d	9,400	65
38	Foresters & conservationists	2,997	4,873	7,900	63
39	Surveyors	2,773	4,486	7,300	62
40 °	Architects	5,509 c	8,868 c	14,300 c	61
40 °	Personnel & labor relations workers	4,754 c	7,669 c	12,300	61
42 °	Osteopaths	6,458 c	10,279 c	16,300 c	59
42 °	Technicians: medical & dental	2,908	4,614	7,300	59
44	Farm & home management advisors	4,059	6,159	9,400	52
45	Radio operators	4,016	5,975	8,900	49
46	Dancers & dancing teachers	2,385	3,483	5,100	46
47	Religious workers	2,316	3,241	4,500	40
48	Recreation & group workers	3,155	4,395	6,100	39

° Indicates a tie ranking.
[a] Median incomes for 1949 and 1959 and the percentage increase from 1949 to 1959 were prepared by Professor A. T. Finegan for the Industrial Relations Section of Princeton University. (Memorandum, May 21, 1964, "Income of Men in 48 Professional Occupations: 1949 and 1959.")
[b] Incomes were projected for 1969 by assuming the 1949 to 1959 rate of income growth for each occupational group would continue in the next decade. Thus it is a purely mechanical extrapolation which certainly is *not* intended to pose as a forecast.
c Indicates an average income higher than for college faculty, deans, and presidents.
d Weighted average of medians for component subgroups.
SOURCE: *United States Census of Population, 1960: Occupational Characteristics* [PC(2)-7A], Table 25; *United States Census of Population, 1950: Occupational Characteristics* [P-E No. 1B], Table 19. The same source provides similar data for women which were omitted here because of smallness of sample and problems of comparability.
This table is reprinted from AAUP Bulletin, Vol. 51, No. 3, June, 1965, with permission of the American Association of University Professors.

that optometry as a profession is succeeding in establishing itself among other recognized professions in the rapidity of its growth economically.*

Optometrists can work productively at their profession for a long time. Table 3 shows a ranking of professional occupations by median age and the income of twelve occupations. Optometrists reach the peak of their income after age 65. Thus, those optometrists who continue to work after 65 do very well indeed. The age 65 group shows optometrists out-producing dentists, osteopaths, and veterinarians. Moreover, we know that a higher percentage of optometrists can continue to work after age 65 than is the case in other health professions.

Professional income by age groups varies with the profession because of the status of the profession and the type of skill involved. The optometrist's income proceeds slowly the first three to five years, gradually increases the next ten years, and reaches a peak between the 14th and 18th year of practice. This peak continues for another 15 years and begins to level off after the 28th year, but a surprisingly high level of income continues into the 40th and even 50th year of practice.

Optometric income varies in different parts of the country, but the degree of variance is not very great. Some changes in income have taken place recently that bear further consideration. Surveys made by the American Optometric Association (1959, 1966a) show a shift in top income areas from the mountain states to the east south-central and south Atlantic areas.

In 1958, the highest average income was earned by optometrists in the mountain states ($11,850); the next highest was earned in the central states ($10,670); and the Pacific and south-central states were tied for third place ($10,230). Six years later, in 1964, neither the mountain states nor the Pacific states were among the three sections of the country with the highest incomes. The east south-central area (Kentucky, Tennessee, Alabama, and Mississippi) had the highest average income ($16,097). The average income in the south Atlantic states was second ($15,940), followed by the east north-central states ($15,555), and the west north-central states ($15,417).

---

* There are defects in all economic surveys. Those with extremely high or extremely low incomes probably do not report. Many successful men do not have the time or inclination to report, although it is probable that they would report with greater frequency than those with extremely low incomes. One does not mind telling people when he is doing well, but is somewhat hesitant to put down poor results even in a confidential survey.

Another point often overlooked in surveys of median income is the relatively high earnings of a few professional men. Elmstrom (1963) reports that nearly 60 percent of the entire optometric income was enjoyed by only 22 percent of the optometrists.

TABLE 3

RANKING OF PROFESSIONAL OCCUPATIONS BY MEDIAN AGE—SPECIFIC INCOME

Median Male Income in Professional Occupations by Age Level, Selected Occupations, 1959 [1]

AGE 25–34		AGE 35–44		AGE 45–64		AGE 65 AND OVER	
Osteopaths	$12,595	Phys. & Surgeons	$15,000+ [2]	Phys. & Surgeons	$15,000+ [2]	Phys. & Surgeons	$13,228
Dentists	10,745	Dentists	15,000+	Lawyers & Judges	15,000+	Lawyers & Judges	13,212
Elec. Engrs.	9,152	Osteopaths	12,793	Pilots & Nav.	14,918	Soc. Scientists	12,750
Aero. Engrs.	9,005	Pilots & Nav.	12,778	Dentists	13,318	Optometrists	11,220
Optometrists	8,264	Lawyers & Judges	12,645	Chem. Engrs.	12,675	Elec. Engrs.	9,656
Chem. Engrs.	8,200	Aero. Engrs.	11,856	Architects	12,113	Academics	9,040
Veterinarians	8,178	Veterinarians	11,466	Osteopaths	12,076	Aero. Engrs.	9,000
Lawyers & Judges	7,480	Chem. Engrs.	11,057	Aero. Engrs.	11,687	Dentists	8,986
Architects	7,283	Optometrists	10,208	Elec. Engrs.	11,445	Osteopaths	8,667
Soc. Scientists	7,242	Elec. Engrs.	9,933	Soc. Scientists	11,006	Chem. Engrs.	8,500
Pilots & Nav.	6,975	Architects	9,900	Veterinarians	10,343	Architects	8,040
Academics	5,813	Soc. Scientists	9,110	Academics	9,664	Veterinarians	7,488
Phys. & Surgeons	5,225	Academics	8,446	Optometrists	9,384	Pilots & Nav.	5,000

1 Median incomes calculated from U. S. Department of Commerce, Bureau of the Census, *U. S. Census of Population, 1960, Characteristics of Professional Workers*, Table 7.
2 Well over $15,000.

This table is reprinted from AAUP Bulletin, Vol. 51, No. 3, June, 1965, with the permission of the American Association of University Professors.

The shift of high median income to the southeastern United States is undoubtedly a reflection of the shift in industry and improved economic conditions that are taking place throughout the south. Nonetheless, the increase in income in a six-year period from $10,230 to $16,000 in the Atlantic and south-central states is truly dramatic. All surveys show this area to have the fewest clinicians relative to the population, and this fact has influenced the results. It is probable that industrialization and increasing education in this area have led to increased utilization of the optometric service and a more pronounced shortage of optometric manpower. The phenomenon occurring in this area is further demonstration of the thesis advanced earlier in this book: the optometric service becomes increasingly important (and apparently profitable) with industrialization and augmented education.

Optometrists have traditionally settled in smaller communities. Moreover, the financially most productive optometric practices are usually located in the smaller cities. In 1964, the median income for optometrists in small cities (under 50,000 inhabitants) was $14,954. The next highest income, $14,234, was earned in the large cities (over 500,000 inhabitants); the lowest median income, earned in the medium-sized cities (50,000 to 500,000 inhabitants), was $12,018. Earlier studies showed that the highest incomes are earned in towns of 25,000 to 50,000, and that towns of 10,000 to 25,000 run a close second. Quite amazingly, all these studies show a high level of income in towns of 5,000 and under. In many rural areas, successful optometric practices are often maintained in towns of 1,000 or less. Usually, these towns have a good drawing territory and are several miles from larger cities.

One of optometry's unique contributions to the health care field is the wide distribution of its members and their willingness to practice in the smaller communities. Hofstetter (1963) wrote:

> Unlike many other highly specialized personnel, including others in the eye field, optometrists are not naturally restricted to large cities, communities with hospital facilities, or major health care centers. They are distributed in almost constant ratio with the population, from towns of less than 2,500 to the largest metropolitan centers.

As long as optometry remains a profession of general vision care, the wide distribution of its members in the smaller communities will continue. It is interesting, however, to speculate on whether this trend may not be reversed in the future. With maturity and increased education, optometry may follow the pattern of other health professions and engage in specialization. Specialty practices can rarely be afforded by the smaller communities. Also, the majority of optometrists today are solo practitioners. It is estimated that between 85 and 90 percent of optometrists practice alone. However, the trend in other health professions is toward group practices with several men sharing an office. If optometrists follow this trend toward clinic practices common in other health professions, they will also tend to move to the large communities.*

Most surveys show that partnership practices result in higher income for each man. The most recent survey (American Optometric Association, 1966b), for example, shows that optometrists associated with other optometrists average $16,722; those in individual practices, $14,832; and those associated with physicians, $11,525. With nearly two thousand dollars' difference between men in associated practice and those in individual practice, it is obvious that there must be many possible advantages in this type of arrangement. The other advantages to the optometrist and to the patient of group practice are discussed in Chapters 9 and 11.

The median income of optometrists does not tell the entire story of optometric economic status. Along with income, one must consider the number of hours that the optometrist must work each week to obtain his income. In assessing the attractiveness of a profession for those who consider entering it, there are three important considerations not usually included in income surveys: (1) the number of hours worked in order to produce the income, (2) the number of years an individual can continue to practice, and (3) the inconvenience of emergency hours. In all three areas, optometrists are extremely fortunate.

Hours: According to all surveys, it is not necessary for the optometrist to work extremely long hours in order to receive a relatively good income. The 1964 survey (American Optometric Association, 1966c), for example, shows that optometrists who spent an average of 30 to 39 hours per week with patients had a median income of $14,500 per year; those who spent 40 to 49 hours earned $14,906; those who worked 60 to 69 hours per week had an average net income of $18,400. The majority of those reporting in this survey were in the office and available to patients between 35 and 45 hours per week.

It is interesting to compare the income of $14,500 for 30 to 39 hours per week with the income of only $4,000 more for a work week almost twice as long. On the basis of a 50-week year, it can be shown

---

* An interesting compromise between practice in large and small communities is made by many practitioners in western Canada. Several optometrists will have a large city clinic type practice, and then each member of the group will cover one or more small towns which he visits periodically.

that optometrists earn about $8.25 per hour for the first 35 hours each week, but only $2.65 per hour for the work after that. One wonders if this additional time might not be spent more productively in study or recreation or if more efficient utilization could not be made of the time at work.

Years worked: Optometrists earn a good income into their seventies and those who wish to work beyond the usual retirement age of most professions are assured of a good income for an added ten to 15 years. Optometry is not taxing on physical stamina. Extra hours are not required as they are of the family physician; not as much manual dexterity is required as it is of the dentist. Many optometrists enjoy practice so much that they prefer to continue working. Their lifetime earnings usually equal or surpass those of many dentists or physicians. Many business and professional men who have tried retirement have found that it was not the utopia they had anticipated. This ability to continue working on a part-time basis with working hours and days one chooses and a comfortable income well into the later years makes optometry attractive to prospective professional men.

Emergency hours: Most of the optometrist's working time is scheduled by appointment. Seldom are emergency calls necessary. Proper patient indoctrination eliminates the need for most optometric emergencies. Patients who require lenses for constant wear because of blurred distance vision or inability to perform work without lenses should always have an emergency pair of spectacles. The doctor who properly performs his complete service informs the patient about the necessity of providing for such an emergency.

Even the emergencies that arise in contact lens wearing are greatly reduced by proper instruction. Problems of insertion and removal of contact lenses rarely arise for patients who have been properly informed. A properly designed fee system puts extra pairs of contact lenses or spectacles within reason. The time required of the optometrist to deliver a pair of duplicate lenses, contact or spectacle, is so short that this service should be financially feasible for most optometric patients.

Legitimate emergencies occasionally do arise when optometric patients experience sudden changes in vision or in ocular conditions, as in injuries, infections, or sudden loss of vision. Some patients screen these problems themselves and consult an ophthalmologist, but others prefer to have their family optometrist do this screening for them. This case is similar to that of the patient who believes he needs surgery, but still consults his family physician first, rather than the surgeon.

Screening patients who have an ocular emergency is part of the family optometrist's professional responsibility. Office assistants must be trained to allow all patients who experience sudden changes in vision to see the optometrist at once. In areas where ophthalmologists' appointments are scheduled long periods in advance, it is possible for the optometrist to assist both the patient and the ophthalmologist in deciding how soon the patient should be seen for medical attention.

Thus, the optometrist, like every other health profession practitioner, must be prepared to have some night calls and some emergencies; his dinner plans will occasionally be altered by a patient in need of his services. But emergencies occur far less often in optometry than in medicine or dentistry. This is partly because optometry's main concern is with healthy eyes; even more, it is due to the fact that eye emergencies are rare. Aside from accidents, few eye and vision disorders appear suddenly. The optometrist's working hours are among the best in the health professions.

SOCIAL STATUS

A profession's place or image in society changes constantly. The more nearly a health profession is related to the life and death of an individual, the more highly it is regarded by society. In such professions as teaching or law, the importance of the profession determines the regard with which society views it. As education has become more important in modern society, teachers have become more highly regarded; as the laws of our society have become more complex, the legal profession has become more highly regarded. Clearly, as the general health of the nation becomes more important, health professions will be even more highly esteemed; as technology advances and the need for clearer, more comfortable, efficient vision becomes more imperative, the profession of optometry will continue to increase in stature.

The importance of a profession to society is not the only factor determining its prestige or social status. Many subtle changes take place over a period of time that influence the public attitude toward a profession. Some of these changes are unavoidable and are not necessarily for the betterment of either the profession or the public. For example, the family doctor who literally devoted his life to the care of his patients has been replaced to quite a degree on the American scene. The general practitioner has still an important place in the American social picture, but increased prestige and income have shifted to the specialists within the field. Many physicians deplore this turn of events and wonder if these changes and attitudes are for the best. Fewer and fewer medical students go into general practice. Whether this change is commendable or whether the trend needs to be reversed remains to be seen. The facts are, however, that the general profession of medicine has felt some lowering of prestige as a humanitarian profession dedicated to the people; the prestige has been transferred to the medical scientist or surgeon who is sometimes more interested in his technique than in the person he serves.

The dentist, because of his educational background and dedication to his profession, has established himself on the American scene. Little obvious commercialism exists, the educational standards are high, the income of the dentist is up, and in general, he is well accepted as a professional man.

Dentistry has one obvious advantage over all other health professions. It is the one health profession that has no competition from outside the profession. Medicine has had inroads constantly from other healing professions such as osteopathy, chiropractic, and podiatry. Dentists, however, from the time they staked out their jurisdiction, have had a monopoly on their field. Physicians do not practice dentistry in any form, and there has been no other professional group attempt to invade this area. There are both advantages and disadvantages to the public in this lack of competition among professions; but the fact remains that dentistry has attained high public esteem with no outside competition to degrade it.

Optometry, on the other hand, gained professional status only after considerable struggle, and in constant competition for both prestige and economic security. The field of vision care was split many years ago; optometry emphasized vision, and medicine stressed the physical care of the eye. However, overlap existed; both groups were interested in refraction. Prestige can be an economic weapon; the withholding of prestige can be a competitive advantage. Thus, optometry's overlapping interest with an established, strong, existing profession and the resultant economic competition has led to difficulty in attaining prestige. As in other aspects of optometry's success story, its willingness to accept increased educational requirements supplied an answer to the problem. Optometry attained not only professional status, but social acceptance and prestige as well, primarily through the academic acceptance of optometry.

Despite continually increasing recognition by the academic community, optometry has had a difficult time in attaining social acceptance. Part of the problem was due to the great rapidity with which optometry evolved as a profession. Even today, there are many people living who can remember the itinerant optometrist, the jewelry department store optometrist, and the optical storekeeper. On the other hand, ophthalmology, the established profession with which optometry competed for the field of refraction, had all of the prestige of the medical profession.

The optometrist, because of his training and interest, develops a very personal interest in comprehensive vision care. Refraction, with the total service allied to it, *is* the optometrist's interest. The ophthalmologist, on the other hand, because of his interest in medicine and surgery primarily, and refraction only secondarily, develops a different attitude toward vision care. A successful ophthalmic surgeon will frequently delegate a great deal of the optometric services in his office to technicians. Thus, the very service offered by the optometrist is deprecated. The ophthalmologist, with all of the glamor of surgery and miracle drugs to cure disease, not only performed the same service as the optometrist, but often relegated it to relative unimportance.*

In its struggle for social acceptance, then, optometry has had not only to demonstrate its own competence in the field of vision care, but also to convince the public of the importance of the service itself. Moreover, optometry has to overcome its own early history and the reputation of some of its members who were reluctant to advance with the times. It is therefore remarkable that optometry has attained the social acceptance it has in recent years. The impact of academic improvement and acceptance has been a major factor. Competence in performing its task has been another of optometry's strong points.

Although the competition with an existing profession of great public acceptance and glamor has been a difficult obstacle in optometry's quest for social acceptance, it has also been a boon. Faced with competition of this sort, optometry was forced to professionalize in a very short period of time. Faced with competition, optometrists have had to study harder, expand the educational process,† and produce satisfactory results with patients. The struggle for existence has served to unite the profession. Competition has had its desirable effects as well as its problems.

The faith of optometrists in their profession and in the importance of the service they render has also had its effect on social status.

---

* In Chapter 11, the importance of increasing the utilization of the optometric service is discussed; it is stated that under-utilization is due in part to inability to pay but also to the public's lack of understanding of the nature and importance of good vision care. Clearly, the attitudes of the professions involved in vision care have a marked effect on public feeling and understanding.

† One of the remarkable aspects of optometry's amazing growth has been the willingness of practitioners to endow colleges. The money for the building at the University of California was raised by the practitioners of that state. Texas optometrists helped build the department at the University of Houston, and Indiana optometrists contributed for the department at Indiana University. Every school receives great help from practicing optometrists.

At the time that optometrists did not *appear* as professional men, both the group and its service were not highly regarded. When most optometrists practiced as shopkeepers, it took great faith and courage for the first men to change their environment and begin to act like professional people. Twenty-five years ago, a fourth of the optometrists practiced in professional surroundings; today, three fourths do so. This reversal of the professional/commercial ratio in so short a time span is remarkable; it is also a great tribute to the faith of optometrists in their chosen calling.

The preceding broad overview does not tell the whole story of optometry's struggle for acceptance. Overall social acceptance and prestige have been dependent on many factors. The optometrist derives his present social standing from: financial recognition, academic recognition, legal recognition, interprofessional recognition, community status, governmental recognition, and opinion molders' recognition.

FINANCIAL RECOGNITION

As mentioned previously, the American people have a tendency to relate income to occupational success. The less they know about the occupation, the more this is true. Kahl (1957) rates it as one of the most important measuring tools that the public uses. If this criterion is true, optometry is well on its way toward professional recognition.

Optometry in 1960 was the third most rapidly advancing profession in income. Although it has a long way to go to equal the medical and dental professions, it seems to be well on its way; there are enough optometrists who are on equal footings economically with other professional men to influence attitudes in most communities.

Financial success is a criterion that must be watched constantly by any profession. When a profession places monetary gains ahead of its contributions to society, it can tarnish its image quite easily. When the profession of medicine began to attract some men because of its income status instead of its service status, the image of the American physician began to decline. Optometry must never lose track of this hazard in its professional training, postgraduate education, and future goals. The fact is, however, that optometrists who are practicing professionally are earning sufficient income. This is one measure of the public's acceptance.

ACADEMIC RECOGNITION

The regard of educated people toward optometry is important. With over half of all American students receiving some higher education, a man's social status is directly related to the amount of his education in America. This is a healthy indicator of American values and one in which optometry has made great strides.

As long as optometry was taught in a trade school atmosphere, it was not regarded as a major health care profession. The first step toward recognition was the abolition of proprietary optometry colleges. The establishing of optometry as part of the university curriculum was another major step. The training of optometric educators in optometry departments of major universities was yet another important step. The granting of the doctorate degree from fully accredited, independent schools and major universities gave optometry acceptance as a learned profession.

It will be some time before the average person realizes that optometry's education is now on a par with that of other established health professions. Most patients are interested only in the type of attention that they receive and the results of that attention in the doctor's office. The establishing of the six-year doctorate program for optometry, however, does increase its status in the minds of the educated citizenry of America.

LEGAL RECOGNITION

America is a country run by laws. Law has always been an important concept in the American way of thinking. From the establishment of the first colonies and their intense desire to do away with the capriciousness of the rules of the kings of Europe, rule by law has been crucial in the American tradition. Every aspect of the American way of life is influenced by the legal system.

Optometry grew up in this framework of legal control. (See Chapter 6.) The legal acceptance of optometry in all 50 states has helped to raise optometry to its present professional status. However, one cannot legislate a group into professional stature unless it is worthy of that recognition. As soon as the members of such a group are worthy of that recognition, they must be circumscribed by law in their activities and their professional behavior. This is the course optometry has taken.

Optometry was quite insistent about defining itself as a profession in its early legal battles. Many states have such a definition in their statutes. Such a definition was necessary for optometry to regulate itself as a profession. In time, as optometry is accepted by its appearance and actions, to spell this definition out in the law in so many words will probably not be necessary. The right of self-control will be given to the profession as it deserves the right, regardless of how the profession is defined. Optometry was able to establish itself legally in all states, often against medical opposition. If, as it claimed, medicine should have had complete jurisdiction over this field because of prior interest, such recognition of optometry would not have been possible. Optometry, however, by virtue of its birthright, was able to convince legislatures and judiciary that it should have professional recognition.

As optometry has matured, it has spent less time seeking legislation to regulate is own members and has become more concerned with the inroads into its jurisdiction being made by other groups. Optometry, in this respect, is following the pattern of most professions in the United States. As a profession becomes established, it becomes more jealous of its rights; it dislikes having any of its activities usurped by other groups. This phenomenon in itself indicates that optometry is now established, for this concern with the intrusions of fringe groups is a major characteristic of established professions (Wilensky, 1964). Today, a major part of optometric legislative or judicial activity is in the field of protecting the presently delineated scope from encroachments by fringe groups.*

INTERPROFESSIONAL RECOGNITION

The desire for approval or recognition is deep in the hearts of all people. One of the most satisfying aspects of professional life is the recognition given to the professional man by his patients. Of equal importance to him, however, is the recognition by colleagues in his own profession and in associated professions.

Optometry has long enjoyed excellent relations with the academic community. A scientist is judged by what he knows and by the research he contributes to the body of knowledge rather than by the discipline in which he was trained (Chapter 5). As optometry was integrated into the university educational system in the United States and as visual scientists who were also optometrists made scientific contributions, they and their profession received recognition. Thus, psychologists, physicists, and other scientists have for many years judged optometry on its merits.

Among other health professions also—dentistry, podiatry, pharmacy, and clinical psychology—optometry has been held in high regard. Many of these professions' members took their basic science courses in the same university classes with optometrists. Many of these

---

* As this is being written, one optometric premise is being tested in the courts of several states. Opticians claim the right to sell contact lenses to any person as long as they do not determine the power of the lens. Optometrists contend that determining how a contact lens will rest upon the delicate eye tissues must be done under the personal supervision of a trained professional man. Clearly, the optometrist has financial gain and prestige at stake; more important here, however, is a strong belief that vision care suffers and the public is endangered by the practice of untrained persons in any area of optometry.

professions' members might have obtained vision services themselves as students in university optometry clinics. As optometry progressed at the academic level, those with an academic background gave optometry recognition. There is also a mutual bond felt by most professions outside of the medical guild. Medicine has made it clear that it feels all health professions should be under direct control of the medical profession. This attitude brings other health groups closer together in many of their areas of planning. This has been noticed in the armed services whenever health professions tried to secure commissions and in the federal government when attempts were made by professions to obtain their rightful position in the health care field. The cooperation of and recognition by dentistry and the other independent professions in the health care field have been most gratifying to optometry.

Individual physicians, particularly those in general practice, have also often held optometrists in high regard. This is particularly true in smaller communities where the local optometrist may have been the only vision care practitioner within a wide geographic area. Clinic building situations in which an optometrist and a group of physicians have practiced in the same building have led to closer ties (Chapter 9). The only major interprofessional lack of recognition of optometry has come from some (but by no means all) ophthalmologists. Even here, the lack of recognition has been by organizations or spokesmen for organizations rather than from individuals. In the light of the supposed economic competition of this group with optometry in the vision care field, it is surprising that there has been as little strife as there has been. However, that little strife has had an effect on the status of optometry. Often optometrists encountered more difficulty with those trained or indoctrinated by the medical profession (nurses or opticians for example) than from physicians themselves.

Many optometrists have received recognition in their local community from individual physicians, although at the same time this acceptance was denied to the profession as a group. One answer offered by medical friends to this paradoxical situation has been revealing. Medicine feels that it must remain faithful to members of its own guild or union. Ophthalmologists and physicians realize that fully qualified and competent optometrists are available. They have seen the results of the optometrist's work both in referral of pathology and in general optometry. They have worked with optometrists in the armed services, and they realize they are taking the same basic science courses in the universities. The main opposition to optometrists is based on the fact that they are not members of the same union as physicians. Attempts are being made to heal this rather sick way of thinking that adversely affects interprofessional relations and can only result in substandard vision care to the public.

In spite of the opposition of political medicine and a few eye physicians, optometry has continued to enjoy increased recognition from individual physicians. Optometry's acceptance as a profession by medicine has been due mainly to the advanced educational requirements of the modern optometrist and to the fact that this education has often been received in the very universities attended by the medical men. Perhaps the next most important area where recognition has been accorded optometrists by physicians is in the armed services, where the two professions have had a chance to work side by side. This chance to become acquainted with one another's work has resulted in mutual respect in almost all instances.

Optometric leaders are the first to admit that criticism of some optometrists is justified. The less than 25 percent obviously commercial element in optometry has brought on most of this criticism.

Criticism of a few optometrists who have failed to recognize diseased conditions of the eye has been offered. This approach will not help interprofessional relations. Optometrists are fully aware that some members at times miss conditions that they should not miss. But equally, ophthalmologists have improperly diagnosed many eye conditions, and official records have been made of hundreds of these mistakes; these records are on file in the office of the American Optometric Association. Constant referral by either profession to this type of error will do nothing to help interprofessional relations and will only bring on more distrust. Man is fallible, and in all health professions mistakes are made. Keeping score of who makes more errors has never solved the problem.

Optometric leaders have recognized that closer cooperation between medicine and optometry is necessary. Fry (1957) offered some very pertinent comments on the division of labor between optometrists and ophthalmologists. He does not argue against the *right* of the ophthalmologist to do some refracting, but says: "The basic argument is simply that it is a waste of expensive training for an ophthalmologist to spend a large part of his time refracting eyes." This premise, because of its importance, will be discussed in detail in Chapter 12.

Fry stresses the importance of having ophthalmologists train optometrists in pathology. He states that "Such teachers can be replaced by optometrists who hold Ph.D. degrees in Physiological Optics, but it is a great waste of human effort to have these men turn around and become experts in another field in which they are not primarily interested." Fry observes that optometrists are willing to accept whatever training and guidance ophthalmologists give them in detecting diseases of the eye and setting up criteria for referral.

Many ophthalmologists have sought to improve the mutual recognition by optometry and ophthalmology of each other's role. Walter B. Lancaster (1928) wrote:

> Just as the dentists have succeeded in organizing a subdivision of medicine into a satisfactory specialty, so the optometrists will in time. A hundred years ago dentistry was a part of the field of the practice of medicine and a setting up of a separate branch of limited practice by men without a full medical training, i.e., with a training limited to dentistry was strenuously opposed by general physicians who declared only those who had a full medical training should extract teeth. A modus vivendi has been established between dentists and physicians to their mutual advantage. There have always been those who deplore the progress of professionalization. Nevertheless, the wheels of evolution roll on inexorably.

The "wheels of evolution" did continue to roll for optometry. Sixteen years later Conrad Berens (1944), one of the best known ophthalmologists of his day, stated his position in a positive fashion:

> Having served as secretary of the American Committee on Optics and Visual Physiology and as a director of the National Society for the Prevention of Blindness, I have gradually accepted the conclusion that lack of cooperation between ophthalmologists and all others concerned with vision and eye health is the most serious unsolved problem in the prevention of blindness today.
>
> Those who have been closely associated with this problem believe almost to a man that optometrists should be taught by those best qualified to teach subjects which would aid in preventing blindness. A recent vote taken by the American Ophthalmological Society and by this section indicates a similar opinion among a large and growing group of ophthalmologists. I believe that a careful unbiased study of the reasons why so many men are now in favor of cooperation by those who hold opposite views would lead to a change of opinion in many cases.
>
> The Armed Forces have used optometrists under the close supervision of ophthalmologists, and in the great majority of instances of which I have personal knowledge, the arrangements have been mutually satisfactory to the ophthalmologist and to the optometrist. Because of this ophthalmologists have asked whether a similar arrangement would not be satisfactory in private practice, as this association has also proved useful in some of the nation's municipal and private hospitals. This is one problem that a special committee of the American Medical Association might well study to the mutual benefit of all concerned.

Today's optometrists would agree with Berens' statement of the importance of mutual regard; they would differ on the need for close supervision. In the past quarter of a century since Berens wrote these words, optometry has developed into a six-year university course.

Optometry has proved itself capable of recognition and referral of patients with pathological conditions. However, Berens' major thesis is proven by the fact that in all communities where optometry and medicine have cooperated with each other, the public opinion of the entire eye care field has improved, and better vision care has been made available to the individual patient.

In general, optometry has been recognized by the academic community in fields allied to vision, by all other health professions, and by many physicians and ophthalmologists. The only strife has come from some of the official medical organizations, from their spokesmen, and from some physicians and medical technologists who followed the "official line" closely. As this is being written, the resolution of this problem seems to be imminent, and the time is close at hand when serious dialogues can begin on the role optometry and ophthalmology must play as separate, independent professions cooperating to enhance total vision care.

COMMUNITY STATUS

Professional men traditionally have realized that they have a contribution to make to their communities beyond their professional activities. Having spent many years in schools, they are familiar with the educational processes. It is only natural, therefore, that they should be interested in the educational processes in their own communities. School boards have always attracted professional men as an outlet for community activities. For years physicians and lawyers have made valuable contributions to the school boards in their areas. Since vision is one of the most important tools in education, optometrists naturally become interested in this area of endeavor. Each decade during this century, more and more optometrists have served on school boards.

A recent check of one of the national optometric organizaions showed that three out of four of the executive officers of the organization had taken a leading part in the community activities of their area. These activities were in the local government, school boards, or business and professional organizations of the community. The profession of optometry demands the optometrist's time during daylight hours, but leaves much free time for community activities in the evening. Optometrists can assume positions of leadership in the community, and they have done so to a very large extent.

Many optometrists belong to a service club,* but this is not the

* Although optometrists are represented in all of the major service clubs in the United States, the majority are members of Lions International. This is due to the fact that Lions' major service endeavor is its Sight and Blind Committee an undertaking with which the optometrist has a great affinity.

only way in which they discharge their obligation to the community. Increasingly, optometrists are participating in little theater projects, sketch clubs, lecture or book club groups, and other cultural activities. Each participation enables the optometrist to make acquaintances in his community. Much more important, however, individuals with an optometrist's educational background have an obligation to contribute to the cultural growth of society.

In the past, optometrists were often left out of many community projects. It was not unusual, even ten years ago, for optometrists to be omitted from school vision programs or ignored in other community activities which pertained to vision. This is no longer the case. Optometrists are now consulted in communities before any vision projects are undertaken. In all communities where optometrists have accepted social responsibility and have taken active parts in citizens' committees, on school boards, on city councils,* and in business and professional group activities, they have been recognized as professional men.

Optometrists are taking an increasingly important part in government on the state level. Public health departments of many states have optometrists on their staffs. Most states now have optometrists in an advisory capacity to help establish vision programs. State officials recognize that no extensive program of vision care can succeed without the cooperation of optometrists. Optometrists, as the general practitioners, see the majority of patients requiring vision care. It is to be expected, therefore, that they would be consulted in arranging any type of health care plans concerned with vision.

In addition to filling appointed and paid positions at a state level, optometrists have become active in state legislatures. † At the time optometrists took part in the battles to attain legal recognition, they were attracted to the groups that write the laws. It was a natural step, therefore, for some optometrists to seek elective office. In this type of activity, as in all other community and social activities, it is essential that the optometrist put the welfare of the people he represents above his own gain or the gain of his profession. This is not

---

* In one local optometric society in California (Tri-Counties) , within an eight-year period, four of the fifty members had achieved election to city councils in four different communities; simultaneously, three of these members held the office of mayor or vice-mayor in their communities.

† Several optometrists have been elected to the state legislatures. Dr. Harold W. Oyster was for many years state senator in the Ohio legislature, rising to the chairmanship of the very important Finance Committee. As this is being written (1967) , there is one optometrist serving in a state senate, the Hon. Edward Swanz of Montana. In addition, four optometrists are serving in the lower houses of their respective state legislatures: the Hon. Donald J. Mitchell, New York; the Hon. Jason D. Boe, Oregon; the Hon. Gordon Duffy, California; and the Hon. Arthur Dorman, Maryland.

always easy, since the welfare of the public and of the profession often are closely related. Personal selfishness can greatly weaken any public official's contribution, and it is to optometry's credit that its elected state and city officials have always served with distinction.

The cultural background of the optometrist, along with his interest in people as individuals and his desire to contribute to the welfare of all society, even beyond his professional abilities, has brought the optometrist to the forefront in all community affairs. These activities have probably been as effective in obtaining recognition for optometry by society as any other aspect of professional behavior.

GOVERNMENTAL RECOGNITION

Legal recognition of optometry during the early twentieth century occurred in the state legislatures. In recent years, however, there has been a shift of emphasis toward the nation's capital. With the increased interest of the federal government in every aspect of public health, education, and welfare, an active national program became imperative. Most professional associations have offices in Washington, and optometry has followed their lead; the American Optometric Association, with its central office in St. Louis, Missouri, in a building owned by the Association, now also maintains a well staffed office in Washington. The federal government has become an employer of optometrists and a leading purchaser (for citizens) of the optometric service.

The American Optometric Association (1965), in discussing the present-day utilization of optometrists, stated:

> The Veterans Administration as well as all three branches of the Armed Forces employ civilian optometrists in various research and service capacities. Optometrists are also utilized in a variety of advisory and product testing capacities, by such agencies as the Department of Agriculture, the Bureau of Standards, Civil Aeronautics Authority, and the Bureau of Public Roads. Full-time employees are under civil service in the professional category. Many optometrists who serve in an advisory capacity to various government agencies may maintain a private practice.

Because of the rapidity of optometry's emergence as a profession, there was a knowledge gap in governmental circles. Officials knew little about optometry and the contributions it could make to vision care. One of the major functions of the Washington office of the American Optometric Association has been and continues to be educational. Department heads, planners, legislators, and all others who have to do with establishing criteria for vision care or for purchasing it for large segments of the population are informed about optometry.

The Washington office is consulted daily by one or another branch of government on problems pertaining to vision care. The knowledge gap is rapidly being closed. Optometrists are being called to testify as experts before congressional hearings with increasing regularity. Many congressmen look to the Washington office for information about optometry and the role it can play in making vision service available to many segments of the population.

Within recent years, the federal government has taken the leadership in helping to solve many social problems. Important citizen conferences have been organized and promoted by the federal government. Notable among these conferences have been the White House Conference on Children and the White House Conference on Aging. Several thousand people were invited to Washington, D.C., for these meetings. In all instances, optometrists had an important part in planning the program, conducting it, and helping to implement the recommendations of these conferences.

Many governmental health care programs have been inaugurated in the last few years. Most of these programs, however, include only major medical care; dental and vision care have been omitted. It is certain, nevertheless, that these programs will be expanded, and vision care will have an increasingly important part in them (Chapters 11 and 12). The fact that optometry as a profession has been recognized by most governmental agencies and is consulted whenever help is needed marks an important forward step in professional recognition.

In Washington, optometry is using the same philosophy of legislation that it used previously in the various states. All legislation is watched carefully for possible application to vision care. Since optometry is the only profession devoted exclusively to vision care, the profession has a responsibility to see that all aspects are properly considered for the good of the profession, and even more, *for the welfare of patients it serves.* This philosophy of public service resulted in legislative recognition in all 50 states; it is now establishing optometry's image in the nation's capital. Optometry has not blindly opposed government's entrance into the health care field. Rather, optometry has taken the position that each program must be judged on its own merits; the major criterion has been whether or not the proposed program would help the public. Many branches of government have appreciated optometry's outlook on the broad field of public health and its judicious approach to suggestions for improving the nation's health.

The largest segment of the population for which the federal government purchases vision care is the military. Through service corps in the Army, Navy, and Air Force, the federal government purchases vision care for all personnel and frequently for their dependents; it also supplies vision care for many veterans. At the time of World War I, vision services were not nearly so complete as they became in later years. By World War II, however, many servicemen required optometric care. Nonetheless, because of the knowledge gap, there was little provision for optometric services on a professional basis. Physicians, dentists, and veterinarians were commissioned in the various branches of the service; optometrists were not.

During World War II, many optometrists did serve in their occupational capacity; they were not recognized as professional members of the health team, however. Optometrists at base hospitals in the United States and abroad served as non-commissioned officers. Many optometrists in this period, because of their years of college training, were offered commissions—but not as optometrists. These commissions were mostly refused; the men served as optometrists without recognition. Since other professional men were serving as commissioned officers, this was a bitter pill for optometrists in the service to swallow. Eventually, the excellent job done by these optometrists and the obvious slights that they had received were recognized. The example set by the optometrists who served as enlisted men and the struggle of optometric associations were finally successful; today, optometrists serve in all branches of the military as commissioned officers.

Army: The Army Medical Service Corps is the largest of the various branches of the service; the present authorized strength of the optometry section is 315 commissioned officers. Greene (1966), an optometrist and senior optometry officer in the Army with the rank of lieutenant colonel, states that a third of the Army's active personnel currently wears lens prescriptions. The need for optometric officers is great.

Originally, optometrists are assigned to posts in the United States in the larger training center hospitals and dispensaries. Like other members of the health team, optometric officers, if they remain in the army as career officers, are sent all over the world.

Hamrick (1966) pays tribute to the optometry section with these words:

> With the exacting requirements of today's modern Army for clear and effective vision, the importance of the Optometry Section and the dedicated group of officers who comprise that Section, cannot be over-emphasized. Vision is frequently the basic skill upon which other skills and abilities depend. Maximum visual performance is essential for the longer periods of intensive study required in the development and employment of the modern Army weapons

systems. A tremendous burden of responsibility is thus placed upon the shoulders of Army Optometry Officers. This responsibility is consistently discharged with professional competence, dignity, and a sense of purpose unsurpassed in the Army Medical Service.

Navy: The Navy pioneered in the struggle for commissions for optometrists. Long before the establishment of the Medical Service Corps in the Army, recognition was given by the Navy to the special training of optometrists. In the early 1940's, optometrists were granted commissions in the Navy; they were to assist in establishing training procedures for improving the speed and accuracy of recognition of aircraft and ships by Navy personnel.

Brown (1966), a Navy admiral in the Surgeon General's office, described the present significance of optometric officers in the Navy:

> The standards for induction and retention in the Naval Service have long reflected a recognition of the importance of good vision to the performance of the multitude of complex tasks required in the fulfillment of the Navy's world-wide commitments. The Navy Medical Department is proud of the splendid optometric services which it provides and which are so important to the accomplishment of its mission.

Air Force: The Air Force has recently changed the organizational status of its optometry section. Morris (1966), a lieutenant colonel and optometrist who is Associate Chief of the Biomedical Sciences Corps for Optometry, reports:

> Approximately one year ago the Air Force Biomedical Sciences Corps was created. This new Corps numbering approximately 800 men and women is comprised of: optometrists, bio-environmental engineers, clinical laboratory officers, psychologists, psychiatric social workers, entomologists, pharmacists, dieticians and physical and occupational therapists. With a more homogeneous corps of officers than existed in the former Medical Service Corps, it is anticipated that more emphasis will be placed on career development and the improvement of promotional opportunities.

The clinical workload of optometrists in the Air Force is approximately 30,000 refractions a month in the continental United States. As in the other services, optometrists are also utilized in preventive health measures and research. Recently, an optometry officer has been selected to serve on a loan basis from the Air Force as the Chief of the Crew Vision Section of the Manned Spacecraft Center of the National Aeronautics and Space Administration.

An Air Force colonel and Chief of the Biomedical Sciences Corps of the Air Force noted that the vision problems of the Air Force, as in the other services, are varied and interesting (Meyer, 1966). He cited problems of pilots operating high-speed aircraft at low altitudes and of eyestrain encountered in repairing electronic equipment. Eyestrain was also a problem for those performing clerical tasks and administrative duties and for the instructional personnel. The possible effects on vision of new systems and materials, as well as the problems of vision in space, hold challenges for the future. Meyer goes on to say that "our goal in the Biomedical Sciences Corps of the Air Force is to provide for an environment which will attract and then retain the high caliber of professional optometric skills needed for the military medical requirements and at the same time, insure professional development, recognition and self-satisfaction in a job well done. In this effort we will continue the present close relationship with the American Optometric Association."

Industrial Vision in Cooperation with the Armed Forces: Industrial civilian employees are associated with all of the services. Civilian employees, for example, work in Navy shipyards. The nature of the work performed by many of these civilian employees is often hazardous to vision. As a result, all branches of the service, Army, Navy, and Air Force, play an active role in industrial vision programs. The Navy has been particularly active for a number of years in this area. Even during World War II, a few optometrists were commissioned in the Hospital Corps to work with Naval employees in industry.

Optometry has a present-day role in the naval industrial establishment. The Bureau of Medicine and Surgery for a number of years has had a Sight Conservation Program for its civilian employees that attempts to eliminate eye injuries, to eliminate accidents resulting from faulty vision, to increase production and eliminate waste resulting from defective vision, and to foster and improve employee morale (Newman, 1966).

To implement this program, the Navy supplies safety spectacles in all large industrial programs and has called upon the services of many optometrists, both civilian and military. Of importance also is the large scale vision screening program to help industrial workers adjust to their jobs. Newman (1966) describes the Navy's policy of adapting workers to the job. He states, "We try to keep in mind that there is no such thing as 'perfect vision.' We are familiar with the fact that some workers will excel in visual skills valuable for one type of job, while some are superior for another." The Navy's attempt to match the visual abilities of workers to the visual requirements of jobs is indeed commendable. Newman goes on to say that, "Even the blind can meet the requirements of output, efficiency and safety in the right type of job."

The optometric industrial consultant, in addition to the many necessary visual studies and recommendations, works on such problems as lighting recommendations, reduction in glare, and utilization of certain colors to reduce accidents. To illustrate the variety of experience encountered, Newman cites two problems.

1. The Chief of Naval Air Training had ordered that training aircraft be painted on wingtips and certain other areas with a bright, orange-colored, high visibility paint. The sprayers engaged in this task noticed nausea, dizziness, and inability to keep at their jobs for any length of time. The paint used had very little odor or fume-producing properties. A tinted lens with proper absorptive quality, when worn in the painters' safety spectacles, completely eliminated the employees' symptoms.

2. One visual requirement of inspectors in an overhaul and repair department of an aircraft re-assemblage line is good depth perception. These workers were screened at regular intervals and referred for more complete examination when it was needed. All of these men, with one exception, had 20/20 unaided acuity and no symptoms. Even though the refractive errors present were minor, the necessary correction was supplied whenever professional judgment so indicated. An immediate improvement was noticed in the depth perception scores and in the workers' attitude toward their jobs.

Optometry has contributed appreciably to the national health in the vision care field. As the federal government enters into this field more and more, optometry will be called upon to contribute its skills. Through the educational program of the American Optometric Association Washington office, and through the performance of optometrists in the military, government has learned what optometry can contribute to a vision program. All welfare programs that provide health care for the public and that include vision services now utilize optometrists. The role of government in expanding these services will be discussed in Chapter 11.

Some improvements in the status of optometrists in the armed forces remain to be made (Lang, 1966). Optometrists should obtain the same rank for their academic degree and education, the same obligated duty time, and the same incentive pay that the members of other health professions now receive. These goals will very likely have been attained between the time this manuscript is being prepared and the time it sees publication. For example, optometrists now receive the rank of first lieutenant (Army) or lieutenant J.G. (Navy) by administrative action; a bill is before Congress that would make this entrance rank permanent by statute.

Overall, optometry has made tremendous strides toward achieving recognition as a health profession by the federal government in the past 20 years. Optometry earned the right to participate in welfare programs, and thereby to help the less fortunate, through its performance in the military.* Optometry and the contributions it can make to vision care programs are now recognized by the federal government. This recognition has added materially to the status of the profession.

OPINION MOLDERS

The social status of the optometrist has improved steadily during the present century, and with increasing rapidity during the past quarter century. One factor that determines status is public opinion. Newspapers, magazines, books, and other media of communication mold public opinion.

Public knowledge of the inner workings of a professional group is limited. People are interested in a profession only when it affects them personally. The word "optometrist" has had a vague meaning to the average person. Surveys 30 years ago revealed that most people had no idea of what an optometrist was. A random sampling taken 12 years ago revealed quite a change in this attitude; about 70 percent of the people questioned knew what an optometrist was. Present-day surveys reveal that almost everyone is familiar with the word "optometry" and realizes that it has something to do with eye care and glasses. They do not know details of the interprofessional squabbles that exist—nor do they care about them. They cannot help but see commercial optometry; they are not aware of organized optometry's problems in eliminating commercial practices. These are the profession's problems and ones that optometry itself must solve.

The public is constantly bombarded with educational (and propaganda) material. An examination of what the communication media were saying about optometry 30 years ago and what they now say about optometry will be revealing. For the optometrist's status *is* what the public thinks about optometry.

Thirty years ago in the pages of a national magazine—the *Reader's Digest*—optometry was severely criticized in a series of arti-

---

* Optometry's participation in military affairs, resulting in its being recognized in government programs, is especially interesting to one author (MJH); this is the second time in 20 years that he has observed a beneficial and serendipitous side-effect of the otherwise destructive business of making war. In the foreword to his doctoral thesis on depth perception, Hirsch (1947) wrote:

In the period between the two World Wars no important advances [in depth perception research] occurred. It seems ironic that it requires wars to advance the knowledge of such an eminently peaceful organ as the eye and that . . . the first information [about depth perception] came through art, the most recent through testing young men for military service.

cles under the title "Optometry on Trial." The author of the series, Riis (1937), claimed to have made a survey of the profession. Optometry in that era was partly business, partly profession. The schools were doing all they could to raise the standards, but too many of the exempt optometrists were still in practice; too many men with trade school education still were practicing optometry in stores.

Any reporter attempting to survey the profession would tend to go to the stores. Here were the practitioners who did the advertising, who attracted their "patients" into their place of business by window displays. To the man on the street they represented optometry. Riis claimed that optometrists sold him glasses when none were needed; that optometrists, although claiming to be professional men, advertised in newspapers, shop windows, street cars, and buses; and that optometrists were incompetent to perform vision examinations. More damaging to optometric morale even than these claims were the statements from eye physicians that optometrists could not diagnose eye disease. Riis claimed that evidence had been collected wherein optometrists had missed the diagnosis of glaucoma, brain tumors, and other diseases. In general, professional standards were sadly lacking according to Riis. Although the entire tone of the article was such as to bring discredit upon optometry, Riis did conclude the article by saying:

> Is there any remedy? Clearly, the standards of the optometrists—both in their education and practice—must be raised. The optometrists must clean their own shop if they expect to enjoy the continued confidence of the public. There are within the ranks of optometry a considerable body of men who wish to raise the standards of their craft, to route out flagrant commercialism, and unethical practices. In the high councils of optometry these men aware of their responsibilities are advocating reforms. . . .

Although the survey conducted by Riis was obviously unfair and not at all comprehensive in scope, and although it covered only the commercial elements, and was written as a sensational piece of journalism, it did serve to jolt optometry in official circles. The *Reader's Digest* magazine was an accepted news medium of the time with a very large circulation; several years passed before the effect of this publicity wore off.

About five years before the Riis article, a committee, headed by the Chairman of the United States Department of the Interior, was appointed to survey the cost of medical care. In a report published by the University of Chicago Press, Reed (1932) gave the results of this survey. In it, midwives, chiropodists, and optometrists were grouped together.

Although this report was less sensational than the Riis article and the study was probably competently conducted, there were some glaring omissions. The committee consisted of 50 people. Public health, educational institutions, special interest groups, economics and sociology, the general public, physicians, dentists, nurses, pharmacists, accountants, and attorneys were represented; but not one optometrist was on this committee.

However, as a result of this study, some important recommendations were made. Reed realized the difficulty involved in trying to obtain accurate figures concerning the work done by optometrists and eye physicians. He stated:

> In this country two groups of practitioners, optometrists and eye physicians, divide between themselves the work of refracting eyes and prescribing glasses. These two groups are economic rivals; their statements regarding each other should be considered in the light of this fact.

Reed was critical of the optometrist's training; yet he did assess the profession of optometry fairly. He recognized that it was developing toward professional maturity. He wrote:

> While the use of eye-glasses for the improvement of vision dates back many centuries, it is only within the past decades that techniques for the accurate determination of refractive errors and their consequent correction through lenses have been developed. The present-day optometrist, whose work is founded on these techniques, is also, therefore, a newcomer on the medical stage.
>
> Both the chiropodist and the optometrist, . . . are earnestly striving to raise the standards of their callings. Both groups, through legal regulation of their practices and through improvement of their schools, have raised the competency of their practitioners. Both believe that their ultimate destiny is to be accepted by the public and the medical profession as recognized practitioners of a medical specialty, possessing a status akin to that of dentists. Both consider that as professional groups they are in a developmental state and would ask that in any comparison with the professions of medicine and dentistry the comparison be made with these professions not as they are but as they were say, thirty or forty years ago.

The professionalization Reed recognized has come to pass. He was skeptical of greatly increasing optometric educational standards, for he felt it would produce optometrists too highly trained for simple refraction. He felt the solution to the problem was in cooperation between ophthalmologists and optometrists and in the division of labor between them. He said:

> . . . for example, in a clinic a group of optometrists might work along with a group of ophthalmologists, the ophthalmologists

first examining all patients and then passing on to the optometrists those patients with no pathological ocular conditions. The optometrist would then refract the eyes of these patients, prescribe the proper lenses and possibly fit the glasses.

Reed's final observation was that group practice might open the way for cooperation between optometrists and physicians. That cooperation today, however, does not rest so much on the division of supervised labor, recommended then, as it does on a mutual respect of the physician for the optometrist and of the optometrist for the physician.

An idea of how far optometry has advanced in public acceptance may be gained by considering a present-day article in a popular magazine of national circulation. Kenneth Alden (1963) reviewed the vision care field in *Coronet* magazine. An interesting aside on Alden's article is that he was not employed or sponsored by any group to gather the material. He started out to write a brief report on eyes and became so involved in it that his investigation took him to many parts of the country. The conclusions published by Alden in *Coronet* magazine are almost exactly the opposite of those of Riis in the *Reader's Digest* a quarter century earlier. Alden's main concern was that interprofessional squabbles between optometry and ophthalmology might affect vision care and should not be tolerated. Alden wrote:

> The accusation that optometrists are ignorant of pathology doesn't seem to hold up. Today, at leading schools of optometry, students spend more time than do medical men on fields of vision care. Their training includes eye anatomy, physiology and pathology, as well as psychological optics, physical optics and the clinical visual sciences. In New York State, optometry students must take a three-hour exam in pathology before they can earn a license.
>
> In contrast, medical students specializing in ophthalmology concentrate on eye surgery and medicine, spending little time on the vision sciences.
>
> Ironically, it's an M.D. who may overlook a hidden disease.

He goes on to cite instances in which ophthalmologists missed general pathology that was affecting vision. Although some optometrists and ophthalmologists occasionally miss eye pathology, reviewing cases like this in the public press results in loss of confidence by the public in both professions.

Several instances of patients with strabismus who were cured by optometrists through visual training are reviewed in the Alden article. These patients had been seen previously by eye physicians without satisfactory results. Alden stressed that it is high time that the eye professionals cooperate and work as a team. He says the fact that it can be done is shown in the Army and Navy programs, which seem to work to the benefit of everyone. In the closing summary in the *Coronet* magazine article, Alden flatly states what he thinks of the interprofessional squabble and the professional ability of members of each of the professions:

> Until peace is declared in the sight-saving professions, you and I will have to be on guard. The best objective advice is this: If you think you may have an eye disease or may need surgery, consult an eye physician—an ophthalmologist recommended by the family doctor you trust. Despite reaching out for other fields, the ophthalmologist can diagnose and treat functional disorders of the eyes, and is often a consultant on diseases which show themselves in the eyes, such as diabetes, cancer, tuberculosis, hypertension. But if you are certain that all you need is glasses, go to a reliable optometrist.

A comparison of the articles of Riis (1937) and Alden (1963) shows how far optometry has come in a quarter of a century. Both articles, insofar as they were critical of the eye care professions, tended to undermine public confidence. However, whereas the first article was a bitter denunciation of optometrists, the later one was much fairer; it praised and criticized ophthalmology and optometry equally.

The appearance of the profession in the communications mass media in a favorable light has helped to elevate the status of the optometrist today. The favorable impressions that members of the public receive in their individual dealings with the optometrist are reinforced by favorable comment in the communications media.

GENERAL SOCIAL STATUS—*Summary*

Optometry has now reached the point in its development where it is practiced successfully as an independent profession. The educational development has kept pace; optometry is recognized in the field of education as an established profession. The legal recognition that must accompany any professional advancement has been quite satisfactory. Gradually, most government bureaus and the armed forces have come to realize that optometrists are important members of the health care team.

Optometry's professional prestige among other professions has greatly improved. Only organized medicine still has reservations, and it will eventually recognize optometry for its valuable contributions to society. The professionalism of groups outside medicine is acknowledged first on the local level and eventually reaches the political level in organized medicine. Optometrists have gained the respect of other health professions and of practicing physicians—and eventually will earn the respect of official medicine too.

Optometrists have increasingly participated in community affairs. Most of this participation has resulted in optometry's further acceptance as a profession. Many valuable contributions have been made to the community by optometrists willing to devote their time and efforts to general community improvement.

As optometry progresses with its professional program, and the final 25 percent of practitioners become more professional in their appearance and behavior, optometry will make further advances. The recognition of this progress is apparent in national magazines, other press media, and the attitude of the public in general. Optometry is still a young profession, however, and must continue to set even higher standards of professionalism. By this means, complete professional recognition will be assured.

CHAPTER 11

PROVIDING THE OPTOMETRIC SERVICE

One characteristic of a profession is its members' concern with making the service available to all persons, regardless of their ability to pay. It has been traditional for members of the health professions to serve without charge rather than to allow any patient to go unattended. The first *printed* book on the eye, *De Oculis* by Benevenutus Grassus (Benevenutus of Jerusalem), published in 1474 from a manuscript written several hundred years earlier, makes reference to the practice of donating one's services to those who cannot pay. Benevenutus described his method for removing straws or barbs of wheat from the eye. He then added:

> I have cured many cases in this manner, especially in Sicily, where they are more common than in other sections of the country, for which I have been well paid. May you do the same; but do not forget the poor; in which case, God will give you grace to operate with success.

Health profession practitioners have usually heeded the advice to "not forget the poor." However, charity is not necessarily the best way to make health services available to the poor. All health professions have tried in one way or another to make their services available to everyone; all have recognized the problem as one that a profession must help to solve. The code of ethics of every professional group accepts for the profession the responsibility of care for all people. The code of ethics of the American Optometric Association (Appendix E) states that it is a duty of all members to "see that no person shall lack for visual care, regardless of his financial status."

Optometry today faces the same challenge as all other health professions—that of increasing the utilization of its service without impairing the quality.* Although the quality of optometric service today in the United States is excellent, not all people can obtain this

---

* In February 1967, President Johnson suggested that the Department of Health, Education, and Welfare hold national conferences to "discuss how we can lower the costs of medical services without impairing the quality." Coincidentally, this subject is essentially the content of the present chapter.

257

service for themselves and their dependents. The sociological problems of increased utilization of the service constitute the phase upon which the profession is just now embarking. Several methods have been tried to make the service more widely utilized.

For many people in the world, no optometric service or a very primitive form of service is still the only vision care available (Chapter 8). Even in the United States—the richest country in the world and the country in which optometry has reached its highest state of development—many people still receive no service. Many others receive care similar to that available several hundred years ago (ready-made spectacles sold by the present counterparts of the earlier peddler or haberdasher). Even those who do receive optometric service of a modern type often do not receive the service as frequently as they should. Just how under-utilized the optometric service is in the United States can be determined from a study by the United States Department of Health, Education, and Welfare (1966a). Interviewees were asked what health services they had obtained during the period of July 1963 to June 1964; the results were expanded to estimate the percentage of persons in the United States who received various health services during a year.

The age group 45 to 64 is of special interest because practically all persons in this age group require optometric service for presbyopia. Had the subjects in this age group received optometric service every two years (the recommendation of most optometrists for optimal care), then 50 percent should have reported having received vision care during any given year. Actually, 13.4 percent of the 45 to 64 age group visited an optometrist, and 8.1 percent visited an ophthalmologist. Many of these latter patients undoubtedly required medical eye care; however, even if it is assumed that all received optometric care, the total number who visited an optometrist or ophthalmologist is only 21.5 percent of the population. Comparison of this figure to the ideal of approximately 50 percent gives some indication of the degree of under-utilization of the service in the richest country in the world during a period of its highest economic development. People either received no optometric service or received the service much less frequently than at the recommended interval of every two years.

In the same study, 9.0 percent of children between the ages of 6 and 16 visited an optometrist, and 6.9 percent visited an ophthalmologist. Thus, 15.9 percent of this age group received some vision care in a one-year period. For optimal vision care, every child in this age group should have at least one vision examination some time during this period (that is, ten percent of the group in any given year). About 20 percent of this age group (by conservative estimate) have a vision problem; such children should receive care annually. Thus, if everyone were receiving optimal care, in any given year at least 30 percent of the children between the ages of 6 and 16 would receive optometric service; actually, 15.9 percent of the children did receive the service.

From the figures in the United States Department of Health, Education, and Welfare study (1966a), it would seem that optometric service is being utilized at approximately half the optimal rate. The problem is not solely one of economics. In England, where the optometric service is available to all people at little or no cost, utilization of the service differs little from that in the United States. One cause of under-utilization is economic; another is cultural. People must understand what constitutes optimal vision service and must have a desire for such service. If this service is to be utilized fully by all who need it, there must be recognition of the need, knowledge of what constitutes good care, willingness to seek care, willingness to accept care, availability of the service, accessibility to the service, and ability to purchase the service. We shall deal primarily with the last aspect of the problem, the ability to purchase care.

OPTOMETRIC ECONOMICS—*A Brief Overview*

Before an optometric profession evolved, there were several hundred years during which spectacles were sold. The traditional payment for this form of optometric service was the price paid for the spectacles. The seller added a profit or mark-up to the cost of the spectacles to reimburse him for supplying the spectacles and for incidental services. Surprisingly, the amount of profit for supplying a pair of spectacles bore the same relationship to the cost of the materials over a period of several hundred years. The traveling spectacle sellers of Continental Europe in the sixteenth century charged three times as much for the spectacles as they cost; the same three times mark-up was characteristic of the sale of spectacles in the early twentieth century in the United States.

At the turn of the century, when some opticians began to test vision, a few had the foresight to begin charging for the service. Opposition by physicians to this fee, in fact, was one factor which led Prentice to seek legal recognition of the new profession (Chapter 6). The fee-for-service concept was adopted early by at least one optometric organization; a requirement for membership in the originally formed American Academy of Optometry was that the optometrist charge his patients a fee for service.

The traditional view that the consumer should pay the cost of services in the form of profit on the spectacles was challenged at the very beginning of the emergence of the optometric profession. Although the idea of a fee for the services separate from the cost of spectacles was advanced very early, most optometrists and the public continued to expect the optometric fee to be tied in to the cost of the spectacles. The public, long used to paying for the spectacles and receiving "free" services, continued to expect this form of economics into the 1940's.

In the early 1940's, Carel C. Koch advanced thinking on optometric economics another step. He suggested that the patient should be billed by the optometrist for *two* different types of service in addition to the materials. Koch (1941) suggested that the optometrist charge one fee for the tests that he performs and for his professional advice; a separate fee would be charged for those services that apply to supplying the spectacles, that is, a "material service" fee. The spectacles themselves were to be supplied to the patient at cost. This system is based on the idea that optometrists perform two different types of services—those professional tasks of vision testing, interpretation, and advice *and* those technical services incidental to the supplying of spectacles.

It had taken a quarter of a century or more for the suggestion of Prentice to attain any degree of acceptance among optometrists and the public; the suggestion of Koch is just now beginning to be followed by the profession and understood by patients. In the meantime, a new concept in fees is developing. Many optometrists have pointed out that there is no such thing as a "routine examination." Different patients require different items of the total service that an optometrist can render. The various services that the optometrist offers should be catalogued and each patient should pay for those services (and only those) that he receives.

The newer concept is to charge individual patients for the items of service that each receives; the older system is to charge all patients the same overall average fee. The system of a total average fee has been used in many health services. Obstetricians have traditionally charged an average fee for "a baby." The obstetrician presented a fee that covered an average amount of pre-natal care, the delivery itself, and some post-natal visits by the mother. Some patients received far more service than others; all paid the average fee. Dentists also often used an average overall fee for a "set of teeth."

At present, several optometric leaders have offered suggested lists of the individual services that optometrists offer; these systems differ from each other in their degree of complexity. However, the broad concept, that of itemizing the parts of the service and charging only for those that the patient receives, seems to be the concept of the future in optometric economics. The public and many optometrists may be slow in adopting the newer thinking, but it is clear that it will prevail.

With the development of a fee scale in which each of the many services is considered, two other concepts have developed—the unit of relative value fee scale *and* the fee slip.

In a unit fee scale, each service is listed and is assigned a unit value rather than a dollar value. The number of units assigned to any procedure is *relative* to the values assigned to others. If, for example, twice as much time, skill, and equipment is needed to perform tonometry as is needed to adjust a pair of spectacles, the former procedure will have a value of twice as many units as the latter. If the minimal task performed by the optometrist, adjusting a pair of spectacles, for example, is assigned a value of one, then all other services can be assigned values of one or more units; if the performance of a preschool screening examination on a child requires five times as much time and skill as spectacle adjustment, then it receives a value of five units. There will be disagreement among optometrists as to what the relative values are in fact. However, those who propose such a system suggest that time, skill, and cost of instrumentation be considered in arriving at values and that these be agreed upon through consensus.

All optometrists who use the same relative value fee scale will not have identical fees; the final step of assigning a dollar value to each unit is a matter of the individual practitioner's choice. In the examples just used, where adjusting spectacles is one unit, tonometry is two units, and preschool screening is five units, an optometrist who assigns the value of $1.00 to each unit would charge $1.00, $2.00, and $5.00, respectively, for these three different services. However, another optometrist who considers a unit to be worth $1.50 would charge $1.50, $3.00, and $7.50, respectively, for these three services. The fees of the two optometrists would differ, but within each practice the *relative* values of the services would bear the same relationship to each other. The value of a unit will differ in various parts of the country, but the relative values should be the same.

If optometrists can agree upon and adopt a uniform relative value scale, the profession will be in a much better position to negotiate with those outside agencies that contract for optometric services. In reaching an agreement with a governmental agency purchasing vision care for a group of people, the only points of negotiation would then be the dollar value assigned to the unit and the items that might be excluded. It would not be necessary to negotiate a price for each service that the optometrist performs. Moreover, if cost of living changes are the cause of renegotiating an agreement between optometry and any agency, then only one item—the remuneration for one unit—need be discussed. It would not be necessary to renegotiate item by item. In most unit fee systems, the materials are furnished at cost.

The other major concept associated with unit fee scales is the fee slip or receipt given each patient listing the various items for which he has been charged. Many optometrists are using fee slips on which many of the services are described so that the patient may know just what parts of the optometric service he has received and how much he has paid for each. Many of the procedures described in Chapter 2, such as ophthalmoscopy, retinoscopy, tonometry, and visual field and subjective testing, are listed. They are also described in a brief statement designed to tell the patient of each item's importance and to enable him to identify that item's part in the total procedure. The fee slip informs the patient of the services he has received and of the cost to him of each. It also informs him of the scope of vision care, enabling him better to recognize other services sold as a bargain but actually cheaper only because they are less inclusive.*

There have been many variations on each fee system; however, four distinctly different concepts have evolved over the years. † These four different basic systems may be summarized in tabular form:

Method	First Suggested	Came into Common Use
Profit on materials only; service included	From the earliest date of spectacles	From the earliest date

---

* The complete itemization of all parts of the optometric examination and the assignment of a relative value to each part of the complete optometric service are fairly recent developments in the profession. The method of arriving at the relative value of each part of the service is somewhat involved and would constitute a complete chapter by itself. Optometry has yet to establish on a national basis a relative value scale of all of its services. This subject deserves more comprehensive coverage and will be explored in detail in a forthcoming text on optometric economics by the present authors.

† We are dealing here exclusively with methods whereby vision care has been purchased by the individual in a "free enterprise" system. Some of these methods, particularly the more recent ones, may also be used when vision care is purchased for a group of people by a third party, such as government. There is, however, another system of payment applicable only to groups that has not been mentioned. This is a "capitation" method, or one in which the doctor is paid a set amount for each patient for whom he is responsible. The doctor receives a fixed annual stipend that is based on the number of persons on his roster and for whose care he is responsible. Few health care plans in the United States have been based on capitation, and it has been bitterly opposed by most health profession groups in the country as being incompatible with the general economic and social system. However, when an optometrist works for a salary for a health plan, he is in a sense working on a capitation basis. He is paid a fixed amount for caring for all of the patients assigned to him.

Method	First Suggested	Came into Common Use
Examination fee plus profit on materials	1890 by Prentice; 1925 by American Academy of Optometry	In more or less wide use by the 1940's
a) Examination (professional) fee; b) Materials (technical) fee; c) Little or no profit on materials	1941 by Koch	In more or less common use by the 1960's
No average fee, but a list of all services rendered, each with its own fee. Materials at cost. Unit fee scale based on relative values of services	1960's by several optometrists and organizations	Will gain acceptance in years to come

Each health service has characteristics in common with the other health services; each also has some attributes peculiar to itself. Aspects of the optometric service differing from those of other health services are:

1. Optometrists furnish materials of moderate value, while most other health professions supply few materials. Physicians may use dressings, splints, casts or other supplies; dentists use some materials in the filling of teeth. Most health professionals, however, are required to supply little material. Optometrists, on the other hand, supply most patients with materials and retrieve the cost of the materials from the patient along with the customary fee for service.

2. Part of the optometric service is truly professional in nature, demanding professional judgment and skills; part, however, can be supplied by a technician. Thus, when an optometrist repairs a pair of spectacles, he is doing work which can be performed equally well by a technician (optician). The existence of two types of services leads to problems in economics. Is an optometrist, for example, entitled to the same hourly fee when he repairs spectacles as when he evaluates a vision problem of a patient? Traditionally, optometrists have practiced in one-man offices, performing both professional and technical tasks.

3. The technical aspects of the optometric service—the repair and adjustment of spectacles—are sometimes required long after the original service was performed. A similar situation exists in part of the dental service in that a denture may require servicing (relining) sev-

eral years after it is fitted. For the most part, however, this sort of situation is not a characteristic of the health professions.

4. The prosthetic device used (spectacles) is also an item of style. Most of the agents used in the health professions serve only a therapeutic role. Spectacles, however, cover a third of the patient's face, and are visible to his friends and family. Style is costly. Anyone selling an item in which style plays a part must carry a stock of materials, must accept a loss for those items that do not sell, and must spend additional time helping the consumer make a choice. As more style enters into an item, more profit must be made on that item. The fact that style is involved in spectacles complicates the picture of the economics of optometric service.

5. Optometric service is needed by all individuals in certain segments of the population. Almost all other health services are required by certain people only. Many of the health services are of the emergency type and affect only a small percentage of the population each year. Optometric service, on the other hand, is required by *all* persons over the age of about 45. Therefore, the cost of optometric service is not insurable in the usual sense of the word (Hirsch, 1954). If one person in a group of a hundred will require an appendectomy in any given year, then each person can contribute 1/100th of the cost to an insurance fund to be used by the unfortunate person who requires the surgery that year. But if every person in the group will require the service, insurance is not feasible as a means to pay the bill. Thus, optometric service and dental service are usually not included in health *insurance* plans. On the other hand, they can be included in prepayment plans or in comprehensive health plans.

Optometric economics differs from that of other professions. Despite these differences, however, optometric economics is similar to that of other health professions. The patient pays mainly for the doctor's time and training and for the expenses of the doctor's office. Each patient must pay his share of the total overhead of a health profession office. This overhead includes the salaries of technicians and receptionists, rent, utilities, insurance, supplies, and depreciation on equipment. Year by year, more expensive, complex equipment appears, and each patient must pay his share of the purchase of this equipment. In the health professions, the doctor must keep abreast of recent developments in his field; the costs of postgraduate education must be pro-rated over the total number of patients. Despite the differences that have been mentioned, the economic aspects of optometric practice are quite similar to those of other health professions.

PRESENT METHODS OF PAYING
FOR THE OPTOMETRIC SERVICE

During the last 30 years in the United States, emphasis has been placed on increased utilization of all health services and better methods of payment for each. Technologically, optometric service has arrived at a point of excellence.* Recently, optometrists, public health officers, government officials, insurance companies, and health planners have turned their attention to the problem of making the service available to more people. This trend will undoubtedly increase in the years ahead.

Most of the vision care in the United States is supplied by the individual practitioner in his office. Between 85 and 90 percent of the optometric offices are one-optometrist offices. The fee, set by the optometrist, is usually paid to him by the patient. It is the opinion of many students of health care trends that this traditional method of practice and of payment will ultimately be changed; a trend toward other methods of practice and of payment has been apparent for the past three decades. Whereas in the United States almost all vision care was obtained in the traditional fashion in the 1940's, today substantial blocks of patients obtain care in other ways.

The traditional one-man practice serving patients who pay their own bills from the family budget is so well known that it requires no further description. It is the basic type of practice; it was operative when the optometric profession emerged. It is certainly the basic type from which the new trends will emerge.

Two distinct trends away from the traditional solo practice of optometry are recognized at this time. One of these is toward multi-optometrist offices, clinics, or health center practices. The other is a trend for practitioners to remain in individual practice but to be paid by a third party.† Several such plans of payment are in opera-

---

* Although optometric service has reached a point of technological excellence, it does not necessarily follow that every optometrist in practice is offering the optimal service to his patients. If each optometrist utilized all technological advances and saw to it that his patients receive a service within the total scope of the profession, the service would be improved. This is true in other professions as well as in optometry. The concept of total scope will be discussed in Chapter 12.

† A third party in the health-care payment system may be described as any person or entity that acts as the agent for members of an organization or segment of the population to purchase health services for the individuals in the group. An insurance company, a branch of local or federal government, a trade union's health and welfare department, or an industrial corporation may act as a third party to purchase health care for the group of people whose interests it represents.

tion. In some plans, *both* the multi-optometrist practice *and* third party payment are used.

MULTI-OPTOMETRIST OFFICES

An evaluation of the cost of optometric service shows that cost could be reduced somewhat if offices were not one-man operations; the one-optometrist office is more costly than optometric overhead need be. Savings, ultimately passed on to the patient, may be realized in almost every item of overhead if several optometrists practice as a group.

When two optometrists share an office, the rent they pay is not double what one optometrist must pay. One optometrist may find it difficult to generate enough professional services to make it economically feasible to employ a technician (optician) ; two or three optometrists together can do so. With only one secretary or office manager, a two- or three-man office can be run almost as easily as a one-man office. Costly equipment may be shared by several optometrists. With increased technology, the equipment for all health services becomes more costly. Often an expensive instrument (an electronic tonometer, for example) is used by one optometrist only half an hour or less per day. If several optometrists use the same instrument, the cost may be amortized over a much greater number of patients.

Optometrists who have converted one-man practices to associate-ship practices almost all agree that the multi-optometrist practice is far more economical in overhead. The trend among optometrists to try two- or three-man offices may be expected to continue.

Group practices are occasionally tried in which many optometrists practice in a single office complex (Chapter 9). In a few large cities, optometric centers in which many optometrists practice have been operated with success. Although the trend toward multi-optometrist offices is unmistakably present, the entire concept is too recent for definite conclusions regarding its future. There is probably an optimal size for a multi-optometrist office; after this size is reached, the return for each additional optometrist added to the staff probably diminishes. Certainly the personal nature of the service decreases when a practice becomes too large. On the other hand, group practices have several characteristics, such as peer judgment, that tend to improve the quality of the care. Through trial and error experimentation by individual optometrists in the next decade or two, we shall learn far more about the ideal size for an optometric group, clinic, or practice.

For the present, although no definitive data can be offered for the ideal size of an optometric group, two conclusions are indicated. First, solo practice is uneconomical, and with the attempt to achieve optimal vision care at minimal cost, the trend toward multi-optometrist offices will continue. Second, some aspects of group practice tend to reduce the quality of the service as the group becomes too large and too impersonal, whereas other aspects tend to improve the quality of the service. A great deal of interesting experimentation is being done by optometrists today who try various sized groups. Data on this aspect of optometric practice should be expected to become increasingly available with passing time.

THIRD PARTY PAYMENT PLANS

From earliest times, the optometrist was paid for his services by the individual patient or his family from the patient's personal funds. Most families planned for the professional services that its members would need, and the family budget provided for the service. If the service was too costly for the family provisions, budget plans were utilized in which subsequent payments were made. Patients without money to pay for optometric service at the time they required it made a down payment and then paid the optometrist a fixed amount each week or month until the total bill was paid. Today, this is the way most families purchase automobiles, television sets, homes, and even clothing. Food is one of the few items for which most American families pay their total bill at the time of purchase.

During and after the depression of the 1930's, many people could not afford health services under the existing system. Many new systems of paying for health services were tried. In the present period, experimentation is still being conducted on a huge scale. Although no single system has emerged as *the* answer, the trend toward third party payment schemes is unmistakable. Optometrists in private practice today are usually able to enumerate a dozen different plans through which their patients' bills are being paid. That so many plans are being tried indicates: (1) the need for systems other than the traditional one, and (2) the fact that no single, satisfactory system has yet been devised.

The problem of making health services available through a third party payment plan is not one of economics alone. The relationship between doctor and patient may be affected. For over 2000 years, ethical codes of all health professions have had a provision that the confidences of the patient shall be kept inviolate; if someone else is paying the bill, however, the doctor must give some information to the third party. Another traditional characteristic of good health services has been the right of the patient to choose his doctor; some third party plans, however, hire specific doctors for members of the plan. These closed-panel plans violate the concept of free choice of doctor.

There are several currently used third party payment plans. A few of them will be discussed here.

SERVICE CLUBS

The very poor in society are unable to pay for their own health services. Traditionally, doctors have taken care of such people as a matter of duty. Charitable organizations and service clubs have also attempted to help to make health services available to the poor. Some service clubs have bought optometric services for the poor, and particularly for children. An important activity of Lions International is the work of its Sight and Blind Committee. Individual Lions Clubs often purchase optometric services for needy children. The child usually goes to the doctor of his choice; upon the recommendation of the school nurse, the local Lions Club reimburses the optometrist. The charge to service clubs is often a little less than the usual fee.

INSURANCE PLANS

Most private third party health payment in the United States today is made through insurance companies and plans such as the Blue Cross. The individual or, more often, his employer pays a monthly (or annual) premium to the insuring corporation; the individual and his family are then covered for hospital bills and or surgical services. The success of these programs has been related to the use of group purchasing power and payment through health and welfare trusts, so that the individual *per se* does not pay the premium.

Some plans include drugs, nursing care, ambulance service, physiotherapy, and other auxiliary health services. There are dozens of plans covering large segments of the population today; each differs slightly from the others. Each plan covers slightly different services; each has some exclusions different from those of the other plans. Each has different payment schedules; and the cost of each is slightly different, although, as might be expected, the more items that are covered, the more expensive the health insurance.

Health insurance came as an answer to the need of people to insure against major expenses of hospital and surgeon or against long, costly illnesses. As these plans evolved, each company or group tried to offer the most attractive coverage for the patient's dollar. Often, however, in the desire to add as many items as possible (office calls to family general practitioner or drug bills), true catastrophe insurance was neglected. Today, many people find it necessary to carry two different types of health insurance—one of the ordinary type, and one against *major* catastrophes.

As a rule, optometric and dental services are not covered in insurance plans. The reason is apparent: almost all people past a certain age require optometric service; nearly everyone needs dental service. When optometric or dental services are included in an insurance plan, they are really not insurance but merely prepayment. Thus, although a major percentage of all medical and hospital bills is now paid at least in part by private insurance or group health insurance, only a very few policies cover optometric or dental services. This form of third party payment is of great significance in general medical practice; it is today of only very limited but growing significance in optometric or dental practice.

VISION SERVICE CORPORATIONS

Although it is impractical to insure against the need for vision care, it is possible to plan ahead and pre-pay for the service. Thus, members of a group may pay a small amount monthly into a fund that in turn would purchase the individual's vision care when he needs it. This method is not greatly different from that of an individual buying his services on a budget plan; the major differences are group rather than individual action and budget payment in anticipation of services rather than after the service has been received. Several such plans have become operative during the past decade and have succeeded in making vision care available to large numbers of people.

The vision service corporations are usually established on a statewide basis, and are organized as non-profit corporations. The California Vision Service is an example of a successful plan. Any group may purchase vision care through these vision service corporations, although usually a health and welfare trust associated with a trade union is the purchaser.* An amount determined through actuarial tables is deposited with the service corporation for each enrollee each month. The member may visit an optometrist on the service corporation panel; the optometrist is then reimbursed by the fund.

This plan would appear to entail much paper work to achieve the minor advantage of prepayment or preplanning by the individual. However, it has several other major advantages in our present economic structure. Most unions have entered into the health and welfare aspect of their members' lives and no longer negotiate with employer groups solely for wages and working hours. Unions also work out plans with management for "fringe benefits," that is, for health and welfare services to union members. The employer often pays a portion of the health and welfare needs of his employees as part of the agreement that the union negotiates. Thus, in vision ser-

---

* The health and welfare trust that purchases coverage for its members is usually administered by someone selected by the trustees. The trustees represent union members and employers. Jointly, they determine the type and amount of coverage, negotiate the plans, and set policy on other details of the plan.

vice corporations, a member of a contracting union often does not pay into the fund the total amount that his vision care will demand; the employer pays into the union health and welfare fund a sum of money for each employee, part of which is allocated for vision care.

Another major advantage is that the service is purchased for the group. Thus, the health and welfare trust is in a better bargaining position (has more purchasing power) than an individual seeking vision care. The trust is often in a position to insist on optometric services of the highest quality. Quality control is an essential feature of service corporations—through selection of materials, through selection of the professional personnel with whom they will contract, and through control of the services deemed to constitute good health care.

With vision service corporations, the patient not only receives high quality care but retains the free choice of doctor. Since it is not necessary for him to demonstrate "need," he retains a confidential relationship with his health practitioner. An example of such a plan is the 1966–1967 contract between the Western Teamsters Union and the California Vision Service.

The union member and his employer each pay a sum of money into the health and welfare trust fund. The trust then contracts with the California Vision Service for the latter group to supply vision care for all members of the Teamsters Union and their dependents. The amount that is paid from the health and welfare fund to the California Vision Service is determined by actuarial tables on what it will cost to give service to all members of the union. The individual member who requires service obtains a simple form from his union's health and welfare department, and presents it to the optometrist of his choice. The patient pays a small amount, to insure that he will not over-utilize the service. In this example, the fee is $5.00.* The optometrist renders the complete service; he then bills the California Vision Service for a total fee minus the $5.00 that the patient has paid. In this particular contract, the fee scale adopted by the optometrists, the union, the California Vision Service, and the health and welfare trustees is based on the Koch plan described earlier. The optometrist submits a bill that includes three items: (1) the professional (examination) services; (2) the material services (technical and professional services needed to select and service the spectacles); and (3) the *cost* of the materials.

---

* There are several different types of plans. For example, the deductible portion may be "front end," as this one is, in which the patient pays the first few dollars, the plan the remainder; or it may be "rear end" deductible, in which the fund pays up to a certain amount, the patient the remainder. The scope of this book does not permit a complete description of all of the types of plans.

At present, California Vision Service has contracts similar to that with the Teamsters with several other unions in California. Vision service corporations in other states have similar plans. The method seems to be a satisfactory one for supplying vision services to union workers and their families. It need not be limited to such groups; any organization that is purchasing health services for its members may contract with a vision service corporation to supply optometric care also.

GOVERNMENT AS A THIRD PARTY

There is a difference of opinion as to the function of government in the United States. Some people believe that government should allow the free enterprise system to solve most social problems, subject only to minor rules and regulations concerning monopolies; others believe that government has a duty to provide for most human welfare needs. The thoughts of most individuals range between these two fundamental social beliefs. It is not within the scope of this book to argue which of these approaches to health care is proper. Various agencies of local and federal government *are* involved in paying for health services. Certain trends in governmental involvement must be recognized and understood. Long range plans made by the health care professions must take these trends into account.

When certain problems could not be solved by the free enterprise system, city, county or state governments undertook their solution; if the problems were of sufficient magnitude or complexity, the federal government accepted the responsibility for their solution. Over the years, there has been increasingly stronger federal governmental participation in all health care programs. As specific segments of the population have been unable to obtain health care for themselves, the government has initiated programs to provide such care. Governmental aid has been made available for the indigent, the physically handicapped, dependent children, the blind, and the aged. Traditionally, county and state governments have helped to obtain health care for these people. In the past 30 years, however, the federal government has become increasingly involved in health and welfare programs.

Much of the federal government health and welfare program falls within the legislation of the Social Security Act.* The original Social Security Act of 1935 now has 19 major amendments and goes

---

* Although a major portion of government concern has been with programs under Social Security, other programs, some of them involving sizable sums of money, do exist. Two of these, involving mainly younger members of society, are under the Office of Economic Opportunity (OEO) and the Elementary and Secondary Education Act (ESEA).

far beyond its original scope. It includes such coverage as: old age insurance, survivors insurance, disability insurance, health insurance, grants for aid to the aged, care for the blind and disabled, medical assistance programs, aid to families with dependent children, work experience and training programs, and many child welfare programs, such as day care centers, foster care, protective services for abused or neglected children, services for unmarried mothers, licensing of child care facilities, and adoption service information. Services performed by optometrists are included in many of these programs.

Often the federal government participates in health and welfare plans by supplying funds for specific purposes to be administered by local, state or county agencies. Most welfare programs in the various states include vision care for welfare recipients. These programs are administered by the local agencies, which receive a large share of their money from federal support programs. Today, almost every state program supplying vision care includes the services of optometrists. This is exactly the opposite of the situation in almost all European countries, in which optometrists are not included in the governmental health plans (Chapter 8).

Optometrists are reimbursed for their services according to different schedules in different states. Each fee system used at some time in the past is in use at this time in some state. Thus, in California, optometric services are purchased for welfare recipients (aged, needy children, families of dependent children) by an examination fee, a fee for lenses, and a fee for frames. The last two items are priced somewhat higher than the actual cost of the materials to include the cost of materials *and* the services entailed in prescribing and supplying these materials. This examination fee plus "marked-up" materials is one of the oldest systems. In other states, the more modern system suggested by Koch (1941) is used; the optometrist receives a fee for the examination and analysis, another fee for the material services, and he is reimbursed for the cost of the materials. In still other states, some form of a yet more modern unit fee system is used: each item of a list of services is assigned a unit value (Wick, 1963). The fee schedule is usually arrived at by negotiation between the state welfare department and the vision services corporation representing the optometrists of that state.

With the federal government offering matching funds, few states can afford not to participate. If a state refuses federal matching funds, it must use local funds (not plentiful in most states). It then must curtail service to the underprivileged or else depend on local service clubs, church organizations, or private welfare organizations. Since few states are willing to forego federal aid in welfare programs, federal government participation seems destined to increase in the future.

Some of the most significant health and welfare legislation of the past 30 years has been listed by the Social and Health Care Trends Committee of the American Optometric Association. This list appears as Appendix G.

In the continuing trend toward federal governmental participation in the payment of health expenses for individuals, 1965 was a milestone. The Social Security program has expanded to include hospital and medical insurance for all persons over the age of 65. This program is unique in that it brings health care to everyone in a particular age group regardless of financial circumstances. Although optometric services are not covered in the program at this time, it seems very likely that they will be included in the near future. Moreover, there is a great probability that other age groups in the population will be covered by subsequent expansions of the program; most probably, the next group added to the coverage will be children. Thus, although the Medicare program does not include vision services, it establishes a pattern that will undoubtedly influence the payment for optometric service in the future. With the acceptance of the important concept that government participation does not depend on ability to pay, the possibility that coverage will include more services (such as vision care) and more groups of people (such as children) becomes very great.

Although the Medicare program does not include vision services, it is clearly of sufficient importance to optometrists that they should be thoroughly familiar with it. A description of the services included in the Medicare program appears as Appendix H.

Government's role as a third party in the payment for optometric services includes these salient facts:

1. Government has already participated in the payment for services for the needy, particularly the aged, the young, and the handicapped.

2. Government at one time or another has paid optometrists according to many fee schedules; the trend is toward establishment of unit fee scales.

3. Services to all persons in certain age groups—regardless of financial circumstances—has characterized recent health and welfare planning.

4. As programs are expanded, they will include more age groups and more complete services for the people within an age group.

5. Those who represent optometry in bargaining with government will seek to have optometrists included in all vision care pro-

grams, to keep the quality of the service maximal, and to obtain a fair fee for the services performed.

6. Government participation in paying the bill for optometric services is already a significant part of many optometric practices. It will continue to increase, and the optometrist will find more and more patients having their bills paid through one or another governmental insurance or prepaid plan.

INDUSTRY AS A THIRD PARTY

Sometimes an industrial company acts as a third party and buys partial vision care for its employees. Industry became interested in vision care through safety programs; thus, private companies usually enter into the payment for vision care mainly in safety programs.

There are many different programs. In the typical one, the employee obtains an examination and a prescription or order for a pair of safety spectacles from the eye practitioner of his choice; the spectacles are ordered by the employer. Sometimes they are furnished free to the employee; sometimes he is charged the laboratory cost; sometimes employer and employee each pay half of the laboratory bill.

The concept of vision safety planning is worthwhile, and many industrial companies have adopted such programs hoping to improve safety conditions and reduce accidents. The basic purpose of the programs, however, is *not* total vision care, but is safety. Therefore, it is difficult to evaluate such programs here, where we are discussing third party payment for total vision care for blocks of patients. Safety programs usually supply safety spectacles only. The individual still contracts for the optometric services on a private basis. These plans usually supply only partial vision care.

Safety programs can be misused—and occasionally this has happened in the past. Employees who require no spectacles on their job, but only need them for reading at home, sometimes obtain safety spectacles—particularly if the employer is paying for them. Employees might obtain safety spectacles even though their jobs are not hazardous (bookkeepers, for example); others will obtain safety spectacles for members of their families. Thus, what is intended to be a safety program sometimes becomes a "fringe benefit." Employees obtain spectacles for off–the–job use, for friends, or for families at the employer's expense or at his contracted laboratory cost. The matter becomes completely ludicrous when, as sometimes happens, an employee who works under moderately hazardous conditions and who has obtained safety spectacles uses them for reading at home but wears no lenses to protect his eyes on the job.

Poor communications among employers, their safety engineers, employees, and optometrists are to blame for many of the misuses of safety programs. The misuse of safety programs has also been encouraged by the trend toward making safety spectacles look as much as possible like "dress" spectacles. Initially, safety spectacles looked "different." Year by year, manufacturers of eyewear, arguing that workers would not wear safety spectacles unless they were good looking, have styled safety spectacles to look as much as possible like other spectacles. As a result, some people wear "safety" spectacles constantly, that is, as "dress" or regular spectacles. The spectacles serve their purpose and are free; some employees, therefore, are willing to tolerate the extra weight and the optical disadvantages of a thick lens.

Whether a safety program proves satisfactory or not depends mainly on its administration and the amount of care that goes into its planning. Several excellent safety programs have been in operation in various industrial companies for many years. These usually are ones in which optometrists helped in planning and in setting up the program. Those that are misused are often programs that have been set up without optometric consultation and that are administered by a company's purchasing department, the head of which is often impressed only by "cheap glasses." A few companies have set up total vision programs (as opposed to safety programs), and these will be discussed later in this chapter.

Unlike governmental plans, industrial participation in paying for optometric services (more exactly, for the optometric materials), is not increasing. As vision service corporations and governmental plans increase, the use of industrial plans to obtain vision care will decrease. The plans will become truly safety programs. Optometrists recognize the need for safety programs and have long stressed the need for special lenses for those engaged in hazardous occupations; they are critical of the use of safety spectacles that are not necessary to the patient's occupation but are obtained merely at an economic advantage as a fringe benefit of employment. Even should industrial companies retire from the field of supplying eyewear, optometrists will continue to work toward improved eye safety programs and will recommend and supply safety spectacles when they are required.

Multi-Optometrist and
Third Party Payment Plans

Two trends away from the traditional one-optometrist office, in which the patient himself pays directly, have been discussed: the trend toward multi-optometrist offices and the trend toward third party payment. There are several plans that incorporate both of these features. In some, the optometric service is offered in conjunction with other health services; in others, only the optometric service is offered. To this broad category of plans that incorporate both features, the name *institutional optometry* may be applied.

HOSPITALS AND CLINICS

The optometric service is sometimes supplied in clinic or outpatient sections of hospitals. Those who receive the services in such institutions are usually welfare or indigent patients. Optometrists who work at such institutions may be salaried, may receive a token salary, or may donate their services totally. County hospitals frequently have a vision out-patient section; the refractive work in these sections is sometimes done by optometrists. Often, however, optometric service in hospitals is supplied by young physicians who receive part of their training by serving at hospitals and clinics.

PREPAID HEALTH PLAN CENTERS

In the past quarter century, several prepaid health care plans have become established. In these plans, the participating member pays a fixed amount of money each year that entitles him to receive most of the health services from doctors who are salaried and who work exclusively for the plan. Often, such centers, in the attempt to make their health services complete, have established optometric sections staffed by optometrists who receive a salary and who work exclusively for the plan.

The member who participates in such a plan receives most of his health services from the plan. In addition to his monthly or annual premium, he usually is required to pay a small fee for each visit. When he needs the services of a physician, he visits the center and pays a small amount (one or two dollars). After he is seen by one of the physicians, any required medication is supplied from the center's pharmacy at a lower than usual price. If a member requires optometric service, he is processed in exactly the same manner. For a small entrance fee, he is given an appointment with one of the staff optometrists; any required spectacles are supplied by the plan at some less-than-usual fee. Some plans have a sufficient number of members to have rather large optometric sections. They employ several optometrists who work full time to bring optometric service to participating members and their families.

These plans are usually established as non-profit corporations. Sometimes they are sponsored by a labor union, in which case the clients are members of the union and their families.

INDUSTRIAL HEALTH CENTERS

Some large industrial corporations have established health centers for their employees. Such centers often have optometric departments. These centers are not very different from the prepaid health centers. The only major difference is that the members are employees whose participation is determined by the fact that they work for the company that sponsors the clinic, rather than by the prepayment of a fee.

The optometric section of a company-sponsored health center may also be responsible for the eye safety program of the company. Thus, the employee may be examined by the company optometrist in the company health center and may receive safety spectacles for use on the job as well as "dress" spectacles for general use. The optometric section may also assume the responsibility for visual conditions in the company's plant. It may advise on lighting conditions, eye hazards, and proper working distances; it may perform vision screening of employees to determine their visual suitability to certain types of work.

Although most companies are neither large enough to support, nor oriented toward sponsoring their own health facilities, there are nonetheless enough such health centers in existence to be considered in the total scheme of health care planning. A substantial number of people receive their optometric service, as well as their other health services, from a "company doctor."

OPTOMETRIC CENTERS

In hospitals, clinics, and the prepaid health plan centers, the optometric service is supplied along with other health services. Thus, the patient requiring vision care goes to the same administrative entity as he does for his other health needs. The optometrist or dentist at such a center is one of many paramedical practitioners who work as a health team. Some plans, however, usually for the care of lower income patients, have been established to supply optometric services exclusively and not in conjunction with other health services.

The Optometric Center of New York observed its tenth anniversary in April, 1966; it is the largest optometric center. It has served as a model for optometric centers in California, Colorado, Virginia, Washington, D.C., and Missouri. Several other states and local societies are planning such programs.

The Optometric Center of New York, which took over the staff and facilities of the Columbia University School of Optometry, had an excellent start under the dynamic leadership of Alden N. Haffner, who still serves as director. Many research projects and postgraduate courses have been sponsored by this center. A major function of optometric centers, however, has been to supply the aged, the handicapped, and the indigent with services that often are not otherwise available. With the rapid growth of government health care plans, the place of optometric centers, present and future, needs to be examined.

Optometric centers have the responsibility for the vision welfare of the community. Up to the present, no other agency has made any serious attempt to provide the community vision need on an organized basis. The boards of directors of most centers are broad based, consisting of lay and professional people. Broadly representative of the community, such a governing board assures community contact, helps to locate the community need, assures participation of the community, and helps to obtain donated funds.

As the federal government continues to take over the responsibility for vision care of the needy, a more dependable source of income than donations will become available. Federal projects that assure adequate welfare fees will enable the centers to operate; staff optometrists will be reimbursed for their time at a reasonable fee.

It is possible to establish some form of optometric center in almost any community that has a few optometrists and a local welfare department. Where it is not possible to have a permanent building, temporary facilities can be established in conjunction with the welfare department; donated equipment may be employed. The center can be used on a biweekly or monthly basis. In more heavily populated areas, one or two days a week may be satisfactory. If a center is to develop properly, however, it is necessary to have a director from the beginning and to start out as a non-profit, tax-exempt institution.

COMMERCIAL OPTOMETRISTS

Technically, a discussion of plans through which patients receive professional optometric service in multi-optometrist offices by a form of third party payment should not include commercial optometric practices. Yet, there are similarities (as well as a few differences) that make it necessary to discuss this form of optometric practice here.

In prepaid health plans, company health facilities, optometric centers, hospitals, and clinics, a major divergence from traditional private practice is that the patient does not have the free choice of doctor or optometrist. The patient in any of these plans is assigned to a house doctor or staff doctor. The staff doctor may be salaried, may be donating his time, or may be receiving part of his professional training at the institution. In any case, the patient does not choose his own doctor. The patient is willing to give up his customary choice in order to obtain other advantages. Some plans recognize this shortcoming and try to give patients a limited choice from among several house doctors. Complete freedom of choice, however, is relinquished by the patient at any of these facilities.

In commercial optometric practices, particularly in the commercial "chains," the patient does exactly the same thing; he accepts any of the optometrists employed by the owner-optometrist. In the health center plans, the administration determines which optometrist the individual patient will see; in commercial optometry, the owner makes the decision. In neither case does the patient make the choice.

Another similarity is the patient's belief that he is obtaining the optometric service at a price substantially below what he would pay if he visited an optometrist in the traditional type of practice. The participant of the health plan is, of course, paying for the service in the form of his annual premium; he believes, however, that he is paying less. The employee who visits the company-owned facility has also paid for the optometric service he receives—in the form of work for the employer to earn the fringe benefit. In the commercial optometric practice, although there has been no prepayment, the patient believes that he is obtaining a bargain.

The similarity is even closer. Some commercial optometrists, through a multitude of tricks and ruses, have attempted to assume the appearance of a third party health plan. A commercial optometrist may have his office in a membership "discount" market that charges a registration fee (that is, only members who pay a minimal fee may purchase items at the store) or that caters only to certain employee groups (government employees, teachers, employees of certain industries, or certain occupations). The buyer in such a store believes that he is receiving a special "discount" because he is a member of the group or because his membership fee covered the "bargain." The optometrist in such an operation hopes to benefit by this erroneous conclusion on the part of the consumer. The consumer believes that his small prepaid membership is similar to the fee in a standard health plan.

Commercial optometrists do all that they can to continue to obfuscate the consumer's thinking. The effort is made to convince the patient that he is in fact receiving the service at a reduced rate because he is a member of a certain union or a member of some other specific group. These plans are particularly vicious because they are inherently dishonest. One cannot build sound relationships on basic dishonesty. Nevertheless, as consumers become aware of prepaid systems, they become vulnerable to the commercial optometrist's schemes for camouflaging his commercial practice as a participating health plan. As the public has become more sophisticated, the commercial optometrist has moved out of the jewelry stores; he now tries to pose as the operator of a prepaid health plan.

THIRD PARTY PLANS—*Trends and Evaluations*

The traditional optometric practice, in which an optometrist cares for those individuals who have freely chosen him and who reimburse him directly, is undergoing change. Moreover, it seems apparent that it will continue to change in the future. The major criticisms of the traditional method of practice are: (1) its unavailability to many people, and (2) the fact that some optometrists do not practice total vision care. There is no criticism of the technological aspects of the service, the personal relationship between optometrist and patient, or other phases of the service. On the contrary, the service that many optometric patients receive in the United States today is recognized as excellent. The number of people who do *not* receive this excellent service or who receive only part of it forms the bases for criticism.

The present level of care is of such high quality that we shall wish to weigh the effect of any proposed changes on this quality. Changes that reduce cost without negatively affecting quality are desirable; changes that reduce cost at the expense of some quality are less desirable; changes that reduce cost *only* by reducing quality are false economies. To evaluate any proposal for change from the traditional mode of optometric practice, there must be criteria for quality of the service. Several characteristics of high quality service are:

1. The service must be complete; all branches of the total body of knowledge must be applied to the individual case. Every optometrist need not perform every phase of the service. Every optometrist must, however, know the total field and be prepared to refer patients who require an element that he does not supply. If a patient who requires a special low-vision aid visits an optometrist who does not supply such aids, that optometrist still has the responsibility of enabling that patient to obtain that aid. Optometry is a general practice, and an optometrist *can* perform most of the parts of the service. Most optometrists do not engage in all of the parts within optometry's total scope; such optometrists still have the responsibility of seeing that each patient receives as much of the total vision care service as he requires. This concept of scope will be discussed in Chapter 12.

2. The patient has free choice of the optometrist who will work with him. If the optometric service consisted solely of measurement of the eye and supplying of spectacles, this freedom of choice would not be of such critical importance. But since the total service is best rendered when the optometrist advises, discusses, and enlightens his patient, the patient must have confidence in his optometrist and be able to communicate with him.

3. Providing high quality optometric service is time consuming. The optometrist must spend sufficient time with each patient not only to perform tests and recommend spectacles or vision training, but to communicate with the patient. Some patients' problems can be solved in a very few minutes; others require much more time. If he is to give optimal service, the optometrist must give each patient the amount of time that the individual problem requires.

4. The service must not be fragmented. Part of the excellence in quality of the service today is the result of optometry's premise that the total service should be under the direct control and supervision of one individual. There is a close interrelationship between the various aspects of the total service; the service is best rendered as a total communicative experience between optometrist and patient. If any part of the unified service is removed from the optometrist's direct control, the quality suffers.

5. Optometrists are expert in the selection and inspection of the materials they use. Since the optometrist uses materials of the highest quality, he must be free to choose from all of the materials available.* Optometrists traditionally have used the materials of many manufacturers, choosing the devices best suited to the individual patient and assuming the responsibility for the highest quality. The optometrist acts as the patient's agent and purchases materials on an open market *for* the patient; he is neither a seller of materials nor a representative of any supplier.

6. The doctor must have adequate equipment and the latest knowledge. The patient then receives the most accurate and comprehensive service. This responsibility is best carried out in a professional atmosphere, in which the doctor senses his individual responsibility as a member of the health care team. The environment must be such that the optometrist is stimulated to keep abreast of advances in the ever-increasing knowledge of his profession.

Any proposed change in the system of paying for optometric care should take these criteria of high quality of service into account; only if they are met can an assessment of the savings be made. Many Americans go to commercial optometric practitioners believing that they cannot afford the fees of the professional optometrist. These people, often in the financial bracket between those who receive welfare and those with middle incomes, usually receive an inferior form of optometric service. Far less time is spent with the patient in com-

* One reason why audiologists have never been able to professionalize and why patients requiring hearing aids do not receive a service of anywhere near the satisfactory quality of that received by optometric patients is the absence of this free choice of materials. Hearing aids are supplied by manufacturers' representatives who sell one brand of aid only.

mercial practices; materials of less than top quality are often used; emphasis is placed on the sale of a pair of spectacles at a bargain price rather than on the total communicative experience. The patient does not receive a bargain; he receives poorer service.

The characteristics of optimal service not only are useful in evaluating the quality of the service offered under any plan, but also help to explain why the service costs what it does. High quality costs money. Plans that offer optometric service at reduced cost are in reality offering a poorer service. The various centers and hospitals and prepayment plans, for example, can reduce cost but must deny the patient his customary free choice of doctor. This is not necessarily bad. Some people may be willing to forego this choice to obtain a service comparable in all other aspects at less cost. Each aspect of the service has its own price tag. Patients may be willing to give up some aspects in order to effect a sufficient saving.

The cost of optometric service, however, does not depend solely on excellence. There are some inefficient aspects to the present service; excellence might be maintained at a lower cost if these aspects could be removed. The one-optometrist office, for example, has been mentioned as an unduly costly operation. Group offices could meet all of the criteria of excellence of service and still do so at a reduced cost. There are several ways in which the service can be made more available without reducing its quality.

The cost of the service and the method of payment are different approaches to the problem of making care universally available. In several governmental plans, for example, the service is of the same quality *and cost* as that traditionally received by the patient who pays his own bill; it becomes available to more people because the government pays the bill. The service is *not* offered at a lower price. There are two distinctly different problems here: the reduction of cost through increased efficiency and the payment for the service by someone other than the patient. Both approaches make the service available to more people, but they are basically different.

Many doctors have expressed the fear that, although it is possible for third parties to buy high quality service, they will not do so in the long run. The argument is offered that third parties will constantly seek ways to reduce cost and may ultimately do so through reducing the quality of the service. This is an ever-present danger, but it can be guarded against. If optometrists have a complete understanding of the criteria of good quality, they can insist on optimal service no matter *who* pays the bill. Optometrists can cooperate with health planners through increasing efficiency and reducing costs if it is not at the expense of quality.

The present years are ones of experimentation. Both optometrists and health planners are trying many approaches to the overall problem of increasing the availability of vision care. Although many different solutions to the problem have been offered and tried, the plans all fall into one of five broad categories:

1. Methods that maintain or even increase quality but reduce cost through increased efficiency. In this category are multi-optometrist offices and increased efficiency within offices through the proper use of assistants.

2. Methods that maintain quality but substitute other than traditional methods of payment. In this category would be governmental support programs, vision service corporations, and insurance plans.

3. Methods that reduce cost through only minor reductions in service. In this category would be health centers, optometric centers, and clinics in which patients receive all aspects of good service except for the free choice of doctor. Institutional care received in such plans is for many people a great deal better than they might otherwise obtain.

4. Methods that reduce (or claim to reduce) cost but distinctly offer a less than optimal service. Commercial optometric practice falls within this category. Not only is the choice of doctor lost, but the service is invariably less personal, the materials are frequently inferior, and the time spent with each patient is often inadequate. Furthermore, the reduction in cost is commonly more imagined than real. Some company health plans and health groups and clinics also fall within this category. Although it is theoretically possible for institutional optometry to offer each patient the requisite amount of time and care, the case is usually otherwise; there is some tendency to reduce quality.

5. Methods that are successful in effecting cost savings in the present framework only. These are plans that take advantage of inconsistencies in the existing situation, but are not long-range solutions. The obtaining of general care through a safety program is an example of this method. Through an unrealistic fragmentation of the service, the individual receives care at a lesser cost. He would not do so, however, if prepaid plans were generally accepted, if private practices had increased efficiency and more realistic fee scales, or if the employer insisted that the safety program be limited to safety and cease being used as a fringe benefit.

Most plans for increasing availability by reducing cost fall mainly into one of these five groups.* The first two increase availability without negatively affecting quality. The fourth category is false

* Increasing the availability of the optometric service will also depend on factors other than that of reducing cost. Accessibility of the service (geographic distribution

savings; the fifth is only a temporary solution that depends on inconsistencies that will not always exist. In the third category are centers and clinics that do reduce cost; excellence of service may or may not be retained. Many optometric planners, recognizing the nature of these groups, have recommended that bodies should be set up within the optometric professional organization to evaluate and certify clinics and centers. Such bodies would first establish standards of quality that would be desirable in an optometric clinical department. If these standards were met, the clinic or center would be certified. The certified clinic would be one that did, in fact, offer high quality care at reduced cost.

REDUCING THE COST

In any discussion of the reduction of the cost of optometric services, the assumption is that the quality will remain optimal. Each method for cost reduction proposed in this section could reduce cost with no reduction in quality. In fact, many of the proposals would improve the quality of the optometric service.

The characteristics to be retained are: a personalized service; a comprehensive, up-to-date service; a unified service; a service in which each patient receives all of the time that his problem demands; and a service in which the patient's total vision problem is reviewed and explained to him. In the past, attempts have been made to define excellence of service on the basis of actual time spent with the patient or on the basis of the number of tests performed. Such criteria are naive, and tend to add unnecessarily to the cost of the optometric service. All patients do *not* require the same tests or the same amount of time. The unsophisticated view that we can define quality in terms of

of optometrists) or increasing the awareness of the need and desire for the service have been discussed elsewhere in this book.

Some idea of the importance and nature of other factors may be obtained from a report to the Secretary of Health, Education, and Welfare that was submitted in December, 1966, by an advisory committee. The committee dealt specifically with the problem of relationships with state health agencies, but also listed eight "Obstacles to Better Health." Cost of the services was only one of many obstacles. The list the advisory committee submitted was:

1. Urbanization generates new problems and brings with it environmental stresses.
2. Obsolete governmental structures make advance in the provision of health services difficult.
3. An overly rigid medical care system inhibits new approaches to the provision of health services.
4. Too little emphasis on the application of knowledge delays health advance.
5. The shortage of manpower hampers the delivery of health care to people.
6. Rising costs tend to make better health care unavailable to many people.
7. Lack of public understanding of health care and inadequacy of health services limit advance.
8. Health professionals and their associations have tended to focus narrowly on matters that may affect their own status.

time or tests alone neglects the very essence of the excellence of the service—its personal nature.

Some optometrists have argued that they should have no concern with their patients' ability to pay for vision care. They point out that the seller of automobiles or television sets is not concerned with whether or not all people can afford his product. If the price is "fair," they argue, the consumer can determine whether or not he can afford a product or service. This attitude is wrong because it equates optometry, a profession, with business or trade. The professional man *does* concern himself with the patient's ability to pay or, more precisely, with the responsibility of seeing that all who require professional service are able to obtain it.

Desirable methods for reducing cost, applicable to traditional optometric private practice, offer an alternative to institutional practice. How well the service can be offered and how many people can be served in this manner will, to a great extent, determine the role private practice will play in the society of tomorrow.

The list of methods for reducing the cost of optometric service is by no means complete. It does, however, offer a basis for thinking about the real professional nature of optometry. Some methods worthy of consideration are:

1. The sharing of office facilities by several optometrists for the purpose of reducing overhead is one method of reducing costs. It has already been discussed. This method for reducing cost will not be universally applicable. One of optometry's great contributions has been the geographic distribution of its members. Optometrists have been willing to practice in the smaller communities and to bring the service to areas that would otherwise be without it. Even with improved transportation, many optometric patients prefer not to travel. The child who requires orthoptic or visual training can visit a local optometrist after school several times a week; it would be impractical for such a child to be transported to a larger city. Older patients often do not drive automobiles and dislike having to be transported by friends or family.

Thus, group practice is a useful method of reducing cost in some communities, but not in all. On the other hand, the patient in the one-optometrist community should probably be willing to pay a small amount more than the patient who has access to the multi-optometrist office. This method (like all the others suggested here) cannot solve all the cost problems in all communities. It is merely one method that will help the cost problem in some communities. The trend in the United States for more and more people to live in larger cities makes group practice more important today and in the future than it was in the past.

2. The proper use of associates and assistants can also reduce the cost of optometric care. It is uneconomical for an optometrist paying the high overhead of an optometric office to spend considerable time in performing mechanical tasks. Optometric office overhead can be as high as ten or fifteen dollars an hour. If the optometrist in solo practice spends half an hour repairing a patient's spectacles, he can produce no other income during that period. Therefore, he must either charge the patient whose spectacles he has repaired an inordinately large fee for this mechanical service (which optometrists rarely do) *or* pass on to the next patient part of the previous patient's bill. If a technician could repair the spectacles while simultaneously the optometrist performed professional services, costs could be reduced.

The problem encountered in introducing assistants to optometric practice lies in the degree of delegation that can be attained without disruption of personalized and unified services. The old-time corner grocer claimed (right up to the day he filed bankruptcy) that his clients wanted personal service and would never wait on themselves in a grocery-cart market. But he was wrong. The situation in optometry is different in that optometrists are talking about a total service the unity of which they wish to preserve. But even in optometry, there is a limit to what patients will, can, and should pay. Personal attention, even for minor mechanical services in a solo practice, is extremely costly. Most patients neither can nor will pay for it.

The question is not *whether* to use assistants, but *how* to use assistants and still retain the personal unified service. This is a complex problem, and there are no simple answers. The phrase "under the direct supervision of the optometrist" to describe how assistants shall function is a semantic solution only. Optometrists will have to experiment with different degrees of delegation of authority. The important concepts are: (a) that the optometrist must delegate some of the less skilled tasks to assistants, and (b) that he must learn to do this and still retain complete control of a unified total service.

3. The realization that there is no one optometric examination that all patients should receive at preordained intervals can lead to reduction in cost. An optometrist can perform dozens of tests (Chapter 2). The important concept in private practice is recognition of which testing procedures the individual patient requires *at any given time*. The concept being adopted by more and more optometrists is that of a continuing service. After each visit, the optometrist decides what service the particular *individual patient* will require and when he will require it. For example, a child who is growing nearsighted is told to return in a year (when his nearsightedness may be expected to have increased) for those tests pertaining to his nearsightedness. Another child with a different ocular status may be told

to return in two years for a different series of tests. This is very different from telling all children to return for a complete examination in the same interval of time.

The very nature of a personalized service demands that reappointments and tests be personalized. The concept of a complete examination for all people is old-fashioned, costly, and worst of all, not necessarily optimal care. The patient who follows a plan of service designed for him, his visual system, and his visual requirements will, in the long run, spend less money than the patient who receives a "complete" examination every year or every two years. As optometrists learn the true art of vision care, they will more nearly gear the service to the individual's needs; this process will reduce costs.

The most recent trend in fee systems, that of assigning a unit value to each discrete segment of the total service, is a practical application of the philosophy that the service should be personalized. Not only should each patient receive those tests and only those tests that his vision requires, but he should be charged only for those elements that he requires.

The trend away from *one* examination, *one* average fee, and *one* time interval between examinations will serve to reduce costs *and* to improve the quality of service.

4. Use of a screening procedure can help to reduce costs. It is possible in a short time to determine whether a vision problem exists or not, especially in a symptom-free patient. A series of a few well-chosen tests that will yield such knowledge is called a screening procedure. Many patients require only this sort of service. When optometrists offered only one type of service, the "complete" examination, the cost was unduly high. Many people, if they wanted *any* optometric care at all, had to submit to a long series of tests, many of which were totally unnecessary. Today, many optometrists offer a screening service. Many vision service corporation plans insist on a provision for screening. Since a screening test requires about a fourth of the time of a regular visual examination and analysis, the price is usually proportionately lower.

As in so many other phases of the newly emerging concept of optometry, screening must be used judiciously. Screening is *not* a quick or cheap substitute for a total examination service. It is applicable mainly to symptom-free patients. It separates those who require further care from those who do not. It does not measure degree of problem or offer a definitive diagnosis. Nonetheless, it serves a very useful purpose in optometric practice. One major use is as a brief assessment of the vision of children at frequent intervals as a preventive measure.

In a sense, screening is not greatly different from the procedure of personalizing the service. It is the first step in the personalized service, for a symptom-free individual's first requirement is an assessment of whether he may have a visual problem of which he is unaware. This question is the one that screening is designed to answer.

Sometimes screening is conducted in a public building on large groups of people (school children receiving a school examination, for example). As a result, the term has come to be associated with this form of procedure. As used in the present context, however, screening refers to a procedure used in the office by a privately practicing optometrist.

5. Working in family units reduces costs. Because the optometric service is communicative and personal, much time is spent becoming acquainted with the patient. The family is a conveniently sized unit with which to work in optometric practice, and many optometrists think in terms of family vision care. This system is particularly useful in families with several young children. Since some eye defects are hereditary, an explanation about one child can often help the parent understand the problems of the other children. Optometrists who have tried the system of working with families have found that two or three children can be examined and the parents can be made to understand the problem of each in a much shorter time when they are seen as a family than when each child has an appointment at a different time.

Optometrists who use this system to reduce costs usually instruct the parents to bring in several of the children; they block out sufficient time to give each child the services he requires. The major time (and hence cost) saving is in case histories and later discussions and explanations.

6. Not insisting indiscriminately on "high fashion" styles for all patients will reduce costs. It has already been noted that style can be a costly ingredient of the optometric service. All patients wish to have a good appearance, but many people, particularly those who require spectacles only part of the time, do not wish to pay an undue amount for "high fashion." The optometrist who wishes to cooperate with those patients who desire to keep costs down will have some "utility" frames of good quality, but of modest appearance. There is no reason why all patients must pay for the fashion consciousness of some.

Not all optometrists will agree with all of the methods outlined here for reducing costs. Moreover, there are probably many other methods that can be used to help reduce costs. Optometrists must concern themselves with making optometric care available to all people; cost is one reason people do not receive care. In these days of experimentation, adherence to one plan or another is not nearly as important as the attitudes held by individual optometrists. Certain attitudes are highly desirable:

1. The optometrist must give more than lip service to the pledge in his code of ethics that no person shall go without optometric service. He must recognize that traditional modes of practice with occasional charity are not capable of solving the problem; nor are they acceptable to the populace. He must be responsible to the individual patient *and* to all people. He must think in terms of *public* health as well as of *individual* health.

2. The optometrist must not be overly concerned with who pays his bill. He must cooperate with government, with planners, with insurance companies, and with vision service corporations. His role should be to insist on adequate control of the quality of service; he should try to obtain for every patient whose bill is paid by a third party the same quality of service that he has traditionally insisted on for his private patients. Who pays the bill is not important; the quality of service *is* important. If, through the better type of third party payment plans, the optometrist can retain optimal service for the public, adequate income for himself, and availability of the service to all patients, then he should do so. If he fails to do so, less desirable institutional optometry may be the mode of practice for the future.

3. The optometrist must increase his own efficiency as well as that of his office. He must retain an adequate income for himself and his family; his compensation should be commensurate with that of other health professional people and in accord with his advanced training. However, he must also pass on to the consumer of his services—his patients—the savings brought about by increased efficiency. How well an optometric office fulfills its mission cannot be judged solely by the amount of personal income that it produces. Unless it can produce adequate income *and* attention for its share of the patients who require vision care, it is unsuccessful. Offices that earn relatively high income from a small number of "carriage trade" patients have a limited social function.

In recent years, it has been necessary to add another dimension to the customary definition of a successful optometric practitioner: not only is he one who has the gratitude of his patients, has the respect of his colleagues, and is a good provider, but he is one who attends to his share of the *total* number of patients who require vision care. Both the profession and the individual practitioner will be judged in the future not only by the number of people for whom care is supplied, but by the number of those who go without it.

CHAPTER 12

THE FUTURE

Within the lifespan of one generation, an occupation that had existed for over 700 years has been transformed into a vigorous, independent, health service profession. The major steps in professionalization have been taken, and optometry, like other health professions, now faces the challenge of the twentieth century—that of making its benefits available to all people.

The individual optometrist can solve many of the profession's problems within his own practice and sphere of influence. In a few areas, however, the best thinking of optometric organizations and long range planners is needed. The American Optometric Association and each state optometric association have set up planning committees that are trying to crystallize the profession's thoughts on future goals, attitudes, and actions. This final chapter deals with some of these far-reaching, continuing problems and possible solutions.

EDUCATION

Optometry has attained professional status in so brief a time primarily because of the soundness of its body of knowledge and the excellence of its schools and colleges. Optometric education, following the pattern of other professions in the United States, evolved from the proprietary school to the independent college and finally to the university-affiliated college. As noted in Chapter 7, the final step in optometry's professionalization must be the creation of several additional university-affiliated colleges.

In the history of other health professions, this final step has occurred in every group that has attained professional status. Dentistry, pharmacy, veterinary medicine, and medicine have all passed through a period when the independent colleges played an important role in education; all have seen the slow disappearance of the independent college. In dentistry, the last independent college of the 55 dental schools became affiliated with a university as recently as the present decade.

Optometric leaders have recognized for some time that ultimately optometric education would have to be integrated in the university system. More than a quarter of a century ago, Sheard (1939) noted the importance of university affiliation. He stated: "Optometry can survive only on the basis of adequate educational training in high-grade institutions of higher learning, namely, universities with medical schools."

In June, 1965, the president of the University of California, Clark Kerr, requested that the Universitywide Committee on Educational Policy examine the appropriateness of optometry as a university discipline and optometry's relationship to medical schools in the University. The report was submitted to the Regents in December, 1965, and was signed by M. A. Amerine. It described the academic community's assessment of optometry's role in the University as follows:

> From the viewpoint of public need, subject matter and professional education, it is the opinion of the Committee that optometry is an appropriate university discipline.
>
> It is the opinion of the Committee that optometry is a paramedical discipline. The relationship between schools of optometry and medicine should be similar to that which now exists between schools of pharmacy, dentistry, nursing and schools of medicine. That is, they should operate administratively as independent schools and academically as cooperative schools whose major concern is health care. Sharing of faculty in teaching and curriculum planning is essential to improvement in the quality of professional education in optometry.

When a profession plans for the replacement of its independent colleges by university-affiliated schools, it is in no way deprecating the important contributions that its independent colleges have made. On the contrary, it is clear from the history of professions that each passed through a period during which independent colleges bore the responsibility for most of the education.* Newer health professions like dentistry and optometry could not have evolved without strong independent colleges.

On the other hand, no health occupation that did not ultimately place the great majority of its training within the university framework has ever attained full professional recognition in the United States. The professionalization of optometry is now all but completed. The final step, an increase in the number of university-affiliated colleges, remains to be taken.

---

* The only exception to this rule among health professions appears to be clinical psychology, which had its roots in university departments of psychology from the beginning.

Not only optometric associations and planners need to recognize this clearly delineated path that must be followed, but individual optometrists, too, must see the broad picture. They must be fully cognizant of where the profession stands in the broad pattern of emergence that it is following. Optometrists, more than almost any other health practitioners, have from the beginning been very conscious of the role education would play in professionalization. Individuals have supported colleges by personally contributing funds, by soliciting funds, by urging state legislatures to place optometry schools in state universities, and by acting as teachers (sometimes without pay) to keep educational institutions operating.

The independent college has been slower in disappearing from the scene in optometry than in other professions. There are several reasons, but most of them stem from the opposition of the medical profession to optometry as an independent profession (Chapter 7). This opposition by organized medicine, which in dentistry was dissipated quickly, has remained throughout optometry's history. Thus, if a university contemplates the establishment of a school of optometry, opposition from organized medicine can invariably be expected to follow.* Optometrists have reacted to this situation with a fear of placing optometric education outside the sphere of influence of the profession. Without the independent schools, they argue, it would be possible for medicine to use its tremendous power in the university structure to take over optometry schools.

This fear that many optometrists have is to some extent justified. However, by now, the experience of optometry schools within universities has been long standing and the relationship between optometry and the universities that teach it has been good. While some danger is clearly present, it is a calculated risk that the profession will have to take. The extension of the optometry course to six years and the recognition of the program as being on a doctorate level by all universities that have schools of optometry indicate that the universities are not about to disenfranchise optometry. As university schools thrive and become integrated into the total university systems, the argument that university affiliation by all schools might be dangerous becomes less valid.

One university, Columbia, has within the recent past discon-

* There are indications that this traditional opposition may be decreasing. The *Transactions of the American Academy of Ophthalmology and Otolaryngology* (Vol. 70, p. 89, 1966) reports a request by the president of a Florida county society of ophthalmology that the Academy write to Florida's congressman and convince him that "a school of optometry in Florida would not be in the best interests of the people of Florida specifically and the United States in general." The Academy took no action, deeming it to be not within its province. An optometry school at the University of Florida remains a possibility for the future.

tinued the teaching of optometry. The pattern that emerged when this occurred may prove to be of value in the future thinking of optometric planners. An optometry college, like other professional colleges, has several functions in addition to undergraduate education or the training of new members of the profession. A college also fosters research, postgraduate education, seminars, and public clinics. When the school of optometry at Columbia closed, all functions other than undergraduate education were taken over by the Optometric Center of New York. The research, postgraduate educational courses, and clinic at the Optometric Center of New York today are comparable with those of any college or university.

This pattern, arrived at serendipitously when the Columbia school closed, may prove to be a useful one in optometry; it indicates a role that the present independent optometric colleges could play in the future. There is need in most large cities for optometric centers, and the present independent colleges may be able to fill this need. The present independent colleges, when they give up undergraduate training, may retain their charters and continue as research, postgraduate, and clinical institutions.

Were the evolution of optometric educational institutions to follow a pattern like that just described, several benefits would accrue. The retention of the institutions as centers would fill a social need in many cities. The charter, clinical staff, and organization would remain intact; *if* optometry should encounter difficulties after all optometric schools become university affiliated, the profession would still control institutions that could easily be converted from centers to colleges. Such measures will probably never be necessary; all indications are that optometry will continue to be well received in the university system. There is a much greater danger in *not* placing optometry in the university system than in doing so. However, a step like that suggested here may give the needed reassurance to those optometrists who have spent their entire professional lives in the atmosphere of a cold war with organized medicine.

Optometric planners now speak of the need for ten or more additional university-affiliated colleges of optometry in the near future. To one not actively engaged in the educational process, this seems like a large number of new schools. However, one major difference between independent and university-affiliated colleges has been the size of the class that has customarily been accepted as optimal. A fundamental premise of the university-affiliated colleges is that no more than 60 to 65 students should be in each class if the student is to receive sufficient laboratory and clinical training and sufficient instructor exposure. On the other hand, private colleges have often found it necessary to admit classes of over 100 students; at times in the past,

individual classes have had several hundred students.* Thus, in order
to maintain the same number of graduating optometrists per year,
each independent college will have to be replaced by two affiliated
colleges. If ten university-affiliated schools were to replace the present
five independent colleges, optometric manpower would remain the
same.

The demand for optometrists, however, is increasing; and with
increased activity of public health plans, this demand will be even
greater. If optometric manpower is to be sufficient to fill the need, approximately 20 university-affiliated schools must be in existence in the
future. A problem that presents itself immediately is the source of educators to staff this number of schools. Here again, the importance of
the trend toward university affiliation becomes quite apparent. Of the
ten optometric colleges, only the three large university-affiliated colleges have graduate departments; they supply most of the new teachers. Thus, for optometric teachers to continue to have strong postgraduate training, affiliated colleges must be strengthened to maintain the supply.

The long-range goal of 20 university-affiliated colleges of optometry has been recognized and adopted by most planners for the profession's future. If this goal can be attained in a reasonable time, the
trend which has been apparent in the past three quarters of a century
will be continued, the number of well trained professional optometrists needed to supply the demand will be maintained, and new
teachers will be trained simultaneously.

Education goes beyond the mere training of new practitioners. If
the science is to advance in scope and to improve technologically, research is necessary. Here again, the need for affiliated colleges is clear,
for most research contributions come from university colleges. It is
not a condemnation of the independent colleges to note that the
financial base of their operation is not sufficient to sponsor expensive
research. Government participation in professional education has
helped the situation of the private colleges somewhat in recent years.
However, even with government subsidy, there seems to be little evidence that major research advances will be made in the independent
colleges. Their purpose in the broad scheme of things has been to
maintain the supply of practicing optometrists—and this they have
succeeded in doing. But as optometry becomes more firmly established
in the social order, the need for independent colleges diminishes.

A final consideration of the role of educational institutions in

---

* There were 726 students registered in the five university-affiliated colleges of
optometry in the classes of 1966–1970; the comparable figure for the five independent
colleges was 1247 students or a ratio of 1.7 to 1. In this same period, none of the
affiliated colleges had any class larger than 61 students. Three of the five independent
colleges had one or more classes with over 100 students.

the future involves the extension of optometric service to worldwide availability. It is clear that leadership in the establishment of the new profession has come from the English-speaking countries. The educational institutions in countries where optometry is already established, the United States in particular, should be the fountainhead for world optometry. As an optometric profession emerges in the underdeveloped areas of the world, local educational systems will develop. They will, however, be dependent on such countries as the United States for the training of their educators for some time to come.

Optometric educational institutions in the United States face a great challenge in the years ahead. They must (1) supply a sufficient number of practicing optometrists in a period of increasing utilization of the optometric service; (2) supply optometric educators for an expanding educational situation; (3) foster research, train researchers, and advance both basic information and applied technology; and (4) accept the responsibility of bringing optometric education to the many emerging countries that will require and want an optometric profession.

This is a formidable challenge, and one would be justified in having grave doubts as to the feasibility of meeting it. However, in the light of the tremendous development through which the profession has passed during the present century, the task does not appear nearly so awesome. The optometric profession, its leaders, and its educational institutions have already met similar challenges successfully. There is every reason to believe that they will meet the present educational demand with success.

SCOPE

Since optometry as a profession developed so rapidly, its scope has changed markedly in the past 65 years. As the profession matures, the scope will change less. Initially, the total scope of optometry was the examination of the patient's vision and the mechanical tasks of fitting, adjusting, and repairing spectacles. To this basic service have been added many new elements. Because some anomalies of vision responded to training procedures, orthoptics was added to optometry's armamentarium. As patients with *any* vision problem learned to consult the optometrist first, optometrists became proficient in differentiating the healthy from the diseased eye. New devices such as contact lenses, aniseikonic corrections, microscopic spectacles, and telescopic lenses were developed; the prescribing and fitting of these devices were gradually added to optometry's scope.

Although the scope of optometry has expanded markedly during the present century, optometrists have been careful to exclude areas that rightfully belong to other groups. Optometric scope does not include the performance of surgery or the prescribing of medication; these areas are within the scope of the practice of medicine. Some optometrists in the United States, and all optometrists in England, do use drugs as an aid in optometric diagnosis. However, it is agreed that to offer drugs to the patient for his use in therapy is beyond the scope of optometric practice. Similarly, optometrists are concerned with visual perception and perceptual problems. Although reading is a perceptual act, optometrists in general believe that the *teaching* of reading is not within optometric scope, but belongs to the field of education. Enhancement of perception to make an individual better able to learn to read is, however, within optometric scope.

The American Optometric Association and the planners within the association have been concerned with delineating the scope of optometry. A list of the activities that comprise the total scope of optometry has been compiled and appears as Appendix I. In years to come, undoubtedly there will be additions to this list, and a few items may be removed from it. Additions will be made as new areas are developed through which optometrists may improve their service or make it more nearly complete; items will be deleted if they are found to lack validity or if it is found that another group can perform the same services more effectively.

The delineation of the full scope of optometry is of sufficient current importance that many state associations have had committees studying it. One state, California, has arrived at a statement of the specific scope of optometry. This statement * describes the scope of optometry as follows:

> Design, construction, adaptation and utilization of ophthalmic lenses including contact lenses, subnormal visual aids, aniseikonic lenses, special occupational lenses and associated devices, such as ophthalmic frames and prosthetic devices.
>
> Detection of ocular disease and the ocular manifestations of systemic disease.
>
> Utilization of methods of determining the refractive state of the eye.
>
> Investigation of neuro-muscular processes underlying vision and their treatment by means of lenses, prisms, vision training and orthoptics.
>
> Investigation and evaluation of visual and perceptual abilities such as visual acuity, color vision, light and dark adaptation, visual fields, critical fusion frequency, etc.
>
> The determination of visual readiness for educability.

* Published as an editorial in the *Journal of the California Optometric Association*, Vol. 35 (2), p. 69, March, 1967.

Investigation of preventive aspects of visual care and utilization to their full extent.

The enhancement of visual performance including the integrating of visual information from the other senses for the purpose of developing educability, comfort, enjoyment and efficiency.

Advice regarding environmental and hereditary factors affecting vision, such as, but not limited to, color vision defects, illumination, safety (industrial, highway, etc.), and school and home study areas, individual patients and/or other publics.

In planning for the future scope of the profession, optometry must not limit itself to traditional concepts. Technological advances are being made so rapidly that no one can foresee the exact course of vision care. For example, it may be possible in the future to treat light by means other than lenses so that it will focus properly on the retina. We are just beginning to understand the basic elements of matter, including the behavior of photo-energy. Research may reveal methods of treatment not even imagined in our present-day approach. The effect of vision on human behavior is only beginning to be understood. Basic research in perception may result in concepts entirely different from those of today, both in diagnosis and treatment.

Optometry must have a complete realization of its importance as the general vision care profession. This realization affects plans for the curricula of optometry schools, the definition of optometry in state laws, and the overall thinking of individual optometrists. Only by taking a comprehensive view of vision care can optometry exist in the future. The profession of medicine has staked out its jurisdiction of treatment by medicines and surgery and has adopted the use of lenses from the early optometrists. It has done little in the field of perception, visual performance, coordination problems, vision training, or developmental vision. Optometry must assume the responsibility in these areas and so enlarge its thinking that these services, as well as any others outside of the field of medicine, will be made available to all of mankind.

INTERPROFESSIONAL RELATIONSHIPS

Although optometry is an independent health profession, both the individual patient and patients in general (the public) are best served when there is cooperation and mutual respect between optometrists and members of the other health professions. The relationships between optometrists and most other health professionals are excellent, but traditionally there has been discord between optometry as a profession and organized medicine. Although relationships are improving markedly, and although individual optometrists and individual physicians cooperate with each other for the benefit of the patients both groups serve, the relationship is of sufficient importance to merit inclusion here as an area in which future change may be anticipated.

Even if petty grievances are overlooked, there are basic problems that tend to keep the optometric and the medical groups apart. Perhaps the most serious problem arises from the fact that both optometrists and ophthalmologists perform the same overall service for many patients even though each regards the service differently.

Most ophthalmologists have the treatment of disease by medicine or surgery as their major interest. Optometrists, on the other hand, are primarily interested in the functional disorders of vision, in the correction of anomalies, or in enhancement of vision. The optometrist thinks in terms of a unified service with the various parts inseparable; the ophthalmologist is much more likely to think in terms of fragmentation of the service and the delegation of parts of it to ancillary personnel such as nurses, opticians, technicians, orthoptists, or optometrists. The optometrist traditionally has accepted the role of the general practitioner in the eye field; the ophthalmologist, the role of a specialist.

Over the years, ophthalmology has leveled many criticisms at optometry—some of them justified. Optometric education at the beginning of the century was certainly far from adequate. The idea of men with less than a year of advanced schooling calling themselves "doctor" was justifiably unpalatable to physicians. But this condition has been corrected; the present optometrist completes a curriculum adjudged to be worthy of the earned doctorate. The commercialism in optometry was another valid criticism by medicine. This, too, is being corrected by optometry. Within the next quarter of a century, social trends, if nothing else, will bring this undesirable phase of optometry's development to an end. The criticism that optometrists were incapable of recognizing disease may have been valid in the earliest years, but this has not been true for many years.

The criticisms of optometry by medicine may have been valid, but often the actions of medical organizations were not designed to correct the situation. Optometrists were once insufficiently trained to merit the title of "doctor," but every attempt to increase educational requirements met with opposition from some medical groups. Optometry has been plagued by commercial elements within the group, but organized medicine has not cooperated with professional optometry in any move to remove commercialism from the entire eye field. Rather, medicine has cooperated with opticians whose commercial competition is given as an excuse by commercial optometrists for their own actions. Even in the beginning, Prentice complained that ophthalmologists lent their support to his "less worthy competitors" while leaving him to starve. Optometrists have not always been able to recognize pathology, but at least twice in the past official medicine has passed resolutions making it unethical for physicians to teach optometrists anything about the recognition of disease. Each time, these resolutions, after being in force for several years, were finally rescinded. The most recent such resolution has just been removed; another period of cooperation may be anticipated.

In view of the overlap of services (and the competition for the same patients), of the many valid criticisms, of the different outlooks of the two groups, and of the almost constant animosity of the official bodies, it is surprising that individual members of the two professions have cooperated with each other as well as they have over the years. Optometrists, almost without exception, make a very determined effort to recognize disease and to refer the patient for medical attention; almost all physicians recognize these referrals as being in the patient's best interest and act upon them with good grace. In fact, the basis for these good relationships among individuals from the two professions is the real basis for interprofessional cooperation. Individual practitioners cooperate with each other because they recognize that this is best for the patients. Similarly, the two groups must cooperate, placing the patient's welfare uppermost in their thinking.

Problems such as the overlap of service need examination in an attempt to secure interprofessional relations that are best for the patient's welfare. With increased social pressures and demand for more health services for all people, serious members of all professional groups are beginning to re-evaluate former patterns. Maumenee (1967), taking cognizance of these increased demands, notes that: "We [ophthalmologists] need the assistance of optometrists, for there are not enough ophthalmologists to check the visual acuity and fit lenses for all who require glasses. Thus we should work hard to develop some plan of cooperation." The total question of adequate manpower to serve the American public's visual needs is a major problem of the future.

Maumenee continues his statement of the future relationship between optometry and ophthalmology by saying: "On the other hand, optometrists should not be allowed to 'legislate themselves' into administering medical eye care, including diagnosis when they are not qualified to do so." No optometrist would disagree with this statement; a question would arise, however, as to the definition of "medical eye care" or "diagnosis." The excellence of interprofessional relationships in the future will hinge upon agreement, not only among optometrists, but among physicians, as to the scope of optometry. If recognition of disease for the purpose of referral of patients to physicians is construed to be the practice of medicine, then the two groups will not be able to reach accord. On the other hand, if ophthalmology recognizes the scope of optometry as being similar to what optometrists feel it is, then an era of good cooperation is close at hand.

Maumenee also refers to the fact that it would be disastrous if groups like optometry "split from medicine and attempted to set up individual specialties." Here there will continue to be disagreement, for optometry sees itself as an independent health profession that never was a part of medical practice. Just as dentistry is an independent but cooperating health profession, so is optometry. The basis for harmony between optometry and medicine will be the agreement of both groups on what is the scope of optometry. This scope will have to be of such a nature that optometry can stand apart as an independent health entity. Whatever elements are present in the scope of dentistry that enable it to stand as an independent profession will have to be present in the finally agreed on scope of optometry.

The salient feature of interprofessional relations is that the patient benefits when all those who serve him communicate well and act in his best interests. Since both optometrists and ophthalmologists have a sincere interest in attaining the same end—optimal care for the patient—there is a basis for discussion. As competition between the two groups is reduced through increased utilization by society of all health services and as each group learns to respect the training and scientific validity of the other's special field of endeavor, greater cooperation will result. As this happens, patients will benefit.

MANPOWER

Several professionally and technically trained groups participate in vision care in the United States. A recent survey of manpower connected with vision service (United States Department of Health, Education, and Welfare, 1966b) reported this division of the personnel:

Professional Services		
Optometrists	17,000	
Ophthalmologists	8,500	(including 1,115 trainees)
Technical Services		
Opticians and Optical Technicians	23,000	
Orthoptists	400	
Total	48,900	

Thus, a group of just under 50,000 people care for the visual needs of the populace of the United States. This group, in number both of professionally trained personnel and of technicians, has increased very little in recent years. The increase has not kept up with the growth in population and the demand for services.

The four occupations that play a part in the total eye care picture will be discussed in the reverse order of their appearance in the table.

The number of orthoptists, 400, is so small as to make almost no dent in the overall annual patient load. Moreover, so small a number of technicians cannot be distributed geographically so as to care for the many patients who require vision training. Optometrists, geographically distributed as they are and believing that orthoptic training must only be given under the direct supervision of one who understands the intricacies of the visual mechanism, carry out the bulk of the vision training in the United States.

The American Association of Certified Orthoptists has 350 members, most of whom are employed by ophthalmologists. A few are employed by hospitals and clinics. Most of the orthoptists specialize in postoperative squint training; they rarely do any work in perception training, which is more in the province of optometry. Training in orthoptics is available to persons with two years of college. The training may involve one year at one of eleven institutions on a ten- to twelve-month period of practical work in a training center under the supervision of a certified orthoptist, combined with the basic two-month course of the American Orthoptic Council.

Visual training, including orthoptics, is an important part of optometric practice. Most optometrists do some form of visual training; they do it personally or closely supervise the work of an assistant. Most optometric technicians are trained in optometric offices, in special courses in optometric colleges, and by extension courses.

Of the 23,000 opticians and optical technicians, 15,000 are technicians, 10,000 of whom are employed by prescription departments of wholesale optical laboratories and therefore have no direct contact with patients (United States Department of Health, Education, and Welfare, 1966b). The remaining 5,000 technicians are employed by retail optical shops, optometrists, or ophthalmologists. Of the 8,000 opticians, 1,500 are employed by optometrists or ophthalmologists, 500 are employed by manufacturers or wholesalers, and 6,000 work in retail optical shops. The distribution of opticians and technicians may be tabulated:

	Technicians	Opticians
Work for Optometrist or Ophthalmologist	1,000 *	1,500 **
Manufacturing, Wholesaling, Industry	10,000	500
Retail Optical Shops	4,000 *	6,000 **

The 7,500 opticians indicated with double asterisks (**) work directly with patients. Some of the 5,000 technicians indicated by single asterisks (*) work with patients; others do not. Thus, between 7,500 and 12,500 opticians are engaged in performing part of the service that optometrists also perform.

Dispensing opticians are licensed in 17 states. The independent optical stores, as they did at the beginning of the century, still continue to fill ophthalmic prescriptions and to sell other optical devices directly to the public. Some states now require licenses for these retail optical stores and the optical technicians they employ, as well as for the opticians who manage them.

Optometrists and ophthalmologists, in recent years, have joined with the American Board of Opticianry to encourage higher standards of training for opticians. Most opticians obtain their training by an apprenticeship that may last four or five years. This is still in keeping with the traditional methods of the guilds of Europe. There are now five opticianry schools, three of them accredited by the American Board of Opticianry; in 1965 they graduated a combined total of 88 students.

An interesting development in recent years has taken place in the hiring of opticians by ophthalmologists. Many ophthalmologists realize that the complete optical service as performed by the optometrist is superior to the division of responsibility as practiced in the past by the ophthalmologist and optical store. According to estimates, in 1966, between one third and one half of the recently certified ophthalmologists were employing opticians in their offices.

Some ophthalmologists oppose the trend toward dispensing. Maumenee (1967) says that physicians should not dispense drugs or appliances for a profit. He notes that: "The small aid that this [dispensing] gives a very few patients who could not obtain products elsewhere as conveniently as they can in the physician's office is far outweighed by the tarnish this practice places on physicians in general. . . ." The relationship of physicians to the dispensing of spectacles has received considerable attention from those interested in public health and from a United States Senate committee headed by Senator Hart. Ophthalmologists are divided between the views expressed by Maumenee and by those who advocate the hiring of opticians by ophthalmologists.*

---

* The difference in evaluation of the role of dispensing in professional practice remains a basic one between optometrists and ophthalmologists. Part of this difference in viewpoint undoubtedly stems from the fact that ophthalmologists tend to practice in cities where other health services, such as dispensing opticians, are also located, whereas optometrists often are the only member of the eye care group in smaller communities. However, there is also a philosophical difference. The optometrist regards examination, prescribing, ordering, fitting, and adjusting of spectacles all as part of a single service. The ophthalmologist tends to make a sharp distinction

Optometrists also have begun to hire more opticians to assist in the technical work of vision care. The direct, personal supervision of the technologist by the professional man is more in keeping with the traditional methods of physicians and dentists in their relations with all ancillary personnel.

Many more opticians and ophthalmic technicians are needed to assist ophthalmologists and optometrists in their work. For some years, dispensing optical shops may continue in existence to fill the prescriptions of ophthalmologists and of a few optometrists who send out their work. The trend at present, however, is toward the direct personal supervision of the optician and technician in the office of the ophthalmologist and the optometrist. In various states, this trend is being escalated by legal rulings on contact lens prescribing. Most rulings and state laws now specify that the responsibility for the fitting of a contact lens rests with the professional man who does the prescribing. This is as it should be; and it is resulting in increasing direct, personal supervision of contact lens prescribing and servicing.

With regard to the professional personnel, optometrists and ophthalmologists, the geographical distribution of practitioners is important. Appendix J shows the distribution of licensed optometrists and certified ophthalmologists in the United States as related to population. It is obvious from this table that optometrists are the family vision care profession in communities of all sizes and not just in the larger cities. Ten states, for example, have less than 15 ophthalmologists.*

A closer view of the number of ophthalmologists shows even more of a manpower shortage than is apparent at first glance. The health manpower survey of the United States Department of Health, Education, and Welfare (1966b) shows the following breakdown:

Total active	Private practice	[Other Practice] Non-Federal	Federal	Training programs	No. of D.O.'s in private practice
8,380	6,672	324	269	1,115	146

between the determining of the lens formula and all of the other steps necessary to obtain proper spectacles for a patient.

* This same phenomenon is observable within states. Of California's 58 counties, 4 with populations under 6,500 have neither an optometrist nor an ophthalmologist; 13 counties, with populations between 6,500 and 25,000, are served by 22 optometrists (at least one in each county) but no eye physicians. Two counties with over 25,000 people are served by 4 and 6 optometrists, respectively, but no eye physicians. Thus, only 4 counties have no eye care at all; 19, or a third of the total number of counties, have no medical eye care facilities. The geographic distribution of the two professional eye practitioner groups may be illustrated by comparing the ratio of optometrists to ophthalmologists in different sized counties. In the 32 least populated counties (population under 100,000), the ratio is 4.35:1; in the 26 higher density counties (population over 100,000), the ratio is 2.55:1.

There are 4,798 certified ophthalmologists in the United States (Appendix J). Part of the nearly 2,000 difference reflected in the two surveys of ophthalmologists in private practice is due to the number of eye, ear, nose, and throat practitioners who never have been certified, but practice a limited form of eye medicine.

The number of optometrists presently in practice is estimated to be no more than 17,000, although Appendix J shows 20,610. The discrepancy arises from the fact that: (1) all registered optometrists are not engaged in active practice, some having retired; and (2) some optometrists are registered in two different communities, having a branch office in an area that requires only a part-time practitioner. In view of the ever increasing demand for optometric services, this number is not sufficient for the future.* It was estimated (Chapter 11) that the service is presently only half utilized. Even if most optometrists could increase their patient load by 20 or 30 percent through increased efficiency, there would still be an insufficient number of optometrists were the service fully utilized.

The required number of optometrists is dependent on the number of patients seeking the service, the scope of the service that is offered, the frequency with which patients will seek care, and the number of patients an optometrist can care for annually without reducing the excellence of the service. It is estimated that at present half of the people have vision problems requiring optometric service. Since these patients should be seen every other year (on the average), it may be assumed that, in any given year, a fourth of the population would use optometric service if the service were fully utilized. Thus, the present population of the United States—200,000,000—would require 50,000,000 annual patient visits for full utilization of the service. Estimates of the number of patients that an optometrist under ideal conditions can care for annually vary from 1,200 (Osias, 1967) to 1,372 (Birchard and Elliott, 1967). Therefore, the number of optometrists required by the present population for complete utilization of the service is between 35,000 and 40,000. The more conservative figure of 35,000, when compared to the number of optometrists (17,000) in active practice, lends credence to the figure of half utilization arrived at earlier (Chapter 11) by another form of calculation. Birchard and Elliott (1967), using less rigid criteria for the amount of service that the people will need, but taking population increases into account, arrive at the figures of a need for 27,258 optometrists by 1970

---

* The number of optometrists is not even sufficient for the present, since supply is not keeping up with population growth. In California, for example, the number of optometrists was 2,397 in 1955 and 2,768 in 1964. However, because of population growth, the ratio of one optometrist per 5,424 people in 1955 dropped to one optometrist per 6,587 in 1964.

and 31,342 by 1980. Even if the approximately 5,000 ophthalmologists performed only optometric service together with the 17,000 optometrists, there still would not be sufficient manpower for all the patients who require care.

Delegating too much of the service to technicians will cause the quality of care to decrease. The time consuming aspects of a personalized service were discussed in Chapter 2. Increased efficiency in offices and increased utilization of technicians for part of the service would probably enable the present professional personnel to increase their patient load by up to 25 percent. Beyond that, quality would probably be negatively affected. No matter how one deals with the manpower figures, more than one step will have to be taken. The choice is not between increasing the number of professional persons *or* increasing efficiency; the problem demands both measures.

A number of questions will have to receive attention in the immediate future. In all of these cases, planners agree qualitatively; only quantity remains to be determined. Thus:

1. There must be increased manpower in all branches of the vision care field, both technical and professional; the question is how much increase is required.

2. There must be increased efficiency in professional offices; the question is how much increase in patient load can professional offices take and still maintain high quality and personal relationships with patients.

3. There must be an increased delegation of tasks to technicians; the question is which tasks can best be delegated without reducing quality.

4. There will be an increase in the number of patients who receive institutional optometry; the question is how to make it as good a service as possible.

UTILIZATION OF MANPOWER

In providing for the eye care of the population, society will utilize diverse personnel: technicians whose training after high school is one or two years, optometrists who have been trained for six or more years, and ophthalmologists whose training is approximately 12 years. In the past, there has been a marked degree of overlap of function. Optometrists sometimes perform jobs that technicians can perform; ophthalmologists sometimes perform tasks that optometrists can perform. Although overlap has existed in the past, manpower and training should not be wasted. For optimal utilization of manpower, members of the team should not perform tasks that another member with less training could do equally well.

The skills of each member of the health team should be used to maximum advantage. Often several different groups are involved. Peters (1966b) has studied the division of services among professions as they now apply to children's vision. His analysis is included here to illustrate the type of thinking that will be used in future studies to attain maximal usage of manpower. Peters lists the responsibilities of various groups for *detecting* vision problems in children.

Vision Problems	Pediatrician	Ophthal- mologist	Optometrist	Educators School Nurse	Psychologist
Disease	X	X	X		
Acuity	X	X	X	X	
Squint	X	X	X		
Refractive error		X	X		
Coordination			X		
Visual performances			X	X	
Developmental			X	X	X
Perception			X	X	X

The *treatment* of children with vision problems also shows an overlapping of several professions. Some of the problems are unique to optometry, and others are unique to ophthalmology. The following table (Peters, 1966b) shows the percentage of children with each type of vision problem.

Tables similar to the ones Peters has used for children will undoubtedly be constructed for the total population. To map out total health care programs, planners will have to know: (1) the extent of the need for services; (2) which members of the team can perform each part of each service; (3) how many members of each group in the team are available; and (4) how long it takes to train each member of the team. Such complete analyses are not now readily available, but new information is being accumulated daily. For maximum utilization of manpower, the most important guide line to follow is that *no member of the team should perform tasks that can be performed equally well by other members with less training.*

The one major exception to this rule is the performance of tasks that bring unity to the total service. Optometrists must do less of the mechanical and technical work, *but* they must continue to do those tasks that are essential to a unified service. Ophthalmologists should continue to perform vision and refractive tests, *but* should do so only rarely. They are overtrained for optometric practice. They will test

INTERPROFESSIONAL RELATIONS IN TREATMENT
OF CHILDREN WITH VISION PROBLEMS

PERCENT CHILDREN			
4%	Organic Problems Congenital Traumatic Disease	uniquely ophthalmology	(100%)
20%	Refractive Error Visual Acuity Squint	shared optometry ophthalmology	(75%) (25%)
10%	Visual Performance Coordination Problems Vision Training Developmental Vision	uniquely optometry	(100%)
6%	Vision Perception as it affects reading	jointly optometry educational psychology	
1%	Visual Rehabilitation Visually Handicapped Brain Injured Mentally Retarded	jointly optometrist ophthalmologist psychologist rehabilitation personnel special teachers	
100%	Visual Environment Lighting Safety	jointly light engineer architect optometrist	
100%	Vision Health Education	jointly optometrist ophthalmologist health educator nurse/teacher	

vision and refraction only when it is in the interest of offering the individual patient a total medical service.

In the past, whenever a more realistic division of labor has been suggested, it has been opposed on the supposition that one group wished to usurp the prerogatives of other groups. But in the present discussion, prerogatives are not involved. Of course, ophthalmologists should test vision when it is essential to their medical diagnosis; of course, optometrists should fit, adjust, or repair spectacles. But the majority of the optometrists' and ophthalmologists' time should be spent in doing the jobs that they alone are specifically trained to do.

It is part of the optometric premise that for some patients optimal service will be received only if the vision tester himself designs the spectacles (Chapter 2) and applies to the design all of the information yielded by the examination. For such patients, the task of designing spectacles cannot be delegated to an optician. Other patients, especially those seeking repairs and replacements, can receive adequate service from an optician. This optometric premise must be carefully examined with the idea in mind of increasing the availability of service and yet still retaining a unified service where needed.

Similarly, it is a medical premise that, since the eye is part of the body, its function is best evaluated by one trained in general medicine. This premise, too, will be found to have validity in certain cases and to lack it in others. This premise, too, will need to be reevaluated, particularly if there are to be enough physicians available for general health care in the United States. An ophthalmologist should perform vision and refractive testing only when it is in fact necessary for the patient's individual problem.

Optometrists believe that technicians, whether opticians, orthoptists, or ophthalmic assistants, should function only under direct supervision. This premise is sometimes challenged by those who point out that it would be equally logical to have optometrists act only under the direct supervision of ophthalmologists. This challenge may be rejected on two counts. First, it has been demonstrated throughout this book that by history, tradition, and content, optometry is *not* a part of medical practice; opticianry is and always has been a part of optometry. Second, optometrists through extended education have the prerogative of exercising the independent judgment granted to those with the requisite education; optometry is an independent profession because its members have the education and training to enable them to function as independent practitioners.

As public health agencies seek to increase the availability of health care, they become interested in the problems of manpower. Manpower and the scope of each of the occupations and professions are closely related. Medical and optometry schools have places for only so many students each year for the training of new professionals. These places belong to society—not to individuals or professions. When an optometrist spends his time in practice performing tasks that an optician could perform, he has wasted one of society's training spots; when an ophthalmologist spends the major portion of his practicing time performing vision examinations and other optometric functions, society has been robbed of a training spot that might have produced a much needed physician to practice medicine. Not only is the conscience of the professions being taken over by government, but the responsibility for manpower as well. The scope and mode of practice of the professional personnel markedly affects the manpower needs of the nation.

The concept that ophthalmologists are overtrained, and yet not specifically trained for performance of the optometric phase of the vision service, is not a new one. Prentice (Chapter 6), in his early statement to the Committee on Public Health of the New York legislature, argued that oculists should confine their work to the recognition and treatment of eye disease. Within the framework of economic competition between the professions and of avowed antagonism, this suggestion has always been rejected violently. However, with a new era, careful planning and cooperation among all professions and interested agencies may be anticipated.

Thus far, in the discussions of making care available to more people, it has been implied that fragmentation is a method of reducing costs. The Nürnberg guild, for example, in the seventeenth century (Chapter 4) reduced the cost of spectacles through this process. The total task was broken down into tiny parts, each of which could be performed by workmen with little skill. The price of spectacles was reduced through this process, but so was the quality. The optical industry in Germany suffered; in England, where skilled craftsmanship was encouraged, it did not. The experience of these guilds would indicate that too much fragmentation results in the loss of persons with overall skill; and this process, in the long run, reduces quality.

There is yet another consideration. Dividing a service into tiny parts that the unskilled can perform does not *necessarily* reduce cost. An example of a divided service being more costly than a unified one is offered by Osias (1967). A large insurance company compared the fees charged to claimants who received the total service from an optometrist with the fees charged to claimants who received part of the service from an ophthalmologist and part from a dispensing optician. The average fees for an examination were $15.94 (ophthalmologist) and $16.34 (optometrist). Thus, the two groups were very close to each other in this service charge. For an examination and lens prescription, the two groups were also very close to each other in their fees. However, when the patient required examination and spectacles, the fees of the unified service administered by the optometrist were much less than those for the service divided between ophthalmologist and optician. The figures obtained by Osias were:

	Optometrist	M.D. and optician
Examination and single vision spectacles	$40.87	$49.03
Examination and bifocal spectacles	51.18	72.68
Examination and trifocal spectacles	57.83	95.50

In this case, the divided service is *more costly* to the consumer than the unified service. Dividing the service will not necessarily reduce costs; planners for public health will want to take a long, hard look at studies of this type.*

In the overall picture of manpower for vision care in the future, optometry has much to offer; its practitioners are well trained to play an important role, but are not overtrained for the service they perform. They are specifically trained to perform the optometric service and are, in fact, better prepared for this function than any other group. Even were there a sufficient supply of physicians to perform the optometric service, and even were cost of training to be of no consideration, there would still be reasons for preferring to have the functions within the scope of optometry performed by a group specifically trained to do so.

In the armed forces, where it is necessary to have vision care at its best, optometrists and ophthalmologists have managed to work together for the patient's welfare; each group has functioned very strictly within its own scope. There is every reason to believe, therefore, that the same situation can, and will, prevail in civilian eye care practice in the future.

* The study by Osias (1967) is used here to illustrate the point that fragmentation does not necessarily reduce cost. It also illustrates another concept, not pertinent to the present discussion, but of some importance. It illustrates the effect on total consumer costs of a "professional fee for service" as opposed to a "mark-up." The materials and laboratory costs of bifocals over single vision spectacles is about $10.00; the optometrist merely added the additional costs to his bill, since he was already reimbursed for the service; the optician, however, added over $20.00, since his fees are based on multiplying the cost of materials by a given factor. The laboratory cost of trifocals is approximately $6.00 or $7.00 more than bifocals. The optometrist merely added this amount to his bill; the optician multiplied this added cost by a factor (probably 3) and added it to his bill. The consumer who requires more costly materials is definitely benefited by a professional "fee for service plus cost of materials" system as opposed to a "mark-up" system.

The figures illustrate another phenomenon that will be of great interest to health planners. The fees for the professional portion of the services were not too different from each other. Unduly high costs resulted *not* from professional services but from that portion of the service performed by the *least* skilled and *least* trained member of the team. The fees that were out of line were those that resulted from the "business" concept. This same phenomenon has been claimed to exist in general health costs. Several studies have shown that the high costs of medical care are not due nearly so much to the physician's service charges as to that part of medical care supplied on a "business" basis—drugs, hospital attention, prosthetic devices, etc. Optometrists, by placing their fees on a "service plus cost of materials" basis, are in fact helping markedly to reduce the overall cost of health care.

OPTIMAL VISION CARE FOR MANY

Optometric service—developed over a 700-year period—has reached a high point of technical excellence. Optometrists have attained professional status in the United States and several other countries within the short period of three quarters of a century. That is the past.

The personalized service offered *to those who can pay for it* in the United States is a highly desirable, beneficial service to the recipient. Its unity and the fact that it is administered by an independent profession enhance its quality. This is the present.

The service is distinctly under-utilized. This is true even in the United States. In much of the world, there is no optometric service at all. The emergence of new nations, increased literacy, and increased industrialization augment the need for optometric services. With increased technology, visual enhancement will be demanded. This, too, is the present—but with consideration for the future.

Optimal vision care should be available to all people. This is the future.

Although the future goal may be stated simply as increased utilization of optometric service without a decline in its quality, the means for attaining this goal are not at all clearly defined. More study will undoubtedly be needed. Several concepts have been developed that will make the goal attainable. The following final comments may serve as a skeleton for the optometry of the future:

THE SERVICE

Optometrists were, are, and should continue to be the general practitioners in the vision field. There is a difference between the examination of a patient in the clinic situation and the management of all of the vision problems of a family over the years. The latter role is the one the optometrist must fill if the care is to be optimal. As the general practitioner, the optometrist will plan the total vision care program for the individual. He will screen patients; he will think in terms of "services that the individual requires" rather than of a "complete" examination periodically. Many parts of the total vision care service the optometrist will perform personally; when he can do so without impairing quality, he will delegate to various assistants tasks that do not require professional judgment. Patients who require the care of specialists and particularly of ophthalmologists will be referred, as they always have been. The optometrist and the ophthalmologist will exchange information and will cooperate with each other in the patient's best interest. Because he is to be the generalist in the eye field, the optometrist will continue to be trained with a strong background in the physical *and* biological sciences; his optometric clinical training will be designed to help him assume the role of generalist.

For increased efficiency, optometric practice of the future will tend to be in multi-optometrist offices. Such offices can be either privately owned or part of a larger, non-profit group. They may be purely optometric, or they may be optometric groups within larger total health centers. Again for efficiency, these offices will make maximal use of technicians and assistants. Throughout this shift to multi-optometrist offices, however, there must be constant, careful appraisal of the nature of the service to assure that efficiency does not destroy the personal relationship and thus the quality of the service.

The multi-optometrist office will also allow for practice that is more nearly representative of the full scope of optometry. Although the fitting of contact lenses, orthoptics, care for the partially sighted, and other phases of optometry can all be practiced by one optometrist, there are advantages to having members of the group especially proficient in various areas as well as in general optometric care. Optometrists today are at a point where they are reconciling their traditional role as the general practitioners in the eye care field with the need for sub-specialties within the profession. The situation in optometry may be resolved much as it has been in dentistry. There is relatively little specialization in dentistry; the majority of dentists practice more or less within the total scope and are generalists. However, there are some specialists, such as exodontists. Most dentists are trained not only to extract teeth, but also to recognize particularly difficult problems in this field and to refer them to a specialist. Similarly, most optometrists not only will fit contact lenses, but also may refer difficult problems to a few optometrists who will specialize in the more difficult areas of this field. The trend toward multi-optometrist offices will help bring the total scope of optometry to more people.

PAYMENT

The question of who will pay the bill will become relatively unimportant to the optometrist. Changes in the United States are occurring in an evolutionary fashion. At present, some patients pay their own bills; some have the bills paid by insurance or vision plans, and some by government. Although the trend is toward the last two forms, it will be many years before all patients are covered by private or government insurance. Therefore, methods of bookkeeping will change. The percentage of income from each source will vary. But no matter who pays the bill, the optometrist must strive to retain the personal nature of his service and its overall high quality. He must seek adequate and appropriate reimbursement—from whatever source of payment—and he must resist attempts to give the public a lower quality service solely on the basis of economy.

Peters (1966a) has discussed the conditions that optometrists should consider as essential if the profession is to develop new roles in comprehensive community health programs. In any social planning, Peters notes, an optometrist, to make a maximal contribution to health care, must: (1) be allowed to join with others to serve the health needs of all; (2) be permitted to provide the highest quality and broadest scope of vision services to all; (3) be respected for his dignity and code of ethics; (4) be subject only to the judgment of his peers in his professional activities; (5) have freedom of professional judgment within his field of competence; (6) have reasonable remuneration commensurate with his education and professional service; (7) have opportunity to enhance his knowledge and skills through continuing education; and (8) participate in the planning process for his own and his colleagues' services.

OVERALL SOCIOLOGICAL CONTRIBUTION

Government may be taking over the conscience of the professions insofar as making care available to individuals, but the professions will retain a conscience on the broader level. Through research, the optometric profession will continue to advance knowledge. Optometric educators will continue to face the challenge of producing the requisite number of optometrists for the expanding needs of society. As the "one world" concept continues to gain acceptance, optometrists in more fortunate areas will accept the responsibility of making worldwide beneficial optometric service available. Optometrists as a group will accept the job of improving the service and of making it available.

The steady improvement in ethical and professional conduct on an individual level will continue as it has in the past. The regressive commercial practices will continue to decrease in number, if for no other reason than that increased third party payment plans will remove the *raison d'être* of such practice. The competition for patients who receive partial service creates an atmosphere in which commercialism thrives; this situation is being replaced by concepts of care within the full scope of optometry for all patients. Professional optometrists do not compete for patients, but rather concern themselves with the arduous task of giving complete vision care to more patients than they might wish to have.

Optometry as an occupation has now passed through the stage of its technological development and has almost completed its evolutionary professionalization phase. As are other health professions, it is becoming deeply involved in the social changes of the present age. Optometrists and optometrists-to-be may view the future with decided optimism based on the history of the profession.

The challenges of the past—those of establishing a new profession—have all been met successfully. The challenges of the future—those of bringing full scope vision care to all people—will be met with equal success.

APPENDIX A

Minnesota Optometry Law of 1901

Chapter 269

Be it enacted by the Legislature of the State of Minnesota:
An act to regulate the practice of optometry.

Optometry

SECTION 1. The practice of optometry is defined as follows, namely: The employment of subjective and objective mechanical means to determine the accommodative and refractive states of the eye and the scope of its functions in general.

When law goes into effect.

SECTION 2. From and after the first day of November 1901, it shall be unlawful for any person to practice optometry in the State of Minnesota, unless he shall first have obtained a certificate of registration and filed the same, or a certified copy thereof, with the clerk of the district court of the county of his residence, all as hereinafter provided.

Minnesota State Board of Examiners in Optometry how appointed, oath.

SECTION 3. There is hereby created a board, whose duty it shall be to carry out the purposes and enforce the provisions of this act, and shall be styled the Minnesota State Board of Examiners in Optometry. Said board shall be appointed by the governor as soon as practicable after the passage of this act, and shall consist of five resident opticians engaged in the actual practice of optometry. Each member of said board shall hold office for a term of three years, and until his successor is appointed. Appointments to fill vacancies caused by death, resignation or removal shall be made for the residue of such term by the governor.

The members of said board, before entering upon their duties, shall respectively take and subscribe to the oath required to be taken by other state officers, which shall be administered by the secretary of state, and filed in his office; and said board shall have a common seal.

Officers, meetings.

SECTION 4. Said board shall choose at its first regular meeting, and annually thereafter, one of its members president, and one secretary thereof, who severally shall have the power during their term of office to administer oaths and take affidavits, certifying thereto under their hand and the seal of the board. Said board shall meet at least once in each year at the state capital, and in addition thereto whenever and wherever the president and secretary thereof shall call a meeting, a majority of said board shall at all times constitute a quorum. The secretary of said board shall keep a full record of the proceedings of said board, which records shall at all reasonable times be open to public inspection.

Who may practice; fees.

SECTION 5. Every person before beginning to practice optometry in this state, after the passage of this act, shall pass an examination before said board of examiners. Such examination shall be confined to such knowledge as is essential to the practice of optometry. Any person having signified to said board his desire to be examined by them shall appear before them at such time and place as they may designate, and before beginning such examination shall pay to the secretary of said board, for the use of said board, the sum of ten dollars, and if he shall successfully pass such examination, shall pay to said secretary, for the use of said board, a further sum of five dollars on the issuance to him of a certificate. All persons successfully passing such examinations shall be registered in the board register, which shall be kept by said secretary as licensed to practice optometry, and shall also receive a certificate of such registration, to be signed by the president and secretary of said board, which shall be filed as hereinbefore provided.

SECTION 6. Every person who is engaged in the practice of optometry in the State of Minnesota at the time of the passage of this act, shall, within six months thereafter file an affidavit in proof thereof with said board, who shall make and keep record of such person, and shall in consideration of the sum of three dollars, issue to him a certificate of registration.

SECTION 7. All persons entitled to a certificate of registration under the full provisions of section six, shall be exempt from the provisions of section five of this act.

Certificate to be recorded with clerk of court, removal.

SECTION 8. Recipients of said certificate of registration shall present the same for record to the clerk of the district court of the county in which they reside, and shall pay a fee of fifty cents to said clerk for recording the same. Said clerk shall record said certificate in a book to be provided by him for that purpose. Any person so licensed removing his residence from one county to another in this state shall, before engaging in the practice of optometry in such other county, obtain from the clerk of the district court of the county in which said certificate of registration is recorded, a certified copy of such record, or else obtain a new certificate of registration from the board of examiners and shall, before commencing practice in such county, file the same for record with the clerk of the court of the county to which he removes, and pay the clerk thereof for recording the same a fee of fifty cents. Any failure, neglect or refusal on the part of any person holding such certificate or copy of record to file the same for record, as hereinbefore provided, for six months after the issuance thereof, shall forfeit the same. Such board shall be entitled to a fee of one dollar for the re-issue of any certificate, and the clerk of the district court of any county shall be entitled to a fee of one dollar for making and certifying a copy of the record of any such certificate.

Failure to make application to board within six months, effect.

SECTION 9. Any person entitled to a certificate, as provided for in section six of this act, who shall not within six months after the passage thereof make written application to the board of examiners for a certificate of registration, accompanied by a written statement, signed by him, and duly verified before an officer authorized to administer oaths within this state, fully setting forth the grounds upon which he claims such certificate, shall be deemed to have waived his right to a certificate under the provisions of said section. Any failure, neglect or refusal on the part of any person holding such certificate to file the same for record, as hereinbefore provided, for six months after the issuance thereof, shall forfeit the same.

SECTION 10. Every person to whom a certificate of examination or registration is granted shall display the same in a conspicuous part of his office wherein the practice of optometry is conducted.

Compensation of board.

SECTION 11. Out of the funds coming into the possession of said board, each member thereof may receive, as compensation, the sum of five dollars for each day actually engaged in the duties of his office, and mileage at three cents per mile for all distance necessarily traveled in going to and coming from the meetings of the board. Said expenses shall be paid from the fees and assessments received by the board under the provisions of this act, and no part of the salary or other expenses of the board shall ever be paid out of the state treasury. All moneys received in excess of said per diem allowance and mileage as above provided for, shall be held by the secretary as a special fund for meeting expenses of said board and carrying out the provisions of this act, and he shall give such bonds as the board shall from time to time direct, and said board shall make an annual report of its proceedings to the governor on the first Monday in January of each year, which report shall contain an account of all moneys received and disbursed by them pursuant to this act.

Annual license fee to be paid before April 1.

SECTION 12. Every registered optician shall in every year after 1901, pay to the said board of examiners the sum of two dollars as a license fee for such year. Such payment shall be made prior to the first day of April in each and every year, and in case of default in such payment, by any person, his certificate may be revoked by the board of examiners, upon twenty days' notice of the time and place of considering such revocation. But no license shall be revoked for such non-payment if the person so notified shall pay before or at such time of consideration his fee and such penalty as may be imposed by said board, *provided* that said board may impose a penalty of five dollars and no more on any one person so notified, as a condition of allowing his license to stand. *Provided, further,* that said board of examiners may collect any such dues by suit.

Revocation of registry certificate.

SECTION 13. Said board shall have power to revoke any certificate of registration granted by it under this act for conviction of crime, habitual drunkenness for six months immediately before a charge to be made, gross incompetency, or contagious or infectious disease; *provided* that before any certificate shall be so revoked, the holder thereof shall have notice in writing of the charge or charges against him, and at a day specified in said notice at least five days after the service thereof, be given a public hearing, and have opportunity to produce testimony in his behalf and to confront the witnesses against him. Any person whose certificate has been so revoked, may after the expiration of ninety days, apply to have the same re-granted, and the same shall be re-granted to him upon a satisfactory showing that the disqualification has ceased.

Violation a misdemeanor, penalty.

SECTION 14. Any person who shall violate any of the provisions of this act shall be deemed guilty of a misdemeanor, and upon conviction, may be fined not less than twenty dollars, nor not more than one hundred dollars, or to be confined not less than one month nor more than three months in the county jail. And all fines thus received shall be paid into the common school fund of the county in which such conviction takes place.

SECTION 15. Justices of the peace and the respective municipal courts shall have jurisdiction of violations of this act. It shall be the duty of the respective county attorneys to prosecute all violations of this act.

Who exempt.

SECTION 16. Nothing in this act shall be construed to apply to physicians and surgeons authorized to practice under the laws of the State of Minnesota, nor to persons who sell spectacles or eye-glasses without attempting to traffic upon assumed skill in adopting them to the eye.

SECTION 17. This act shall take effect and be in force from and after its passage.

Approved April 13, 1901.

New Jersey Optometry Law *

45:12-1. *Practice of Optometry defined.* Optometry is hereby declared to be a profession, and the practice of optometry is defined to be the employment of objective or subjective means, or both, for the examination of the human eye for the purpose of ascertaining any departure from the normal, measuring its powers of vision and adapting lenses or prisms for the aid thereof. A person shall be deemed to be practicing optometry within the meaning of this chapter who in any way advertises himself as an optometrist, or who shall employ any means for the measurement of the powers of vision or the adaptation of lenses or prisms for the aid thereof, practice, offer or attempt to practice optometry as herein defined, either on his own behalf or as an employee or student of another, whether under the personal supervision of his employer or preceptor or not, or to use testing appliances for the purpose of the measurement of the powers of vision or diagnose any ocular deficiency or deformity, visual or muscular anomaly of the human eye or prescribe lenses, prisms or ocular exercise for the correction or the relief thereof or who holds himself out as qualified to practice optometry.

45:12-2.–12.4. *Board, How Constituted, Officers, Compensation, Appoint Agents, Rules and Regulations, Records, Examination.*

45:12-5. *Applications for certificate of registration; qualifications of applicants; examination; issuance of certificate.* A person desiring to commence the practice of optometry shall file with the Secretary of the Board, upon blanks to be furnished by the Secretary, an application, verified by oath of the applicant, stating therein that he is more than twenty-one years of age, of good moral character, has been a resident of the State of New Jersey for a period of at least two years prior to the date of filing of the said application, is a citizen of the United States, or has declared his intention to become such a citizen, has a preliminary education equivalent to a course of at least four years in an approved public or private high school and has been graduated from a school or college of optometry maintaining a standard satisfactory to the Board and which was in good standing in the opinion of the Board at the date of graduation, and shall have received a diploma conferring upon him the degree of doctor of optometry, or what in the opinion of the Board may be considered the equivalent thereof, and shall have taken an examination before the Board to determine his qualifications therefor. If the examination of any applicant for registration shall be satisfactory to the majority of the Board, he shall receive from it a certificate of registration authorizing him to practice optometry. All examination papers shall be deposited in the New Jersey State Library, and remain there for a period of one year, at the expiration of which time they shall be destroyed, and they shall be prima facie evidence of all matters therein contained.

45:12-6. *Fees; numbering and recording of certificates; filing of photograph of registrant.* The fee for such examination shall be twenty-five dollars, and for a certificate of registration, fifteen dollars, to be paid to the Secretary of the Board by the applicant upon filing his application and receiving his certificate, respectively. Before any certificate is issued it shall be numbered and recorded in a book kept in the office of the Board and its numbers shall be noted upon the certificate. A photograph of the person registered shall be filed with the record. In all legal proceedings the record and photograph so kept in the office of the Board, or certified copies thereof, shall be prima facie evidence of the facts therein stated.

45:12-7. *Issuance of license to licensees of other States; fee.* Any applicant for

* These rules and regulations are excerpts from the New Jersey law. Code numbers have been included for reference.

Laws are a constantly changing entity. Exact duplicates of recent changes in regulations can be obtained by writing directly to the optometry board of examiners at the state capital.

license to practice optometry, upon proving to the satisfaction of the Board that he is of good moral character, a citizen of the United States, or has declared his intention to become such a citizen and that he has been examined and licensed by the examining and licensing Board of another State of the United States, and that at the time of the granting of such license the standard of requirements for the licensee to practice optometry in the State where such license was granted was at least substantially equal to the standard of requirements for such license established by this chapter, or upon proof that he has successfully passed an examination conducted by the International Association of Boards of Examiners in Optometry and upon filing with the Secretary of the Board a copy of his license or certificate, verified as a true copy by the affidavit of the Secretary of the Board granting such license, may, in the discretion of the Board, be granted a license to practice optometry without further examination upon the payment to the Treasurer of the Board of a license fee of fifty dollars, and in such application for a license without examination all questions of academic requirements of other States shall be determined by the Commissioner of Education of this State.

45:12-8. *Certificate displayed in office; practitioners' names displayed outside; practice outside office.* Every person practicing optometry shall display his registration certificate or certificates, together with his registration renewal certificate or certificates, in a conspicuous place in the office or offices wherein he practices optometry, but not in such manner that they may be seen from the outside of such office or offices, and, whenever required, exhibit the registration and renewal certificates to the Board or its authorized representatives. Every office where an optometrist is practicing shall have displayed on a sign so as to be read on the outside of the office the name of each optometrist practicing therein. When practicing the profession of optometry outside of or away from the office, he shall deliver to each patient a bill for professional services rendered, which shall contain his full name, home post-office address and address of his principal office in this State, the number of his certificate, and his signature.

Every person practicing optometry in New Jersey, shall notify the Board in writing of any change of address or location of his office or offices at least five days prior to occupying said new office, returning therewith the appropriate registration renewal certificate or certificates and the Board shall issue a new registration renewal certificate or certificates for the new office location or locations.

45:12-9. *Every registered optometrist shall on such date as the Board may determine, annually pay to the Secretary-Treasurer of the Board a registration renewal fee of $10.00, for which he shall receive a renewal of his registration.*

A nonactive registration renewal certificate shall be issued to those not practicing within the State and should a nonactive registrant desire to practice during the registration year he shall notify the Board in writing of his office location, shall pay the required $2.00 fee to the Secretary-Treasurer and shall return the nonactive registration renewal certificate for cancellation. The Board shall thereupon issue an active registration renewal certificate to said registrant.

Every person having an active or nonactive license to practice optometry in New Jersey shall notify the Board in writing of any change of address and pay a fee of $2.00 and return therewith his registration renewal certificate and the Board shall issue a new registration renewal certificate.

Every registered optometrist having a nonactive registration renewal certificate for a period of 5 days or more who desires an active registration certificate shall be required to submit to a practical examination, conducted by the Board, and if the results of the examination are satisfactory to the majority of the Board, he shall then be issued an active certificate of registration authorizing him to practice in this State.

The Board shall have the power to issue, upon proper application and payment of the prescribed fees, branch office registration certificates to active licenses when, in its discretion and after a proper investigation, it determines that a new branch office complies with the provisions of this chapter and the rules and regulations of the Board and that such action serves the public interest; provided, that nothing herein contained shall permit the Board to deny branch office registration certificates to active licensees who have conducted branch offices prior to September first, one thousand nine hundred and forty-seven; and provided, that the Board shall not issue more than two branch registration certificates to any one licensee after January first, one thousand nine hundred and forty-eight.

Every licensee holding an active registration renewal certificate who may practice at any place other than the address for which his active registration renewal certificate is issued shall be required to obtain from the Secretary-Treasurer for a fee of fifteen dollars a branch office registration certificate for each and every location wherein he practices; provided, that nothing herein contained shall be construed to require an active licensee to obtain a branch office certificate for the purpose of serving on the staff of a hospital or institution which receives no fees (other than entrance registration fees) for the services rendered by the optometrist and that the optometrist receives no fees or compensation directly or indirectly for such services rendered; and further provided, that nothing herein contained shall be construed to require an active licensee to obtain a branch office certificate for the purpose of rendering necessary optometric services for his patients confined to their homes, hospitals or institutions.

Every licensee holding a branch office registration certificate or certificates shall, on such date as the Board may determine, annually pay to the Secretary a registration renewal fee of ten dollars for each branch office registration certificate he holds, for which he shall receive a branch office registration renewal certificate or certificates.

In case of default in payment of registration renewal fees by any registered optometrist, his certificate or certificates to practice may be revoked by the Board upon twenty days' notice to said optometrist of the time and place of considering such revocation; but the certificate or certificates shall not be revoked if the person so in default pays such fees before or at such time of consideration named by the Board.

Branch office registration certificates and branch office registration renewal certificates shall be displayed in the offices for which they are issued as provided for in Section 45:12-8 of this title.

45:12-10. *Certification of records of Board as to issuance of licenses; fee; certificate as evidence.* The Secretary of the Board, upon request, shall certify over the seal of the Board whether the records kept by it show or fail to show the issuance of a license to practice optometry or any branch thereof or any other profession or business, the practice of which is licensed by the Board, or the issuance of any annual certificate of registration for such practice. The fee for such certificate shall be three dollars. Any such certificate, whether made on such request or made by said Secretary for use in proceedings in which the Board may be a party, shall be prima facie evidence of the facts therein stated.

45:12-11. *Revocation of certificates; "unprofessional conduct" defined; preferring charges.* The Board shall have the power, and it is hereby made its duty, to refuse to grant, to revoke or to suspend for a specified time, to be determined in the discretion of the Board, any license to practice optometry in the State of New Jersey for any of the following causes:

a. Loaning, selling, or fraudulently obtaining any optometry diploma, license, record, or certificate, or aiding or abetting therein.

b. Gross incompetency.

c. The obtaining of any fee by fraud or misrepresentation or the practice of deception or fraud upon any patient or patients.

d. Chronic and persistent inebriety, or the habitual use of narcotics.

e. Affliction with a contagious or infectious disease which in the opinion of the Board, renders practice of optometry by the licensee or applicant for license dangerous to the public health.

f. Conviction of a crime involving moral turpitude; or where any licensee or applicant for a license has pleaded non vult contendre or non vult to any indictment, information, allegation or complaint, alleging the commission of a crime involving moral turpitude, or where any licensee or applicant for a license presents to the Board any diploma, license, or certificate that shall have been obtained, signed, or issued unlawfully or under fraudulent representation. The record of conviction or the entry of such a plea in any court of this State or any other State or in any of the courts of the United States or any foreign country, shall be sufficient warrant for the revocation or suspension of a license.

g. Conviction in a court of competent jurisdiction of a high misdemeanor.

h. False, fraudulent or misleading advertising of the practice of optometry or of any art, skill, knowledge, method of treatment or practice pertaining thereto. Advertising of the practice of optometry or of any art, skill, knowledge, method of treatment or practice pertaining thereto or ophthalmic materials, the character or durability of services or ophthalmic materials or advertising to perform optometric services or with reference to providing glasses, spectacles, contact lenses, frames, mountings, lenses or prisms free of charge or on credit or installments or anything of similar import to the foregoing, by means of circular, handbills, card, letter, sign, poster, pictures, respresentations of eyes or eyeglasses, advertising matches, mirrors or other articles or by advertisement in newspapers, books, magazines or other publications or by projection by means of light, electronics, crier, radio broadcasting, television or by use of an advertising solicitor or publicity agent or any other advertising media; provided, however, that any person licensed under the provisions of this chapter may issue appointment cards or professional cards to his patients, when the information thereon, is limited to matter pertaining to the time and place of appointment and that permitted on the professional card, or may display the name of the licensee on the premises where he is engaged in the practice of his profession upon the windows or doors thereof and by doorplates, or name or office directory when the information is limited to that of the professional card. For the purposes of this section a professional card shall contain only the name, title, profession, degrees, address, telephone number, office hours of the licensed optometrist, and the words "eyes examined," "eye examination," or "hours for the examination of eyes." The foregoing is not to be construed as prohibiting the publication by an optometrist of his professional card in regularly published newspapers provided his said card and advertisement does not contain any information other than that permitted in the definition of the professional card as is found in this section.

i. Announcing his name in any city, commercial, telephone, or other public directory, or directories in public or office buildings using display or boldface type or type that is in any way dissimilar in size, shape, or color to that used for other practitioners of the healing arts in the same directory. No optometrist shall cause or permit himself to be listed in a telephone directory under any name other than the name in which he is registered with the Board as the holder of a valid, unrevoked, active license to practice optometry in this State.

No optometrist shall cause or permit any listing of any

(1) inactive, retired, removed or deceased optometrist or any other ocular practitioner, except that, for a period of not more than 2 years from the date of succession to the practice of another optometrist, an optometrist may use a telephone listing of such optometrist together with the words "succeeded by," "succeeding" or "successor to."

(2) any trade name or corporate name, or the name of any person, firm, corporation, partnership or association not licensed to practice optometry under the provisions of chapter 12 of Title 45 of the Revised Statutes of New Jersey in which additional listing the address or telephone number is the same as that of the said optometrist.

The listing of an optometrist in a telephone directory shall contain only the name, title, the word "optometrist," degrees, address or addresses, office hours and telephone number or numbers of licensed optometrist, including, if desired, the words "if no answer, call ...."

Any optometrist listed in the classified section of any directory shall be listed only under the classification entitled "Optometrists," at the address or addresses for which he holds a valid, unrevoked, active license to practice optometry in this State.

j. Displaying any spectacles, eyeglasses, eyeglass or spectacle frames or mountings, goggles, lenses, prisms, spectacle or eyeglass cases, ophthalmic material of any kind, optometric instruments, or optical tools or machinery, or any merchandise, material, or advertising of a commercial nature in office windows, or reception rooms or in display cases outside of the offices, where the display of such merchandise, material or advertising would make it visible from the street.

k. Displaying his licenses, diplomas, or certificates in such a manner that they may be seen from the outside of the office.

l. Using the title doctor or its abbreviations without further qualifying this title or abbreviation with the word optometrist.

m. Use by an optometrist of the words, "clinic," "infirmary," "hospital," "school," "college," "university," or "institute" in English or any other language in connection with any place where optometry may be practiced or demonstrated; provided, however, that nothing in this section shall prevent an optometric clinic, approved by the Board, from being conducted on a nonprofit basis by a school or college of optometry or an association of registered optometrists.

n. The continuance of an optometrist in the employ of, or acting as an assistant to any person, firm or corporation, either directly or indirectly, after he has knowledge that such person, firm or corporation is violating the laws of New Jersey concerning the practice of optometry.

o. Any conduct which is of a character likely to deceive or defraud the public.

p. Soliciting in person or through an agent or agents for the purpose of selling ophthalmic materials or optometric services or employing what are known as "chasers," "steerers," or "solicitors," to obtain business.

q. The issuance of appointment cards or the display of the name of the licensee on the premises where he is engaged in the practice of his profession when the information goes beyond that permitted by a professional card.

r. The display of the name and title of the licensee, or other information in lettering larger than four inches in height for street-level offices, or larger than six inches in height for offices above street-level and in no event shall there be more than three such displays, and the illumination of said name and title except during office hours; the use of colored or neon lights, eyeglasses or eye signs, whether painted, neon, decalcomania, or any other either in the form of eyes or structures resembling eyes, eyeglass frames, eyeglasses or spectacles, whether lighted or not.

s. Any violation of rule or regulation duly promulgated by the Board hereunder or of any provision of this chapter.

t. No optometrist shall cause or permit the use of his name, profession or professional title by or in conjunction with any association, company, corporation, or nonlicensed person, in any advertising of any manner.

u. Practicing optometry in any retail or commercial store or office not exclusively devoted to the practice of optometry or other health care professions where materials or merchandise are displayed pertaining to a business or commercial undertaking not bearing any relation to the practice of optometry or other health care professions; providing, however, that any optometrist practicing in premises of this type prior to January 1, 1963, shall be permitted to continue in his present location; but when and if any optometrist who is a lessee or an employee of a lessee, vacates such premises no other optometrist shall be permitted to practice in said vacated premises.

v. Prior to prescribing for or providing eyeglasses or spectacles a complete minimum examination shall be made of the patient to determine the correct lenses necessary for such a patient. The requirements of such minimum examination shall be defined by rule or regulations of the New Jersey State Board of Optometrists.

w. Any person licensed as an optometrist who violates Section 45:12-11 (i), (h), (m), (q), or (r) of this chapter shall, at the discretion of the Board, be subject to a penalty of $50.00 for the first offense and $200.00 for each subsequent offense in lieu of the suspension or revocation of his license.

x. Any person who has been guilty of gross malpractice or gross neglect in the practice of optometry which has endangered the health or life of any person.

Proceedings for the revocation of a certificate or suspension of the right to practice shall be begun by filing with the Board a written charge or charges against the accused. These charges may be preferred by any person or the Board may on its own motion direct its Secretary to prefer the charges.

45:12-12. *Hearing of charges; court powers of Board.* When charges are preferred, the Board, or a majority thereof, shall hear and determine them, and for such purpose the Board, or a majority thereof, shall have the powers of a court of record sitting in the county in which its meeting shall be held, to issue subpoenas and to compel the attendance and testimony of witnesses. A time and place for the hearing of the charges, within the city of Trenton, shall be fixed by the Board as soon as convenient, and a copy of the charges, together with a notice of the time and place when they will be heard and determined, shall be served upon the accused or his counsel at least twenty days before the date actually fixed for the hearing. The accused shall be entitled to the subpoena of the Board for his witnesses. Where personal service or service upon counsel cannot be effected and such fact is certified on oath, the Board shall cause to be published for at least seven times, at least twenty days prior to the hearing, in two daily papers in the county in which the optometrist was last known to practice, a notice to the effect that at a definite time and place a hearing will be held for the purpose of hearing charges against the optometrist upon an application to revoke his certificate. At the hearing the accused shall have the right to cross examine the witnesses against him and to produce witnesses in his defense, and to appear personally or by counsel.

45:12-13. *Unanimous finding necessary for revocation or suspension of certificates; practice thereafter prohibited.* The Board shall reduce its findings to writing, to be signed by all the members who have heard the charges. If the Board unanimously find that the charges or any of them, are sustained, it may thereupon, in its discretion, revoke or suspend the certificate of registration. No person shall practice optometry after his certificate of registration shall have been revoked or suspended in accordance with the provisions of this chapter.

45:12-14. *Refusal, revocation or suspension of certificates reviewable by certiorari.* All rulings of the Board in refusing to issue or refusing to renew, or suspending, or revoking any certificate of registration shall be conclusive and binding unless the party in interest shall within sixty days of the ruling apply for a review by certiorari or proceeding in the nature thereof to a court of competent jurisdiction and said court is hereby authorized and empowered to review and correct the action of the Board, and the Board shall forthwith carry out the judgment of the court on such review. Such review may be applied for according to the practice of such court and the Board, if ordered so to do, shall transmit to the court all documents and papers on file in the matter, together with a transcript of the evidence, the findings, and the rulings, and all matters pertaining to the same.

45:12-15. *Issuance of new certificate after revocation.* Where the certificate of registration of any person has been revoked the Board may, after the expiration of one year, entertain an application for a new certificate in like manner as original applications for certificates are entertained, and, upon such new application it may, in its discretion, exempt the applicant from the necessity of undergoing an examination.

45:12-16. *Optometrists convicted of crime reported to State Board.* The clerk of every court wherein a person licensed to practice optometry in this State shall be convicted of a crime shall make a report thereof in writing to the Board of the conviction. The report shall state the name and address of the person convicted and the name of the court and the judge presiding therein at the time of the conviction, the date thereof, the nature of the crime of which the person was convicted and the sentence imposed by the court.

45:12-17. 45:12-17.1. *Board, Expenses, Compensation for Examinations.*

45:12-18. *Board, Reports, Receipts and Disbursements.*

45:12-18.1. *Records exclusive property of optometrist.* The record of an optometrist of the examination of a patient, including patient's name, address, age, occupation, and all findings and pertinent facts concerning the patient discovered and disclosed during the course of such examination, as well as the record of professional services rendered and the fees charged therefore shall, because of the confidential nature in the relationship, be the exclusive property of the optometrist who rendered the professional services to the patient. Any unauthorized use by any other person, firm or corporation of the information contained therein shall constitute an infringement of the property rights of the patient and the optometrist, and shall subject the offender to a civil suit for damages by the person aggrieved.

45:12-19. *Illegal practices.* No person, not a holder of a certificate of registration duly issued to him, shall practice optometry within the State, and no person shall falsely personate a registered optometrist of a like or different name, nor buy, sell or fraudulently obtain a certificate issued to another. No person shall directly or indirectly for himself or others do or engage in any acts or practices specifically prohibited to duly registered optometrists by the provisions of Section 45:12-11 of this chapter.

No person shall peddle spectacles, eyeglasses or lenses or practice optometry from house to house or on the streets or highways notwithstanding any law providing for the licensing of peddlers. This shall not prohibit, however, an optometrist from attending, prescribing, and furnishing spectacles, eyeglasses or lenses to a person who by reason of an illness, or physical or mental infirmity is confined to his place of abode, or to a hospital or other institution.

It shall be unlawful for any person licensed to practice optometry under the laws of the State of New Jersey to advertise, practice or hold himself forth as being entitled to practice under a name other than his own, unless he be an associate of or any assistant to an optometrist licensed under the laws of the State of New Jersey, and it shall be unlawful for any unlicensed person, or any association or corporation directly or indirectly to engage or undertake to engage in the practice of optometry by utilizing the services, upon a salary, commission basis, or by any other means or method, of any person licensed to practice optometry in the State of New Jersey. It shall be unlawful for any optometrist to engage or undertake to engage in the practice of optometry in behalf of any unlicensed person, association or corporation, by or the formation of partnerships between except that this shall not prohibit the employment by optometrists or physicians duly licensed in the State of New Jersey.

It shall be unlawful for any person, association or corporation to issue cards offering free eye examinations or eye examinations for any price, or eye examinations at a discount or offering special rates or discounts for eyeglasses.

45:12-20. *Penalty for illegal practice, court proceedings for recovery.* Any person who violates the provisions of this chapter, or obstructs or interferes with any duly authorized agent of the Board in the performance of any duty under this chapter, or any person who employs or gives aid or assists any person not authorized to practice optometry within the meaning of this chapter, to practice optometry in this State, shall be subject to a penalty of two hundred dollars for the first offense and five hundred dollars for each subsequent offense, to be sued for and recovered by and in the name of the Board. Every district court and every court of common pleas in any county is hereby empowered, upon the filing of a complaint in writing, duly verified, which verification, when made by a member of the Board, or by a member of any incorporated optometrical society of this State or any county thereof, may be made upon information and belief, that a person has violated any provision of this chapter, to issue process at the suit of the Board as plaintiff. The process shall be either in the nature of a summons or a warrant, which warrant may issue without any order of the court or judge first being obtained against the person so charged, which process, when in the nature of a warrant, shall be returnable forthwith, and when in the nature of a summons shall be returnable in not less than five nor more than fifteen entire days; and such process shall state what provision of law is alleged to have been violated by the defendant. The officers to serve and execute all process under this chapter shall be the officers authorized to serve and execute process in said courts.

45:12-21. *Judgment; commitment of defendant for nonpayment; defendant to be detained, unless bond filed, upon adjournment of trial.* Upon the return of such process, or at any time to which the trial shall be adjourned, the court shall proceed summarily to hear the testimony and to determine and give judgment in the matter without a jury and without the filing of any pleadings for the plaintiff for the recovery of the penalty, with costs, or for the defendant, and shall, if judgment be rendered for the plaintiff, cause any defendant, who refuses or neglects to forthwith pay the amount of the judgment rendered against him and all the costs and charges incident thereto, to be committed to the county jail in the case of a first offense for a period not less than thirty nor more than sixty days, in the discretion of the court, and in the case of a subsequent offense to be committed to the county jail for a period not less than sixty nor more than one hundred and twenty days for each subsequent offense in the discretion of the court. The court shall have power to adjourn the hearing or trial in any case from time to time, and in such case, except in cases in which the first process was a summons, it shall be the duty of the judge thereof to detain the defendant in safe custody, unless he shall enter into bond to the Board, with sufficient surety in double the amount of the penalty claimed, conditioned for his appearance on the day to which the hearing shall be adjourned, and thence from day to day until the case is disposed of, and to abide by the judgment of said court. The bond, if forfeited, may be prosecuted by the Board.

45:12-22. *Titles not authorized.* Nothing contained in this chapter shall confer upon any person practicing optometry the right to add, affix, or attach to his name the title, designation, character or letters of M.D., surgeon, doctor, unless qualified by the word optometrist, ophthalmologist, or to indicate in any way that he is engaged in the treatment of injuries of the human eye, or to use any therapeutic measures or agencies other than those included in the practice of optometry as defined in Section 45:12-1 of this chapter for the treatment of the human eye, unless he is authorized to do so by the Board, body or persons empowered by law to award such right or title.

APPENDIX C

Schools and Colleges of Optometry

ILLINOIS COLLEGE OF OPTOMETRY
3241 South Michigan Avenue, Chicago, Illinois 60616

INDIANA UNIVERSITY—DIVISION OF OPTOMETRY
Health Center Building, Bloomington, Indiana 47405

LOS ANGELES COLLEGE OF OPTOMETRY
950 West Jefferson Boulevard, Los Angeles, California 90007

MASSACHUSETTS COLLEGE OF OPTOMETRY
178 Newbury Street, Boston, Massachusetts 02116

THE OHIO STATE UNIVERSITY—SCHOOL OF OPTOMETRY
338 West Tenth Avenue, Columbus, Ohio 43216

PACIFIC UNIVERSITY—COLLEGE OF OPTOMETRY
Forest Grove, Oregon 97116

PENNSYLVANIA COLLEGE OF OPTOMETRY
6100 North Twelfth Street, Philadelphia, Pennsylvania 19141

SOUTHERN COLLEGE OF OPTOMETRY
1246 Union Avenue, Memphis, Tennessee 38104

UNIVERSITY OF CALIFORNIA—SCHOOL OF OPTOMETRY
Berkeley, California 94720

UNIVERSITY OF HOUSTON—COLLEGE OF OPTOMETRY
Cullen Boulevard, Houston, Texas 77004

APPENDIX D

Typical Optometry Curriculum
University-Affiliated School

PREPROFESSIONAL SCHEDULE

FRESHMAN YEAR

Fall		Winter		Spring	
Course	Units	Course	Units	Course	Units
English 1A or Speech 1A	5	English 1B or		Foreign Language III.	4–5
Foreign Language I	4–5	Speech 1B	5	Mathematics 16B	4
Chemistry 1A	4	Foreign Language II	4–5	Psychology 1	4
	13–14	Chemistry 1B	4	Elective	4–5
		Mathematics 16A	4		16–18
			17–18		

SOPHOMORE YEAR

Course	Units	Course	Units	Course	Units
Foreign Language IV	4–5	Statistics 2	5	Elective	4
Chemistry 8A	4	Chemistry 8B	4	Poli. Sci. 5	4
Physics 2A	4	Physics 2B	4	Physics 2C	4
Biology 1A	5	Biology 1B	5	Biology 1C	5
	17–18		18		17

PROFESSIONAL CURRICULUM

FIRST YEAR

Fall		Winter		Spring	
Course	Units	Course	Units	Course	Units
Optometry 100	1	Physiol. Optics 101	5	Optometry 104	3
Anatomy 102	4	Physics 106B	4	Physiol. Optics 102	5
Physics 106A	4	Physiology 112	4	Physiology 113	4
Elective	4–5	Bacteriology 103	4	Physiology 113L	2
	13–14		17		14

SECOND YEAR

Course	Units	Course	Units	Course	Units
Optometry 105	3	Optometry 128	3	Optometry 131	3
Optometry 127	5	Optometry 130	5	Optometry 133	5
Physiol. Optics 125	5	Physiol. Optics 129	5	Physiol. Optics 132	5
Elective	3–4	Elective	3–4	Elective	3–4
	16–17		16–17		16–17

THIRD YEAR

Course	Units	Course	Units	Course	Units
Optometry 150A	3	Optometry 150B	3	Optometry 150C	3
Optometry 152	5	Optometry 158A	4	Optometry 158B	4
Optometry 453	3	Optometry 454	4	Optometry 455	4
Physiol. Optics 151	5	Physiol. Optics 160	5	Optometry 161	5
	16		16		16

FOURTH YEAR

Course	Units	Course	Units	Course	Units
Physiol. Optics 199	3	Physiol. Optics 199		Physiol. Optics 175	1
or Optometry 499	3	(or Optom. 499)	1	Optometry 486B	2
Optometry 178	2	Optometry 185	4	Optometry 177	4
Optometry 480A	5	Optometry 486A	2	Optometry 480C	5
Optometry 483A	5	Optometry 480B	5	Optometry 483C	5
	15	Optometry 483B	5		17
			17		

PREPROFESSIONAL COURSES

FRESHMAN YEAR

Chemistry 1A–1B. General Chemistry. (4–4)

    1A. Stoichiometry and introduction to structural chemistry. The laboratory takes up stoichiometry and thermochemistry.

1B. Reversible reactions, equilibrium constants and their dependence on temperature and pressure, and electrical cells. The laboratory takes up equilibria of weak acids and sparingly soluble salts, and electrical cells.

Psychology 1. General Psychology. (4)

Three 1-hour lectures and one 1-hour section meeting per week. Introduction to the principal areas, problems, and concepts of psychology.

Mathematics 16A–16B. Analytic Geometry and Calculus. (4–4)

Three 1-hour lectures per week. Elements of analytic geometry, differential and integral calculus. The exponential, logarithmic, and trigonometric functions. The algebra of matrices and systems of linear equations. Convexity and systems of linear inequalities. Statistics 16 is intended to follow 16A–16B.

Speech 1A–1B. First-Year Reading, Writing and Speaking. (5–5)

Three 1-hour lecture and discussion periods and one 1-hour individual conference period per week. Written and oral composition, based upon readings and discussions of major works of literature, philosophy, and science.

History 17A. United States History (5).

Three 1-hour lectures and one 1-hour section meeting per week.

SOPHOMORE YEAR

Chemistry 8A–8B. Survey of Organic Chemistry. (4–4)

Two 1½-hour lectures and one 3-hour laboratory per week. A survey of the important classes of organic compounds, with emphasis on materials of interest to students of the biological sciences.

Physics 2A–2B–2C. General Physics Lectures and Laboratory. (4–4–4)

Three 1-hour lectures, one 1-hour discussion section, and one 3-hour laboratory period per week. Elective in the College of Letters and Science. Required for premedical students and students in architecture. Mechanics, properties of matter, heat, sound, light, electricity and magnetism, atomic and nuclear physics.

Biology 1A–1B–1C. General Biology. (5–5–5)

Three 1-hour lectures and one 3-hour laboratory per week with an additional discussion section, field trip, or laboratory per week. *Prerequisites: Chemistry 1A (semester system) Chemistry 1A–B (quarter system).* Intended for students majoring in biological sciences, but open to all qualified students. Sequence beginning in the fall.

Statistics 2. Introduction to Statistics. (5)

Three 1-hour lectures and three 1-hour laboratories per week. *Prerequisite: high school algebra.* Elementary treatment of basic ideas in probability and statistical inference. Models; conditional probability; measures of location, spread, and association; binomial distribution, normal approximation. Sampling; point estimation; some standard significance tests; power.

Political Science 5. American Institutions. (4)

Two 1½-hour lectures per week. A survey of the powers, structure and operations of government, primarily at the national level.

PROFESSIONAL COURSES

FIRST YEAR

Fall Quarter

Optometry 100. History of Optometry. (1)

One 1-hour lecture per week. The profession of optometry, its history and present status.

Anatomy 102. General Human Anatomy. (4)

Two 1½-hour lectures and one 4½-hour lab. Prepared human dissections, models, and microscopic slides.

Physics 106A. Geometrical Optics. (4)

Three 1-hour lectures and one 3-hour lab. Geometrical methods applied to the optics of mirrors, lenses, and prisms.

Elective. See section on electives.

Winter Quarter

Physiological Optics 101. Anatomy of Eye and Orbit. (5)

Three 1½-hour lectures and one 2-hour laboratory per week. The macroscopic and microscopic anatomy of the orbit, its content and adjacent structures. The cranial nerves associated with vision and their cortical connections. The blood supply to the eye and orbit. The embryology of the eye.

Physics 106B. Physical Optics. (4)

Three 1-hour lectures and one 3-hour laboratory. Phenomena of diffraction, interference, and polarization of light, and their application.

Physiology 112. General Physiology. (4)

Three 1½-hour lectures. Cellular mechanisms underlying biolectric, secretory and contractile phenomena in living organisms.

Bacteriology 103. Biology of Host-Parasite Interactions in Infectious Disease. (4)

Three 1-hour lectures and one 1-hour recitation per week. *Prerequisite: Biology 1A–1B–1C.* The study of infectious disease as an aspect of ecology; symbiosis and parasitism; evolution of the germ theory of disease; mechanisms of microbiol pathogenicity and host resistance; interaction of genotype and environment in host-parasite relationships.

Spring Quarter

Physiological Optics 102. Dioptrics of the Eye. (5)

Four 1-hour lectures and one 2-hour laboratory per week. The eye as an optical instrument; image forming properties, optical defects, and image quality; dimensions; optical constants, schematic eyes, cardinal points, ametropia, accommodation, retinal image size, blur circles, diffraction, aberrations, scatter, and absorption.

Optometry 104. Ophthalmic Optics. (3)

Two 1-hour lectures and one 3-hour laboratory per week. History of the development of lenses and spectacles; optical properties of lens materials; the theory and design of spectacle lenses. Laboratory exercises in lens cutting, edging, beveling, drilling, mounting, neutralization, and frame fitting and adjusting.

Physiology 113. Mammalian Physiology. (4)

Three 1½-hour lectures. Function of organ systems in man and other mammals.

Physiology 113L. Mammalian Physiology Laboratory. (2)

One 4½-hour laboratory.

Second Year

Fall Quarter

Physiological Optics 125. Vegetative Functions of the Eye. (5)

Three 1-hour lectures and two 2-hour laboratories per week. Consideration of the physiology of the cornea and lids; formation and function of lacrimal fluid; formation, function and drainage of the aqueous humor; intraocular pressure; metabolism and circulation in the eye; physiology and biochemistry of the lens; iris and pupil; accommodation, photochemistry. The characteristics of drugs producing miosis, mydriasis, cycloplegia, accommodative spasm, and anesthesia of ocular surfaces.

Optometry 105. Ophthalmic Optics. (3)

Two 1-hour lectures and one 3-hour laboratory per week. Continuation of Optometry 104.

Optometry 127. Refraction of the Eye. (5)

Three lectures and two 2-hour laboratories. Optical and biological variables determining the refractive state of the eye. Lectures and laboratory assignments on subjective, and objective techniques of measurement and methods of correcting refractive anomalies: skiametry, keratometry, ophthalmoscopy, visual acuity, subjective refraction, amplitude of accommodation.

Elective. See section on electives.

Winter Quarter

Optometry 128. Introduction to Pathology. (3)

Two 1½-hour classes per week. Basic pathological processes in human development, senescence and disease. A correlated survey of disturbed function in disorders of visceral systems, including disturbances of electrolyte and fluid balance and of metabolism.

Physiological Optics 129. Motility of the Eye. (5)

Three 1½-hour lectures and one 2-hour laboratory per week. Detailed consideration of ocular movements; specification of direction of regard, line of sight, visual axes, center of rotation, primary position; kinematics of the eye, Listing's Law; action of the extraocular muscles; types of movements, reflex, saccadic, pursuit, versions, vergences; accommodation; accommodative convergence; convergence accommodation.

Optometry 130. Optometric Analysis. (5)

Three 1-hour lectures and two 2-hour laboratories. Routine examination and case analysis; interrogation and case history, motility, phorometry, versions, vergences, relative accommodation and the various techniques for the analysis of optometric data. Introduction to clinical observations.

Spring Quarter

Optometry 131. Clinical Manifestations of Disease and Pharmacological
Influences on Disease and Function (3)

Two 1½-hour classes. A survey of disease processes and systemic disorders with special reference to ocular implications and manifestations. The role of modern drugs in therapy and side effects of drug use, especially as they relate to the eye and vision.

Physiological Optics 132. Visual Stimuli. (5)

Three 1½-hour lectures and one 2-hour laboratory per week. Study of visual stimuli, their nature and specification; radiometry; photometry; colorimetry; illumination; light sources; atmospheric scatter; effects of radiation. Color vision.

Optometry 133. Anomalies of Binocular Vision. (5)

Four 1-hour lectures and one 2-hour laboratory. Detection, measurement, classification, etiology, symptomatology, signs and prognosis of the latent and manifest disorders of binocular fixation, both comitant and noncomitant; orthoptics and visual training. Clinical observations.

Elective. See section of electives.

Third Year

Fall Quarter

Optometry 150A. Ocular Disease. (3)

Two 1-hour lectures and one 2-hour laboratory. Introduction to ocular diseases and their optometric detection; symptomatology and signs of ocular disease. External examination of the eye, pupillary reactions. Internal examination of the eye, ophthalmoscopy, biomicroscopy, tonometry; visual fields.

Physiological Optics 151. Monocular Sensory Processes of Vision. (5)

Three 1½-hour lectures and one 2-hour laboratory. Action of visible light on the retina, visual pigments and electrical phenomena. Light sense: sensitivity, threshold, differential thresholds, luminosity curves. Effects of stimulation: single and periodic, critical frequency of flicker, light and dark adaptation, after-images, spatial and temporal induction. Form sense: visual acuity. Perception of motion.

Optometry 152. Advanced Geometric Optics. (5)

Five 1-hour lectures. Gaussian optics. Aberrations and methods of correction, chromatic aberration and dispersion, oblique astigmatism, "corrected curve" lenses, design and characteristics of ophthalmic instruments.

Optometry 453. Optometry Clinic. (3)

One 1-hour lecture, one 4-hour clinic, and one 2-hour Dispensary. Optometry Clinic. Examination and prescribing of lenses to clinic patients. Dispensing of eyewear.

Winter Quarter

Optometry 150B. Ocular Disease. (4)

Two 1-hour lectures and one 2-hour laboratory per week. Systematic study and classification of ocular diseases, their differentiation, and ophthalmological management.

Physiological Optics 160. Binocular Vision and Space Perception. (5)

Three 1½-hour lectures and one 2-hour laboratory per week. Binocular integration; horopter, correspondence, figure-ground relations, perception of size, shape, direction, distance, motion, time and complex patterns; information theory.

Optometry 158A. Visual Rehabilitation. (4)

Three 1-hour lectures and one 2-hour laboratory. Aniseikonia, subnormal vision and geriatric optometry.

Optometry 454. Optometry Clinic. (4)

Two 1-hour lectures, one 4-hour clinic, one 2-hour dispensing per week. Examination and prescribing of lenses to clinic patients, special problems in ophthalmic optics.

Spring Quarter

Optometry 150C. Ocular Disease. (3)

Two 1-hour lectures and one 2-hour laboratory per week. Continuation of Optometry 150B.

Optometry 158B. Visual Rehabilitation. (4)

Three 1-hour lectures and one 2-hour laboratory per week. Orthoptics, pleoptics, and pediatric optometry.

Optometry 161. Contact Lenses. (5)

Three 1-hour lectures and two 3-hour laboratories per week. Historical development, physical and optical properties of contact lenses and their adaptation to the human eye, with emphasis on the anatomical and physiological implications.

Optometry 455. Optometry Clinic. (4)

Two 1-hour lectures, one 4-hour clinic, one 2-hour dispensing. Continuation of Optometry 454.

FOURTH YEAR

Fall Quarter

Optometry 178. Applied Psychology for Optometrists. (2)

Two 1-hour lectures per week. Patient management and communication, oral and written; suggestion and hypnosis.

Optometry 480A. Advanced Optometry Clinic. (5)

Three 4-hour clinics and one 3-hour dispensing. Optometric examination of patients in the clinic performed independently by student clinicians under supervision of the clinic staff: refraction and dispensing.

Optometry 483A. Special Clinical Practice. (5)

Clinical practice in contact lenses, aniseikonia, subnormal vision, strabismus, orthoptics, and the detection of ocular diseases.

Physiological Optics 199. Independent Study. (1–5)

One 1-hour class per week. Independent study in physiological optics. Students will elect either Physiological Optics 199 or Optometry 499.

Optometry 499. Special Study. (1–5)

Independent study in optometry.

Winter Quarter

Physiological Optics 199 or Optometry 499. (1)

Optometry 185. Practice Management. (4)

Three 1-hour lectures per week and two field trips per quarter. Laws governing the practice of optometry. The establishment and management of an optometric practice; economics, taxes, insurance, accounting methods, office design, mode of practice, practice administration, and patient relations; professional organizations and societies.

Optometry 486A. Clinical Colloquia. (2)

One 2-hour seminar per week. Analysis and discussion of representative cases encompassing diagnosis, etiology, prognosis, treatment, referral, consultation and professional communication.

Optometry 480B. Advanced Optometry Clinic. (5)

Three 4-hour clinics and one 3-hour dispensing per week. Optometric examination of patients in the clinic performed independently by student clinicians under the supervision of the clinic staff: refraction and dispensing.

Optometry 483B. Special Clinical Practice. (5)

Six 2-hour clinics per week. Clinical practice in contact lenses, aniseikonia, subnormal vision, strabismus, orthoptics, and the detection of ocular disease.

Spring Quarter

Physiological Optics 175. Recent Advances in Physiological Optics. (1)

One 1-hour class per week. Recent advances in physiological optics and optometry.

Optometry 177. Public Health Optometry. (4)

Two 1½-hour lectures and field trips. Vision performance: screening methods, establishment and evaluation of standards, importance in industry, schools, and vehicle operation; eye safety programs; methods of supplying vision care by means of government assistance, in the armed forces, in health clinics and hospitals, group practice and prepaid and insurance programs.

Optometry 486C. Clinical Colloquia. (2)
Continuation of Optometry 486.

Optometry 480C. Advanced Optometry Clinic. (5)
Continuation of Optometry 480.

Optometry 483C. Special Clinical Practice. (5)
Continuation of Optometry 483.

ELECTIVES

A student's electives should be chosen so as to broaden his knowledge and ability. Normally, the electives should be chosen from the following list of courses, designed to give the student an appreciation of the health care problems and the social structure of communities.

Anthropology 140. The Nature of Culture. (4)
Anthropology 141. Comparative Society. (4)
City and Regional Planning 110. Introduction to City Planning. (5)
City and Regional Planning 121. Urban Aesthetics. (4)
Political Science 111. Urban Government and Politics. (5)
Political Science 160B. Political Behavior, Parties, and Interest Groups. (5)
Psychology 152. Behavior Disorders and Their Modification. (5)
Psychology 160. Social Psychology. (5)

Public Health 106. Introduction to Human Ecology and Health. (4)
Public Health 110. The Hospital in Contemporary Society. (4)
Public Health 134. Community Health Education. (2)
Public Health 175. Introduction to Epidemiology. (3)
Social Science 1A. Introduction to Social Science. (4)
Social Welfare 100. The Field of Social Welfare. (4)
Sociology 117. American Society: A Comparative Analysis. (5)
Sociology 129. Industrial and Occupational Sociology. (5)

The student may, if he prefers, pick electives designed to broaden his scientific background from the following list:

Biochemistry 102. Principles of Biochemistry. (4)
Biochemistry 102L. Laboratory. (4)
Engineering 180. Biological and Economic Feedback Systems. (3)
Genetics 101. Principles of Genetics. (5)
History 130A. Ancient and Medieval Science. (5)
History 130B. Scientific Revolution. (5)
History 130C. Science Since 1750. (5)
History 131. Topics in the History of Physical Science. (5)
History 132. Topics in the History of Biological Science. (5)
Mathematics. Any course.
Medical Physics 103. Human Biology. (4)
Molecular Biology 110. Molecular Basis of Heredity. (4)

Physics 110A–110B–110C. Electromagnetism and Optics. (3–3–3)
Physiology 101. Cell Physiology. (4)
Physiology 123. Comparative Physiology. (4)
Physiology 132. Environmental Physiology. (4)
Physiology 152. Physiology of Human Development. (4)
Physiology 153. Physiology of the Aging Process. (4)
Physiology 162. Physiology of Sensation. (4)
Physiology 162L. Laboratory in Sensation. (2)
Psychology 104. Theory of Psychological Measurement. (5)
Psychology 110A–110B. Biological Psychology. (4–4)

Psychology 123. Sensory and Perceptual
  Processes. (4)
Psychology 140, Developmental
  Psychology. (5)
Zoology 113. Normal and Abnormal
  Growth. (4)

Zoology 135. Animal Behavior. (4)
Zoology 150. Genetics. (5)
Zoology 151. Human Genetics. (5)
Zoology 185A–185B–185C. Optics and
  Metrology in Biology. (3–3–3)

APPENDIX E

American Optometric Association Code of Ethics

It Shall Be the Ideal, the Resolve, and the Duty of the Members of The American Optometric Association:

TO KEEP the visual welfare of the patient uppermost at all times;

TO PROMOTE in every possible way, in collaboration with this Association, better care of the visual needs of mankind;

TO ENHANCE continuously their educational and technical proficiency to the end that their patients shall receive the benefits of all acknowledged improvements in visual care;

TO SEE THAT no person shall lack for visual care, regardless of his financial status;

TO ADVISE the patient whenever consultation with an optometric colleague or reference for other professional care seems advisable;

TO HOLD in professional confidence all information concerning a patient and to use such data only for the benefit of the patient;

TO CONDUCT themselves as exemplary citizens;

TO MAINTAIN their offices and their practices in keeping with professional standards;

TO PROMOTE and maintain cordial and unselfish relationships with members of their own profession and of other professions for the exchange of information to the advantage of mankind.

Adopted by the House of Delegates of the American Optometric Association, Inc., at Detroit, Michigan, June 28, 1944

American Optometric Association Rules of Practice

A. No member shall willfully violate the optometry law or the optometry board rulings of the state in which he practices.

B. No member shall practice in or on premises where any materials other than those necessary to render his professional services are dispensed to the public.

C. No member when using the doctor title shall qualify it in any other way than by the use of the word "optometrist." He may, however, when not using the prefix, use after his name the "O.D." degree designation.

D. No member actively engaged in the practice of optometry shall in any manner publicize or hold himself forth as an optician.

E. No member shall display his license, diplomas, or certificates in such manner as to be seen and read from outside his office.

F. No member shall hold himself forth in such a way as to carry the slightest intimation of having superior qualifications or being superior to other optometrists.

G. No member holding an official position in any optometric organization shall use such position for advertising purposes or for self-aggrandizement.

H. No member shall display any sign containing other than name, profession, and office hours; same to be used only on office windows or at entrance to his office. Letters must not be luminous or illuminated and must not be more than 4" in height for street level and 7" in height for office above street level.

I. No member shall display eyeglass signs or painted or decalcomania eyes anywhere.

J. No member shall use other than his professional card on or in any publication or in any public display; said card shall not exceed two (2) columns by two (2) inches, and it shall not contain any more than his name, profession, address, telephone number, office hours, eye examinations by appointment, practice limited to .... (any one optometric specialty). Educational material may be published only when it has been specifically approved by the executive committee of the respective state association.

K. No member shall use bold-face type or in any other manner attempt to attract special attention to himself in any telephone or other public directory.

L. No member shall display any merchandise, ophthalmic material or advertising of any kind in windows or in any room of his office for the purpose of inducing patronage.

M. No member shall do anything inconsistent with professional standards of the optometric and allied health professions.

N. No member shall fail to observe scrupulously the code of ethics and other provisions of both his own state association and the American Optometric Association.

Enforcement of the provisions of the Rules of Practice shall be the duty of the various state associations. It is recommended that when a member is doubtful of the ethics or advisability of any action he contemplates, he shall submit a detailed statement to the proper committee of his state association for approval. This committee, if in doubt as to the point involved, shall in turn submit the question to the executive committee of the state association for final opinion. Logically, the trustees of the American Optometric Association will give an opinion if asked by the state association.

Passed Unanimously by the A.O.A. House of Delegates, June 28, 1950.

APPENDIX G

"SERVICES TO PEOPLE"

DEPARTMENT OF HEALTH, EDUCATION AND WELFARE PROGRAMS

ADMINISTERED IN COOPERATION WITH APPROPRIATE STATE AND LOCAL AGENCIES *

Legislation	*Programs—Purposes or Provisions—Special Features*

Social Security Act of 1935 As Amended Titles II & XVIII	Social Security—Old Age Survivors, Disability and Health Insurance Programs
	1. Old Age Insurance—workers' retirement plan—financial protection for old age
	  a. Benefits for retired workers—65 and over—reduced benefits if at age 62
	  b. Benefits for retired workers' families—wife and/or dependent children
	  c. Benefits for uninsured workers and others 72 and over
	2. Survivors' Insurance—protects families against total loss of income if wage earner dies
	  a. Benefits for widows or dependent widowers of beneficiaries
	  b. Benefits for dependent children of beneficiaries
	  c. Benefits for dependent parents of beneficiaries
	3. Disability Insurance—protects disabled workers and families (not workmen's compensation)
	4. Health Insurance—"Medicare Program"—pays for medical care—those 65 and over
	  a. Hospital Insurance—pays hospital bills primarily—some related expenses
	  b. Medical Insurance—voluntary $3 monthly premium plan—primarily for doctor bills

Federal Credit Union Act of 1934 As Amended	Credit Union Program—Federal staff provides advice and technical assistance to groups that wish to organize a Credit Union—also performs supervisory examinations (annual audits)—provides instructional materials and advice to Credit Union staffs and committees
Social Security Act of 1935 As Amended Titles I, IV, X, XIV, XVI & XIX Econ. Opp. Act PL 88-452-Title V	Public Assistance Programs—provide for general welfare of specific groups of needy persons 1. Grants for Aid to Aged, Blind or Disabled—financial aid and social services to persons 65 and over; the blind (all ages) and disabled over 18 years of age 2. Medical Assistance Program—provides medical care for public assistance recipients and for medically indigent persons who can provide their own maintenance 3. Aid to Families of Dependent Children—financial aid and social services for needy mothers and children—because of death, desertion or unemployment of wage earner 4. Work Experience and Training Program—trains unemployed ADC parents and others (including potential indigents) to be employable—job training and education (3 R's)

* *This list shows programs as of January, 1967. It was assembled by the staff at the Office of the Regional Director, Department of Health, Education, and Welfare, Region V, Chicago, Illinois.*

337

Legislation	*Programs—Purposes or Provisions—Special Features*
Older Americans Act – PL 89-73	Programs for the Aged and Aging—provide grants and technical assistance to States, public and private non-profit agencies and groups to develop services for the elderly and train personnel for such work

Social Security Act
of 1935
As Amended
Title V
	Child Welfare Programs—following services plus case finding, referral, follow-up and other care
	1. Day Care Centers—for pre-school children of working mothers and others
	2. Special Programs—providing services to children and mothers, including:
	   a. Foster Care—placement of children in private homes or institutions
	   b. Protective services for abused or neglected children—includes legal
	   c. Services for unmarried mothers—counseling, medical, financial—other
	   d. Licensing of all Child Care Facilities—includes Day Care Centers, Foster Homes, etc.
	   e. Adoption Information Service—actual placement for adoption by Department of Welfare

Vocational Rehabilitation Act PL 83-565 PL 89-333	Vocational Rehabilitation Program—helps handicapped persons to become employable 1. Provides all services necessary to help disabled become employable—diagnosis to treatment 2. Authorizes research demonstration projects and training for careers in rehabilitation 3. Cooperates with Social Security Administration in disability determination program
Public Health Service Act of 1944 As Amended	Public Health Grants—to help State Health Departments provide services and conduct programs for: 1. Cancer Control—screening exams, testing, referral, follow-up and educational programs 2. Chronic Illness and Aging—preventive examination and referral—detection of diabetes and glaucoma—home services for ill and aging—teams of doctor, nurse and social worker 3. General Health—laboratory tests, sanitation, milk and food inspection, health education, etc. 4. Heart Disease Control—prevention and early detection—rheumatic fever registry—free medicine and referral and treatment for coronary disease 5. Radiological Health—registration and inspection of radiation sites—check hazards—etc. 6. TB Control—testing, early detection, referral, registry, follow-up, surveillance 7. Dental Health—improve dental health, laboratory services, screening
Community Health Services and Facilities Act of 1961 PL 87-395	Out of Hospital Health Services for the Chronically Ill and the Aging—special projects such as: 1. Improve Nursing Home services—team of nurse, O.T., P.T.—teach staff better procedures 2. Expand home care program—visiting nurse, homemaker, physician, therapists (O.T.—P.T.—Speech)

Legislation	*Programs—Purposes or Provisions—Special Features*
	3. Home dental care—senior students provide services using portable equipment
	4. "Meals on Wheels"—private agencies provide hot meals to homebound elderly at low cost
	5. Provide artificial kidneys and transplants to those who would otherwise die
National Heart Act PL 80-655	Community Heart Disease Control Programs—combined demonstration and service projects such as:
	1. Home nursing care—additional nurses to care for cardiac patients at home
	2. Rheumatic Fever prevention—dentists take throat cultures and provide dental services
	3. Treatment and rehabilitation of stroke victims—help communities "strike back at stroke"
National Cancer Act PL 87-290	Reduction of Illness and Death from Cancer—special projects and demonstrations such as:
	1. Public health visiting nursing care for cancer patients at home
	2. Detection of cancer and training of physicians and technologists in use of new techniques
	3. Screening for cervical cancer and testing of new "Do-It-Yourself" exam methods
	4. Other special projects—early detection and treatment—services plus training
PHS Act As Amended PL's-78-410; 87-868; 89-109	Communicable Disease Control Programs—immunizations, VD-TB-control measures to:
	1. Eradicate syphilis—case finding, testing, treatment, follow-up, doctors' reports, education
	2. Reduce new cases of tuberculosis by early detection, treatment and follow-up
	3. Immunize—against polio, tetanus, diphtheria, measles, etc.—pre-school children
National Mental Health Act PL 79-487 & PL 88-164	Mental Health Programs—assist States to develop, provide and improve services
	1. Grants for prevention, care, treatment and rehabilitation of mentally ill—includes out-patient clinics and community programs. Grants for initial staffing in some cases
	2. Grants for construction of facilities for mentally ill and retarded—specific conditions
Title V Soc. Sec. Act & 1965 Amendments PL 89-97 & PL 88-156	Maternal and Child Health Programs—to provide and improve services to mothers and children
	1. Prevent or reduce sickness and death of mothers and children—includes diagnosis and treatment
	2. Provide health care to mothers and infants with complicating health conditions—low income
	3. Improve health of pre-school and school age youth in low income areas—includes treatment
	4. Provide special medical and other care to crippled and other handicapped children

APPENDIX H

Services Provided under Medicare *

Inpatient Hospital Benefits Covered

A. Room and board in a semiprivate room (two to four beds in a room). B. Nursing services. C. Supplies, appliances, and equipment, such as splints, casts, wheelchairs, crutches, etc. D. Blood transfusions, except for the first three pints of blood in a "spell of illness." E. Medical social services. F. Therapeutic services, such as x-ray or radium treatments. G. Operating room costs. H. Drugs furnished by the hospital. I. Diagnostic services, such as blood tests, electrocardiograms, etc. J. Services of hospital residents and interns who are in approved training programs.

Inpatient Hospital Benefits Not Covered

A. Physicians' and surgeons' services. (Your medical insurance will help to pay your doctor bills.) B. Private room, furnished at your request, unless it is medically necessary. (If you request a private room, you will pay the difference between the private and semiprivate rates.) C. Private duty nurses. D. Cost of first three pints of blood. (If a donor replaces the blood, the hospital will not charge you for it.) E. Personal comfort and convenience items which you request, such as telephone, radio, or television in your room.

Extended Health Care Benefits Covered

A. Room and board in semiprivate room (two to four beds in room). B. Physical, occupational, or speech therapy. C. Nursing care. D. Medical social services. E. Drugs, supplies, appliances, and equipment ordinarily furnished to patients by the extended care facility.

Extended Health Care Benefits Not Covered

A. Physicians' services. (Your medical insurance will help pay for physicians' services.) B. Services in a facility which is operated primarily for the treatment of mental illness or tuberculosis. C. Private duty nurses. D. Private room, furnished at your request, unless it is medically necessary. (If you request a private room, you will pay the difference between the private and semiprivate rates.) E. Personal comfort or convenience items which you request, such as telephone, radio, or television in your room.

Home Health Benefits Covered

A. Part-time nursing care. B. Physical, occupational, or speech therapy. C. Services of home health aids (in connection with your treatment). D. Medical social services. E. Medical supplies, except drugs. F. Use of medical appliances. G. Any of the above rehabilitation services outside your home which require equipment that cannot be brought to your home.

* Rewritten from the booklet *Health Insurance under Social Security—Your Medicare Handbook,* published by the United States Department of Health, Education, and Welfare. This booklet is available at no cost from any Social Security office, and is recommended for all professional personnel. It includes complete instructions to doctor and patient for the preparation of Medicare forms.
The sections which have been revised by the present author (REW) are: *Outpatient Diagnostic Benefits Not Covered; Medical Insurance* and *Home Health Services Not Covered.*

340

Home Health Benefits Not Covered

A. Physicians' services. (Your medical insurance will help to pay your doctor bills.) B. Full-time nursing care. C. Prescription drugs. D. Personal comfort items. E. Services furnished by a home health agency operated primarily for the treatment of mental illness. F. General housekeeping services. G. Meals delivered to your home (sometimes called "meals on wheels").

Outpatient Diagnostic Benefits Covered

A. Diagnostic x-rays. B. Pulmonary function tests. C. Electrocardiograms. D. Blood tests. E. Kidney function tests. F. Urinalysis. G. Other tests given to determine the nature and severity of an ailment or injury.

Outpatient Diagnostic Benefits Not Covered

A. Physicians' services. (Your medical insurance will help to pay for physicians' services.) B. Tests given as a part of routine physical checkups. C. Services not related to the diagnosis of your condition.

Because of the tremendous scope of this undertaking, many rules and regulations have had to be established. Every effort has been made to simplify the necessary formalities. Without going into detail, it can be said that the arrangements have been made to resemble the traditional care which has been given by hospitalization insurance in the past. There are, of course, some very important differences because this age group has been exempted from most private health insurance programs in the past.

Each patient is given a health insurance card which he uses when admitted to any hospital. The payments are made directly to the hospital or other organization furnishing the services by the private insurance company or Blue Cross, which has been designated by the Social Security Administration to handle such claims.

Following the example of most private hospitalization insurance, the plan involves payment of a deductible fee. The patient pays the first $40.00 for each period of hospitalization services. The insurance covers up to 90 days for each period of illness. The first 60 days of such care, the hospital insurance pays all, except the $40.00 deductible; for the 61st day to the 90th day, the insurance pays all but $10.00 daily for the services covered.

Because long illness is often encountered by the older patient, special extended care benefits have been arranged. Often a patient can be transferred to an "extended care facility" when he no longer needs intensive hospital care. In such an event, the hospital insurance pays for all covered services for the first 20 days and all but $5.00 daily for the next 80 days.

Many communities do not have extended care facilities, but have home health agencies that provide visiting nurse service and other health care. The insurance will pay up to 100 home visits in a one-year period following discharge from the hospital for extended care facility service.

Many times, outpatient hospital diagnostic services are needed. The items covered in this area were mentioned previously. These benefits are paid for "diagnostic study" during a 20 day-period in which the patient receives such services from the hospital. For each 20-day period, the patient pays the first $20.00 and the hospital insurance pays the remaining 80 percent of cost.

It is obvious that years of research and effort went into planning the hospitalization insurance to meet best the needs of our elder population. It is admitted that many details will have to be worked out at a later date, but that this plan is a tremendous advancement in the care of this segment of our population cannot be denied. As mentioned previously, the increased cost of income tax, combined with the cost of living, has made it very difficult for the average family to insure properly against unexpected illness in old age. The majority of our older citizens, about two thirds at present, are capable of taking care of themselves and prefer to do so.

However, unexpected illnesses can wipe out a lifetime of savings, and it is toward this problem that this social legislation is directed.

The program is financed by Social Security contributions collected along with regular Social Security payments, with employees and employers contributing equal amounts. Plans have been made to adjust benefits as needed. The law provides that the $40.00 inpatient deductible, for example, will be examined each year and adjusted as hospital costs change.

Medical Insurance

The medical insurance part of the program is the one that caused most of the difficulty with medical organizations. As a result, several compromises have been worked out, some of which undoubtedly will be changed as the program is developed: one of these compromises is composed of the voluntary program for which participants have to sign up individually. The individual agrees to pay $3.00 per month, and the federal government matches this fee with a $3.00 per month payment. Again, the need for such a program was brought about because most insurance companies did not cover people past 65 at rates that patients could afford for the type of coverage needed. Had this not been the case, it is doubtful that such a program would have been put into effect.

The $50.00 deductible for medical bills is typical of most insurance programs. One fundamental difference in the Medicare program, and a very important one, is that any expenses after the first $50.00 in one entire year are covered. That is, the cost of each recurring illness is paid without the $50.00 deductible, as is not the case with most private insurance carriers.

After the $50.00 deductible, the insurance takes care of 80 percent of the reasonable charges for all additional covered services for the rest of the year. Reasonable charges are based on the customary charges of the doctor and the prevailing rates for similar medical services in the area. The final determination of these charges rests with the organization assigned by the Social Security Administration to pay these claims.

As was the case with hospital insurance, it has been necessary to define carefully which services are covered and which are not under the medical insurance program. Since the original Social Security health plan was set up to take care of major health care problems, routine dental care and optometric care were omitted. Following is a brief summary of the doctor bills covered by the medical insurance.

Doctor Bills Covered

A. Medical and surgical services by a physician wherever they are furnished. B. Services in connection with a physician's treatment, such as diagnostic tests, medical supplies, the services of his nurse, drugs that cannot be self-administered, and similar services ordinarily included in physicians' bills. C. Dental surgery by a doctor of dental medicine or a doctor of dental surgery, but only if it involves major dental surgery, such as an operation on the jaw.

Doctor Bills Not Covered

A. Routine physical checkups. B. Eye examinations for prescribing or fitting glasses. C. Hearing examinations for hearing aids. D. Routine dental care. E. Immunizations. F. Services of practitioners such as chiropractors, naturopaths, chiropodists or podiatrists, optometrists, and Christian Science practitioners.

The medical services and supplies covered in addition to routine doctor bills are as follows.

Other Medical Services and Supplies Covered

A. Diagnostic tests such as x-rays and laboratory tests (unless covered by hospital insurance). B. X-rays and other radiation therapy. C. Surgical dressings, splints, casts, and similar devices. D. Drugs which a doctor administers as part of his personal services (such as a tetanus injection following an injury). E. Rental of medical equipment for use in the home (for example, wheelchairs, hospital beds, oxygen tents, etc.). F. Prosthetic devices (other than dental) to replace all or part of an internal body organ. G. Braces, artificial limbs, artificial eyes, including replacement required by a change in your condition. H. Certain ambulance services, but only when medically necessary.

Other Medical Services and Supplies Not Covered

A. Prescription drugs and drugs that can be self-administered (for example, insulin injections for a diabetic condition). B. Patent medicines (aspirin, cough medicine, etc.). C. Hearing aids. D. Dentures (false teeth). E. Eyeglasses. F. Orthopedic shoes.

In addition to medical services and doctor bills, several home health services are provided for.

Home Health Services Covered

A. Part-time nursing care. B. Physical, occupational or speech therapy. C. Services of home health aids (in connection with your treatment). D. Medical social services. E. Medical supplies, except drugs. F. Use of medical appliances. G. Any of the above rehabilitation services outside your home which require equipment that cannot be brought to your home.

Home Health Services Not Covered

A. Full-time nursing care. B. Prescription drugs. C. Personal comfort items. D. General housekeeping services. E. Meals delivered to your home (sometimes called "meals on wheels")

As mentioned previously, routine dental and optometric care have been omitted in these first health care plans. Certain exceptions are made in the event of dental surgery or the supplying of cataract lenses. It has been decided that, under the coverage of "prosthetic devices to replace all or part of an internal body organ," the coverage should include those glasses that are required to replace the lens of the eye. At this time, optometry's exact status in this program has yet to be defined. It is certain, however, that optometrists will furnish these services under Medicare, and for that reason, they should be familiar with the program.

Method of Payment

Payment to the doctor has been made flexible. As mentioned previously, the first $50.00 of all medical expenses in a given year is not covered by insurance. Also, only 80 percent of the reasonable charges are covered. The doctor may be paid either directly by the patient or by the insurance carrier. If the doctor agrees to accept the money from the carrier, he is obligated to accept 80 percent of what the carrier considers reasonable. In the event that the doctor does not accept the assignment, he can charge whatever he wishes, and the patient is obligated to pay it as he can, the insurance paying the patient only 80 percent of what is a reasonable charge in the community. For example, a doctor might charge his customary fee of $100.00; if the carrier determines that $80.00 is the reasonable fee in the community, the reimbursement will be based on $80.00 and not $100.00. The doctor is under no obligation to accept the assignment.

APPENDIX I

Scope of Optometric Services

The scope of optometric services is an expanding one, going far beyond basic clinical refraction or the commonly termed "eye examination and the providing of glasses." It includes the investigation of individual eye health and abnormalities, dysfunctions of the entire seeing mechanism, research, education, programming, direction, administration, and many other areas of activity. Some of the important services are:

1. *Vision Screening.*

To identify those in a group who require vision care. Adapted to schools, industry, motorists, nursing homes, OEO projects, etc. Optometrists program, direct, and operate professional screening projects, train and supervise technicians in the use of screening devices, and evaluate results.

2. *Investigation of Visual Problems.*

To investigate fully patients with symptoms of ocular discomfort. Such symptoms may be physical, pathological, or of other origin, and may require correction by lenses, orthoptic training, surgery, dentistry, or other means.

3. *Refraction.*

To use lenses, prisms, phoropter, and other instruments to determine the power required for a patient's eyeglass prescription.

4. *Instrumentation.*

To use, in clinical studies of an individual patient, many instruments and procedures which are not required in refraction, but which enable the optometrist more fully to determine the visual status of the patient. These include:

a. *Visual Field Charting.* The perimeter, tangent screen, and other devices give the extent of visual fields. This information is necessary in disease detection.
b. *Tonometry.* Determining the intraocular pressure—necessary in glaucoma detection.
c. *Ophthalmoscopy.* To view the interior of the eye, which may disclose the existence of cataracts, retinopathy, glaucoma, and other abnormalities related to eye health or to general health.
d. *Slit-lamp Biomicroscopy.* To study eye tissues and certain eye functions, and also to insure proper fit of contact lenses.
e. *Isochromatic Charts.* To determine the degree of color-blindness.

5. *Developmental Vision Examination.*

To determine relativity of physical and mental development to vision development, and to prescribe for the visually retarded.

6. *Contact Lens Fitting.*

To provide therapeutic improvement for conical cornea, aphakia, and other conditions. Also, for cosmetic purposes.

7. *Visual Training.*

To develop visual skills for optimal visual performance.

8. *Orthoptics/Pleoptics.*

To train amblyopic, strabismic, and cross-eyed persons.

9. *Care for the Partially Sighted.*

To diagnose the visually subnormal patient and provide correction by telescopic lenses, microscopic lenses, contact lenses or other devices.

10. *Artificial Eyes.*

To fit this prosthetic device when needed.

11. *Retarded Reader Training.*

To develop the visual component, thus enhancing the ability to read more rapidly.

12. *Care of the Physically Handicapped—Rehabilitation.*

To cooperate with and assist other disciplines in the visual rehabilitation of those in physical or vocational programs.

13. *Care of the Mentally Retarded.*

To analyze the visual ability of the mentally retarded and prescribe for their visual needs through visual training, or other means, to lessen the impact of retardation.

14. *Aniseikonic Correction.*

To diagnose and prescribe for disparity of size in the retinal images with use of the eikonometer.

15. *Industrial Vision. Consultation.*

To organize vision care programs in industry for safety and efficiency of employees in a given industry, and to correct environmental deterrents, and to plan, operate, and evaluate such programs.

16. *Highway Safety. Consultation.*

To cooperate with state authorities in establishing vision standards, tests, and procedures for driver licensing and auto and highway safety.

17. *Fabricating and Dispensing Eyewear.*

To determine the appliance the patient will wear for visual correction; the optometrist will procure or fabricate it, and dispense it to the patient at laboratory costs.

18. *Military Services.*

Optometrists serve in the armed forces as commissioned officers in clinical, research, and administrative capacities.

19. *Government Services.*

Optometrists serve in many civil service capacities and are commissioned in the Public Health Service.

20. *Group Health Centers and Clinics.*

Over 200 optometrists are in clinical service with these institutions.

21. *Research.*

Optometrists are engaged in research through all of the optometric schools and colleges, and individually and collectively in many other institutions.

22. *Optometric Centers.*

Optometric centers are in operation in many cities. They serve primarily the indigent and low income patients. Some are "specialty centers," providing services not available in every optometric office.

23. *Education.*

Optometrists are engaged in teaching and administration in the ten schools and colleges of optometry in the United States.

——*AMERICAN OPTOMETRIC ASSOCIATION*

Licensed Optometrists and Certified Ophthalmologists
Related to the Population of the United States
of America
(Peters, 1966b)

State	Population	Certified Ophthalmologists	Population Per Certified Ophthalmologists	Licensed Optometrists	Population Per Licensed Optometrists
Alabama	3,407,000	42	111,905	184	18,510
Alaska	250,000	3	83,333	16	15,625
Arizona	1,581,000	44	35,932	128	12,351
Arkansas	1,933,000	20	96,650	143	13,517
California	18,084,000	669	27,031	2,461	7,348
Colorado	1,966,000	72	27,305	201	9,781
Connecticut	2,715,000	99	27,424	279	9,731
Delaware	491,000	11	46,364	33	14,879
Dist. of Columbia	808,000	64	12,625	182	4,439
Florida	5,705,000	155	36,806	514	11,099
Georgia	4,294,000	57	75,333	287	14,962
Hawaii	701,000	18	38,944	65	10,785
Idaho	692,000	13	53,231	96	7,208
Illinois	10,489,000	269	38,992	1,992	5,265
Indiana	4,825,000	88	54,829	547	8,821
Iowa	2,756,000	38	72,526	359	7,677
Kansas	2,225,000	34	65,441	245	9,082
Kentucky	3,159,000	48	65,812	246	12,841
Louisiana	3,468,000	61	56,852	248	13,984
Maine	989,000	22	44,954	123	8,041
Maryland	3,432,000	73	47,013	195	17,600
Massachusetts	5,338,000	182	29,329	852	6,265
Michigan	8,098,000	179	45,240	786	10,303
Minnesota	3,521,000	88	40,011	425	8,285
Mississippi	2,314,000	21	110,190	130	17,800
Missouri	4,409,000	94	46,904	483	9,128
Montana	705,000	13	54,230	91	7,747
Nebraska	1,480,000	30	49,333	184	8,043
Nevada	408,000	10	40,800	37	11,027
New Hampshire	654,000	12	54,500	78	8,385
New Jersey	6,682,000	175	38,183	732	9,128
New Mexico	1,008,000	19	53,053	74	13,622
New York	17,915,000	735	24,374	1,838	9,747
North Carolina	4,852,000	55	88,218	338	14,355
North Dakota	645,000	13	49,615	82	7,866
Ohio	10,100,000	208	48,558	1,056	9,564
Oklahoma	2,465,000	35	70,429	262	9,408
Oregon	1,871,000	65	28,785	324	5,775
Pennsylvania	11,459,000	301	38,069	1,373	8,346
Rhode Island	914,000	16	57,125	141	6,482
South Carolina	2,555,000	26	98,269	166	15,391
South Dakota	715,000	10	71,500	93	7,688
Tennessee	3,798,000	60	63,300	320	11,869
Texas	10,397,000	220	47,259	844	12,319
Utah	992,000	34	29,176	86	11,539
Vermont	409,000	9	45,444	35	11,686
Virginia	4,378,000	71	61,661	265	16,521
Washington	2,984,000	88	33,909	400	7,460
West Virginia	1,797,000	39	46,077	159	11,302
Wisconsin	4,107,000	89	46,146	454	9,046
Wyoming	343,000	10	34,300	38	9,026

TOTAL   191,334,000   4,798   39,877   20,610   9,283

Sources, Blue Book of Optometrists, 1965–66
    Directory of Medical Specialists, 1965
    Bureau of the Census, Statistical Abstracts, 1965

REFERENCES

Alden, Kenneth: Battle for your eyes, Coronet, 1 (1): 48–52, 1963.

Alexander, Shana: An ordeal to choke a sword-swallower, Life, 60 (3): 17, Jan.21, 1966.

American Optometric Association: 1958 National Economic Survey. St. Louis, 1959.

American Optometric Association: Optometry; a Career with Vision. St. Louis, 1965.

American Optometric Association: 1964 economic survey—report No.1, J. Am. Optom. Assn., 37 (4): 364–367, 1966a.

American Optometric Association: Economic survey—report No.4, J. Am. Optom. Assn., 37 (7): 683–685, 1966b.

American Optometric Association: Economic survey—report No.5, J. Am. Optom. Assn., 37 (8): 781–785, 1966c.

American Pharmaceutical Association Newsletter, Feb. 1966.

Atkinson, Donald T.: Magic, Myth and Medicine. Greenwich, Conn., Fawcett Publications, Inc., 1956.

Attiwill, Keith: The "eye gap" in Australia's health service, Optom. Weekly, 57 (2): 34–35, Jan.13, 1966.

Backman, Howard: Optometry in Western Europe, Am. J. Optom. and Arch. Am. Acad. Optom., 42 (2): 94–108, 1965.

Barnett, Albert: Historical and other articles contributed in *The Optician,* in The Year Book of the New York State Optometric Association, 1943.

Bausch & Lomb Optical Co.: Milestones in Optical History. Rochester, N. Y., 1936.

Berens, Conrad: The making of an ophthalmologist, J. Am. Med. Assn., 126 (11): 671–674, Nov.11, 1944.

Bergin, Dorothy A.: The first decade of the Los Angeles College of Optometry, Optom. World, 52 (4): 16, 19, 22, 1965.

Birchard, Clifton H. and Theodore F. Elliott: Pt. 3. A re-evaluation of the ratio of optometrists to population in the United States in the light of socio-economic trends in health care, Am. J. Optom. and Arch. Am. Acad. Optom., 44 (3): 168–182, 1967.

Boger, Frederick: (Editorial), Opt. J., 1 (1): 13, 1895.

Boring, Edwin G.: Sensation and Perception in the History of Experimental Psychology. New York, D. Appleton-Century Co., 1942.

Braff, Jeffrey D.: Personal correspondence, Sept.17, 1965.

Brown, R. B.: Optometry in the Navy. J. Am. Optom. Assn., 37 (4): 339, 1966.

Champness, R.: A Short History of the Worshipful Company of Spectacle Makers up to the Beginning of the Twentieth Century. London, Roland Champness, 1952.

Clendening, Logan: The Human Body. Garden City, N. Y., Garden City Publishing Co., 1927.

Court, Thomas H. and Moritz von Rohr: On the development of spectacles in London from the end of the seventeenth century, Trans. Optical Soc. (London), 30 (1): 1–21, 1928–1929.

Court, Thomas H. and Moritz von Rohr: Contributions to the history of the Worshipful Company of Spectaclemakers, Trans. Optical Soc. (London), 31 (2): 53–90, 1929–1930.

Cox, Maurice E.: Optometry, The Profession; Its Antecedents, Birth, and Development. Philadelphia, Chilton Co., 1947.

Crombie, A. C.: Early concepts of the senses and the mind, Sci. Am., 210 (5): 108–116, 1965.

Dastoor, S. K.: Eye care in India, Optom. Weekly, 57 (8) : 26–27, Feb. 24, 1966.

Deitrick, John E. and Robert C. Berson: Medical Schools in the United States at Mid-Century. New York, McGraw-Hill Book Company, 1953.

De Lacey, P. R.: Trends in Australian optometric education, Australian J. Optom.. 50 (3) : 62–69, 1967.

Donders, F. C.: On the Anomalies of Accommodation and Refraction of the Eye, translated by W. D. Moore. London, The New Sydenham Society, 1864.

Duke-Elder, W. Stewart: Text-book of Ophthalmology, Vol.1, 2d impression. St. Louis, C. V. Mosby Co., 1940.

Duke-Elder, W. Stewart: Text-book of Ophthalmology, Vol.4. St. Louis, C. V. Mosby Co., 1949.

Dvorine, Israel: Theory and Practice of Analytical Refraction and Orthoptics. Baltimore, Waverly Press, Inc., 1939.

Eglin, Lela: Vision care in Russia, J. Calif. Optom. Assn., 34 (7) : 408–411, 1966–1967.

Elmstrom, George P.: Optometric Practice Management. Philadelphia, Chilton Books, 1963.

Fitch, Albert: My Fifty Years in Optometry. Philadelphia, Pennsylvania State College of Optometry, 1955, 1959. 2 vols.

Flexner, Abraham: Medical Education in the United States and Canada; a Report to the Carnegie Foundation for the Advancement of Teaching. New York, Carnegie Foundation for the Advancement of Teaching, 1910. Bull.No.4.

Flick, C. S.: Great names in optics—Frans Cornelis Donders, Optician, 124: 247–252, 1952.

Fry, Glenn A.: An experimental analysis of the accommodation-convergence relation, Am. J. Optom., 14 (11) : 402–414, 1937.

Fry, Glenn A.: Further experiments on the accommodation-convergence relationship, Am. J. Optom. and Arch. Am. Acad. Optom., 16 (8) : 325–336, 1939.

Fry, Glenn A.: Fundamental variables in the relationship between accommodation and convergence, Optom. Weekly, 34 (6–7) : 153–155, 183–185, 1943.

Fry, Glenn A.: The division of labor between optometry and ophthalmology, Am. J. Optom. and Arch. Am. Acad. Optom., 34 (3) : 150–156, 1957.

Gies, William J.: Dental Education in the United States and Canada; a Report to the Carnegie Foundation for the Advancement of Teaching. New York, Carnegie Foundation for the Advancement of Teaching, 1926. Bull.No.19.

Gifford, Edward S., Jr.: The Evil Eye; Studies in the Folklore of Vision. New York, Macmillan Co., 1958.

Giles, G. H.: World optometry; its development and future, Canadian J. Optom., 28 (1) : 3–19, 1966.

Grassus, Benevenutus: De Oculis Eorumque Egritudinibus et Cirus; translated . . . from the first printed edition, Ferrara, 1474, by Casey A. Wood. Stanford University, Calif., Stanford University Press, 1929.

Greene, Billy C.: [Optometry in the Medical Service Corps, U.S. Army], J. Am. Optom. Assn., 37 (4) : 338, 1966.

Greenspoon, Morton K.: An optometric visit to Japan, Optom. Weekly, 57 (47) : 21–22, Nov.24, 1966.

Gregg, James R.: The Story of Optometry. New York, Ronald Press, 1965.

Grims, Dragan: Optical services in Yugoslavia, Optom. Weekly, 57 (23) : 39–40, June 9, 1966.

Gunkel, Peter C.: Glasses and social insurance in Germany, Optom. Weekly, 57 (24) : 25–26, June 16, 1966.

Haggard, Howard W:. Mystery, Magic, and Medicine; the Rise of Medicine from Superstition to Science. Garden City, N. Y., Doubleday, Doran & Company, Inc., 1933.

Haight, Gordon S., editor: The Autobiography of Benjamin Franklin. New York, Published for the Classics Club by W. J. Black, 1941.

Hamrick, William A.: [The Medical Service Corps and Optometry in the U.S. Army], J. Am. Optom. Assn., 37 (4) : 337, 1966.

Hill, Emory: History of eyeglasses and spectacles, *in* American Encyclopedia of Ophthalmology, edited by Casey A. Wood. Chicago, Cleveland Press, 1915, Vol. 7, pp. 4894–4953.

Hirsch, Monroe J.: A Study of Visual Distance Discrimination: Relation of the Position of Subjective Equality to the Sensitivity and the Effect on Both of Antiseikonic Lenses, the Observers Distance, and the Presence of the Size Cue. A dissertation submitted to the Committee on Graduate Study, Stanford University, 1947.

Hirsch, Monroe J.: The non-insurability of ocular refractions, Am. J. Optom. and Arch. Am. Acad. Optom., 31 (4) : 206–213, 1954.

Hirsch, Monroe J. and Meredith W. Morgan: The measurement and grading of refractive state by the Armed Forces, Am. J. Optom. and Arch. Am. Acad. Optom., 42 (12) : 707–726, 1965.

Hofstetter, H. W.: The zone of clear single binocular vision, Am. J. Optom. and Arch. Am. Acad. Optom., 22 (7–8) : 301–333, 361–384, 1945.

Hofstetter, H. W.: Optometry; Professional, Economic, and Legal Aspects. St. Louis, C. V. Mosby Co., 1948.

Hofstetter, Henry W.: Optometry and children's vision, *in* Vision of Children, edited by Monroe J. Hirsch and Ralph E. Wick. Philadelphia, Chilton Books, 1963, pp.69–77. See page 77.

Hulin, Wilbur S.: A Short History of Psychology. New York, Henry Holt and Company, 1934.

Hutchins, Robert M. and Mortimer J. Adler, *editors,* The Great Ideas Today, Vol. 3. Chicago, Encyclopedia Britannica, 1963, pp.87–88.

Iwasaki, Riichi: National health service in Japan, Optom. Weekly, 57 (10) : 37, March 10, 1966.

Kahl, Joseph A.: The American Class Structure. New York, Holt, Rinehart and Winston, 1957, Chapts. 3 and 9.

Knoll, Henry: A millennium of optical progress; thoughts on the 1000th anniversary of the birth of Alhazen, Opt. J. and Rev. Optom., 102 (7) : 38–40, Apr.1, 1965.

Koch, Carel C.: Agitation unfounded on the consumer costs of ocular service, Am. J. Optom. and Arch. Am. Acad. Optom., 18 (11) : 525–529, 1941.

Koch, Carel C.: "Squint" in the land of the Mayas, Am. J. Optom. and Arch. Am. Acad. Optom., 26 (7) : 315–317, 1949.

Lancaster, Walter B.: The optometry problem, J. Am. Med. Assn., 91 (24) : 1847–1848, Dec.15, 1928.

Lang, Gideon L.: Goals of the Committee on Military Affairs, J. Am. Optom. Assn., 37 (4) : 345–346, 1966.

Lesser, S. K.: Fundamentals of Procedure and Analysis in Optometric Examination, 2d ed. Fort Worth, Texas, Copyright by the Author, 1933.

Lienberger, Ernest: Health regulations in Switzerland, Optom. Weekly, 57 (21) : 20, May 26, 1966.

Maddox, Ernest E.: The Clinical Use of Prisms, 2d ed. Bristol, Eng., John Wright and Co., 1893.

Magoulas, Beatrice: Optometric progress in Greece, Optom. Weekly, 57 (12) : 34–35, March 24, 1966.

Magraw, Richard M.: Ferment in Medicine. Philadelphia, W. B. Saunders Co., 1966.

Manas, Leo: Visual Analysis, 3d ed. Chicago, Professional Press, 1965.

Maumenee, A. Edward: The educational and political structure of ophthalmology in America, Arch. Ophth., 77 (3) : 295–304, March 1967.

Meyer, Alvin F.: [Optometry in the Biomedical Sciences Corps, U.S. Air Force], J. Am. Optom. Assn., 37 (4) : 343, 1966.

Miller, Maxwell: Optometry's historic contributions to science and medicine, Am. J. Optom. and Arch. Am. Acad. Optom., 41 (3) : 154–179, 1964.

Morgan, Meredith W., Jr.: The nervous control of accommodation, Am. J. Optom. and Arch. Am. Acad. Optom., 21 (3) : 87–93, 1944a.

Morgan, Meredith W., Jr.: Accommodation and its relationship to convergence, Am. J. Optom. and Arch. Am. Acad. Optom., 21 (5) : 183–195, 1944b.

Morgan, Meredith W., Jr.: The clinical aspects of accommodation and convergence, Am. J. Optom. and Arch. Am. Acad. Optom., 21 (8): 301–313, 1944c.

Morgan, Meredith W., Jr.: Analysis of clinical data, Am. J. Optom. and Arch. Am. Acad. Optom., 21 (12): 477–491, 1944d.

Morgan, Meredith W., Jr.: Optometry is optometry, Am. J. Optom. and Arch. Am. Acad. Optom., 31 (8): 423–426, 1954.

Morgan, Meredith W., Jr.: Personal communication, 1967.

Morris, Floyd M.: [Optometry in the Biomedical Sciences Corps, U.S. Air Force], J. Am. Optom. Assn., 37 (4): 344, 1966.

Muller, Carl W.: National health service in Norway, Optom. Weekly, 57 (16): 29–30, Apr. 21, 1966.

Newman, B. L., The role of optometry within the naval industrial establishment, J. Am. Optom. Assn., 37 (4): 353–356, 1966.

Nielsen, Jorgen F.: Optometry in Denmark, Am. J. Optom. and Arch. Am. Acad. Optom., 42 (1): 24–30, 1965.

Osias, Leonard: Unpublished data presented to the California Optometric Association, 1967.

Percival, Archibald Stanley: The relation of convergence to accommodation and its practical bearing, Ophthalmic Rev., 11: 313–328, 1892.

Percival, Archibald Stanley: The Prescribing of Spectacles, 3d ed. New York, William Wood and Company, 1928.

Peters, Henry B.: Optometric Service in a Comprehensive Health Program; tenth annual Thomas H. Peters Memorial Lecture, Berkeley, Calif., Oct. 22, 1966a (to be published in 1968).

Peters, Henry B.: Vision care of children in a comprehensive health program, J. Am. Optom. Assn., 37 (12): 1113–1118, 1966b.

Polyak, Stephen L.: The history of our knowledge of the structure and function of the eye, in The Human Eye in Anatomical Transparencies, by Peter C. Kronfeld et al. Rochester, N. Y., Bausch & Lomb Press, 1943, pp.73–92.

Prentice, Charles F.: Legalized Optometry and the Memoirs of its Founder. Seattle, Wash., Casperin Fletcher Press, 1926.

Raphael, Jack: Health services in Israel, Optom. Weekly, 57 (9): 35–36, March 3. 1966.

Reed, Louis S.: Midwives, Chiropodists, and Optometrists; Their Place in Medical Care. Chicago, University of Chicago Press, 1932. Pubs. of the Committee on the Costs of Medical Care, No.15.

Riis, Roger William: Optometry on trial, Reader's Digest, 31: 77–85, 1937.

von Rohr, M.: Contributions to the history of the spectacle trade from the earliest times to Thomas Young's appearance, Trans. Optical Soc. (London), 25 (2): 41–71, 1923–24.

Saunders, J. B. deC. M., and Charles D. O'Malley: The Illustrations from the Works of Andreas Vesalius of Brussels with annotations and translations, a discussion of the plates and their background, authorship and influence, and a biographic sketch of Vesalius. Cleveland, World Publishing Co., 1950.

Shastid, Thomas Hall: The history of ophthalmology, in American Encyclopedia of Ophthalmology, edited by Casey A. Wood. Chicago, Cleveland Press, 1917, Vol.11, pp.8524–8904.

Sheard, Charles: Zones of ocular comfort, Am. J. Optom., 7 (1): 9–25, 1930.

Sheard, Charles: A program for professional optometry, Opt. J. and Rev. Optom., 76 (11): 18–21, June 1, 1939.

Skeffington, A. M.: Differential Diagnosis in Ocular Examination. Copyright by the Author, 1931.

Snyder, Charles: The Rev. Mr. Goodrich and his visual problem, Arch. Ophth., 73 (4): 587–589, 1965.

Southall, James P. C.: Mirrors, Prisms and Lenses, 3d ed. New York, Macmillan Company, 1933.

Tato, Carmen: Ophthalmic optics in Spain, Optom. Weekly, 57 (17): 38–39, Apr.28, 1966.

Tawney, R. H.: The Acquisitive Society. New York, Harcourt, Brace, and World, Inc., 1920.

Taylor, Harry L.: The antiquity of lenses, Am. J. Physiol. Optics, 5 (4): 514–516, 1924.

U.S. Department of Health, Education, and Welfare. National Center for Health Statistics: Characteristics of Patients of Selected Types of Medical Specialists and Practitioners, United States, July 1963–June 1964. Washington, D.C., Government Printing Office, May 1966a. Publ. Health Service Pub. No.1000, Series 10, No.28.

U.S. Department of Health, Education, and Welfare. National Center for Health Statistics: Health Resources Statistics; Health Manpower, 1965. Washington, D.C., Government Printing Office, 1966b. Publ. Health Service Pub. No.1509.

Weymouth, Frank W.: Optometry and the slow diffusion of knowledge, Am. J. Optom. and Arch. Am. Acad. Optom., 38 (5): 260–264, 1961.

Weymouth, Frank W., Paul R. Brust, and Franklin H. Gobar: Ocular muscle balance at the reading distance and certain related factors, Am. J. Physiol. Optics, 6 (2): 184–205, 1925. [Reprinted Am. J. Optom. and Arch. Am. Acad. Optom., 40 (9): 504–519, 1963.]

White, Eugene V.: Behind the scenes of the pharmaceutical center, J. Am. Pharmaceutical Assn., New Series 5 (10): 532–535, 552–554, 1965.

Wick, Ralph E.: The unit fee system for optometrists in public welfare contracts, Am. J. Optom. and Arch. Am. Acad. Optom., 40 (3): 166–173, 1963.

Wilensky, Harold L.: The professionalization of everyone? Am. J. Sociology, 70 (2): 137–158, 1964.

Wiseman, Eugene G.: Chairman's address, *in* Report of the 4th and 5th Annual Conventions of the American Academy of Optometry, 1925. (Vol.1 of the Transactions of the Academy.)

Wood, Casey A.: *in* American Encyclopedia of Ophthalmology. Chicago, Cleveland Press, 1918, Vol.12, p.9102.

Wood, Casey A.: The first scientific work on spectacles, Annals Med. History, 3 (2): 150–155, 1921.

INDEX